Appetite and Food Intake
Central Control, Second Edition

Appetite and Food Intake
Central Control, Second Edition

Edited by
Ruth B.S. Harris

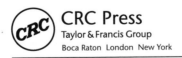

CRC Press
Taylor & Francis Group
Boca Raton London New York

CRC Press is an imprint of the
Taylor & Francis Group, an **informa** business

CRC Press
Taylor & Francis Group
6000 Broken Sound Parkway NW, Suite 300
Boca Raton, FL 33487-2742

First issued in paperback 2021

ISBN 13: 978-1-03-209681-0 (pbk)
ISBN 13: 978-1-4987-2316-9 (hbk)

Library of Congress Cataloging-in-Publication Data

Names: Harris, Ruth B. S.
Title: Appetite and food intake : central control / [edited by] Ruth B.S. Harris.
Description: Second edition. | Boca Raton : CRC Press, 2017. | Previous edition: Appetite and food intake : behavioral and physiological considerations / edited by Ruth B.S. Harris, Richard D. Mattes (Boca Raton : CRC Press, 2008). | Includes bibliographical references.
Identifiers: LCCN 2016045823 | ISBN 9781498723169 (hardback : alk. paper)
Subjects: LCSH: Ingestion--Regulation. | Appetite--Physiological aspects. | Appetite disorders. | Food habits--Psychological aspects.
Classification: LCC QP147 .A66 2017 | DDC 612.3/1--dc23
LC record available at https://lccn.loc.gov/2016045823

**Visit the Taylor & Francis Web site at
http://www.taylorandfrancis.com**

**and the CRC Press Web site at
http://www.crcpress.com**

Contents

Preface

Obesity is recognized as a global health issue that is associated with increased risk for chronic disease and results in increased morbidity and mortality. Excessive weight gain is a significant health issue for all westernized societies, but the United States has one of the highest rates of overweight in the world, with more than two-thirds of the adult population classified as overweight or obese. This means that the number of individuals maintaining a healthy weight is in a minority. Conceptually, it is easy to reduce body weight by lowering energy intake and increasing expenditure; in reality, weight-loss programs that depend upon dietary and behavioral changes have very low rates of success, especially over the long-term. Successful strategies can only be developed if the scientific rationale is reliable, which emphasizes the need to gain a better and more detailed understanding of the complex and integrated mechanisms that influence appetite, food choice, food consumption, and energy expenditure. During the past two decades, gastric bypass surgery has emerged as the most effective treatment for obesity, but this major surgery is associated with multiple risks and emphasizes the need for less invasive treatments and strategies to reverse weight gain or to reduce incidence of weight gain in the first place.

The first edition of this book reviewed knowledge on the intake of micronutrients and macronutrients, food choice, and opposing views on whether or not there are mechanisms that control food intake. An emphasis was placed on perspectives gained from the use of animal models versus human trials, and a large majority of the information remains current, making it unnecessary to simply update these chapters. Therefore, I have taken the opportunity with this second edition to focus on current and emerging areas of interest in the control of food intake and energy balance, spanning the advantages of new and continuously developing technologies in animal and human studies to novel perspectives on which aspect of body composition is being sensed and controlled.

The first section of the book is devoted to some less common models that are being used to investigate the control of food intake. Conservancy of neural circuits and neuropeptides across species allows the use of simple systems, such as *Caenorhabditis elegans* and *Drosophila*, to elucidate the role of specific neurotransmitters in different aspects of ingestive behavior, taking advantage of relatively simple circuitry and in-depth knowledge of the genome of the organism. At a different level, hamsters provide a rodent model for investigating neuropeptides that drive food aquisition, and the data illustrate a striking similarity between hormones and neurotransmitters that influence foraging and hoarding with those identified as important to consummatory behavior, even though these two components of ingestive behavior are under independent control. In contrast to the work with the simple models such as *C. elegans*, group housed nonhuman primates provide a unique opportunity for testing the impact of social environment on food choice and consumption that is directly relevant to the human situation. Although not easily available to all investigators, it is clear that we can learn an enormous amount from animal models other than the commonly used rats and mice.

In the last decade, there have been major advances in technologies that facilitate manipulation of specific central control systems. The ability to induce or knock down expression of neuropeptides in select populations of neurons in adult animals has helped eliminate the possibility of compensation for prenatal genetic modifications. Acute activation or inhibition of neurons based on neuroanatomic location and neuropeptide expression with designer receptors exclusively activated by designer drug or optogentics has resulted in elegant experiments that confirm the functional and anatomic integration of different control systems. The limitations associated with the use of these invasive procedures in humans are partially compensated for by functional magnetic resonance imaging, which identifies brain areas that are activated by food cues and how this is influenced by internal energy status, emotional status, and external environment. These elegant techniques have supported rapid and unprecedented progress in the identification of the neuronal circuitry that drives ingestive behavior.

In parallel with the progress made at the molecular and cellular level, there has been a growing appreciation of the influence of environment on development and on long-term risk for chronic disease, including diabetes and obesity. Grounded in earlier human studies that defined the impact of severe food deprivation during gestation on lifelong risk for disease in the offsping, recent animal studies have explored mechanisms that mediate the effects of the developmental environment, including diet and maternal and paternal energy status, on the physiology and behavior of both the immediate offspring and of future generations. Two chapters summarize current investigations of how energy balance is influenced by epigenetics and by the impact of prenatal and neonatal environment on the development of hypothalamic circuits that influence food intake.

Historically, a majority of research investigating the central control of food intake has focused on the hypothalamus, but now there is a growing appreciation for the critical role played by the hindbrain, which integrates information from higher brain areas with that coming from the periphery to determine an appropriate feeding response. Until recently, investigation of the long-term signals that represent the energy balance status of an organism has been independent of the study of short-term gastrointestinal and sensory signals that influence meal size and frequency. The hindbrain plays a major role in integrating these different types of information and allows changes in body energy stores to influence feeding behavior. Control of ingestive behavior is essential for homeostasis and one parameter that is critical for survival is control of blood and brain glucose. Two chapters address the association between glucostasis and ingestion. One focuses on the identification of brain areas and neuronal cell types that are glucose sensitive. The second reviews new evidence that astrocytes play a critical role in responding to changes in central glucose concentration, representative of a new and growing appreciation for the functionality of glia in physiologic control systems.

Traditionally, it has been concluded that food intake is controlled to maintain body energy stores in the form of fat. A challenge to this perspective is provided based on evidence from past and present studies that fat-free mass may drive day-to-day changes in food intake, whereas body fat correlates with intake over a period of days or weeks. It is proposed that fat-free mass is the primary determinant of resting metabolic rate, which is the major component of energy expenditure under normal conditions and most closely predicts energy intake on a daily basis. Thus, daily energy intake is linked to fat-free mass with the opportunity for modulation by the amount of energy stored as fat. The final chapter reviews current drugs available for treating obesity, focusing on those that influence food intake and food choice with an emphasis on combination therapies. The fairly small number of approved and effective medications illustrates the difficulty in developing a pharmacological treatment for a highly complex system that not only integrates many different types of information associated with food-related decisions but also justifies the exploration of combining drugs with synergystic activity. It also highlights the need for further investigation of the systems that influence food intake so that less invasive, but effective treatments can be developed to alleviate the reliance for body weight control on gastric bypass surgery. This intervention is not covered in this book, primarily because the restraint of food intake is due to imposition of a physical limitation on eating, rather than direct manipulation of a control system that has been implicated in maintenance of energy balance. There is, however, a large and growing literature on the physiological, psychological, and behavioral benefits and limitations of the procedure, which is providing unexpected insight into the influence of the gut on metabolism.

The summary of some of the current trends in research on ingestive behavior in this edition should be considered a companion to the first edition, in which there was an emphasis on the knowledge gaps between basic and applied research. It also should provide a useful, although not exhaustive, reference for students and other professionals who need an overview of aspects of the control of ingestive behavior that are outside their area of specialization. Many of the chapters provide a historic overview of key observations that were made in a specific areas of research, which gives a valuable perspective and context not only to those chapters but also to the field in general. In addition, some of the topics addressed by the authors included in this book should increase awareness of the value of different approaches to common issues encountered in the study of ingestion. As you go through the chapters presented here, it is clear that there is a significant degree of cross-reference and of reliance on similar established observations, emphasizing that no individual area within the study of appetite and ingestive behavior can stand alone.

Contributors

Lori Asarian
Institute of Veterinary Physiology
Center for Integrative and Human
    Physiology
University of Zurich,
    Winterthurerstrasse
Zurich, Switzerland

John E. Blundell
Institute of Psychological Sciences
Faculty of Medicine and Healt
University of Leeds
Leeds, United Kingdom

Sebastien G. Bouret
The Saban Research Institute
Developmental Neuroscience Program
Children's Hospital Los Angeles
University of Southern California
Los Angeles, California

and

Inserm, Jean-Pierre Aubert Research
    Center
University Lille
Lille, France

Audrey Branch
Department of Cellular Biology
Biomedical & Health Sciences Institute
University of Georgia
Athens, Georgia

Carlos A. Campos
Department of Integrative Physiology
    and Neuroscience
College of Veterinary Medicine
Washington State University
Pullman, Washington

and

Department of Biochemistry
University of Washington
Seattle, Washington

Mi Cheong Cheong
Department of Biochemistry and
    Molecular Biology
Virginia Commonwealth University
Richmond, Virginia

Alain Dagher
Montreal Neurological Institute
McGill University
Montreal, QC, Canada

Kristen Davis
Department of Biochemistry and
    Molecular Biology
Virginia Commonwealth University
Richmond, Virginia

Jung-Eun Han
Montreal Neurological Institute
McGill University
Montreal, QC, Canada

Ruth B.S. Harris
Department of Physiology
Medical College of Georgia
Augusta University
Augusta, Georgia

Gerlinda E. Hermann
Pennington Biomedical Research
    Center
Baton Rouge, Louisiana

Mark Hopkins
School of Food Science and Nutrition
University of Leeds
Leeds, United Kingdom

Miranda D. Johnson
Department of Psychiatry & Behavioral
    Sciences
Johns Hopkins University School of
    Medicine
Baltimore, Maryland

Michael J. Krashes
Diabetes, Endocrinology, and Obesity
    Branch
National Institute of Diabetes and
    Digestive and Kidney Diseases
and
National Institute on Drug Abuse
National Institutes of Health
Baltimore, Maryland

Thomas A. Lutz
Institute of Veterinary Physiology
Center for Integrative and Human
    Physiology
University of Zurich,
    Winterthurerstrasse
Zurich, Switzerland

David H. McDougal
Pennington Biomedical Research
    Center
Baton Rouge, Louisiana

Vasiliki Michopoulos
Yerkes National Primate Research
    Center
Department of Psychiatry & Behavioral
    Sciences
Emory University School of Medicine
Atlanta, Georgia

Jason Nasse
Department of Integrative Physiology
    and Neuroscience
College of Veterinary Medicine
Washington State University
Pullman, Washington

Selin Neseliler
Montreal Neurological Institute
McGill University
Montreal, QC, Canada

Ji Su Park
Department of Biochemistry and
    Molecular Biology
Virginia Commonwealth University
Richmond, Virginia

James H. Peters
Department of Integrative Physiology
    and Neuroscience
College of Veterinary Medicine
Washington State University
Pullman, Washington

Robert C. Ritter
Department of Integrative Physiology
  and Neuroscience
College of Veterinary Medicine
Washington State University
Pullman, Washington

Sue Ritter
Department of Integrated Physiology
  and Neuroscience
College of Veterinary Medicine
Washington State University
Pullman, Washington

Richard C. Rogers
Pennington Biomedical Research
  Center
Baton Rouge, Louisiana

Ping Shen
Department of Cellular Biology
Biomedical & Health Sciences Institute
University of Georgia
Athens, Georgia

Lin Song
Department of Psychiatry & Behavioral
  Sciences
Johns Hopkins University School of
  Medicine
Baltimore, Maryland

and

Department of Physiology and
  Pathophysiology
Xi'an Jiaotong University School of
  Medicine
Xi'an, Shaanxi, PR China

Kellie L.K. Tamashiro
Department of Psychiatry & Behavioral
  Sciences
Johns Hopkins University School of
  Medicine
Baltimore, Maryland

Mark E. Wilson
Yerkes National Primate Research
  Center
Department of Psychiatry & Behavioral
  Sciences
Emory University School of Medicine
Atlanta, Georgia

Young-Jai You
Department of Biochemistry and
  Molecular Biology
Virginia Commonwealth University
Richmond, Virginia

1 Appetite Control in *C. elegans*

Kristen Davis, Mi Cheong Cheong,
Ji Su Park, and Young-Jai You

CONTENTS

1.1 INTRODUCTION

1.1.1 *CAENORHABDITIS ELEGANS* FEEDING

Caenorhabditis elegans is a 1-mm-long free-living nematode that feeds on bacteria. The feeding organ of *C. elegans* is a pharynx, a neuromuscular tube responsible for sucking bacteria into the worm from outside, concentrating them, and grinding them up (Doncaster 1962, Seymour et al. 1983). The basic mechanics and the neurons and muscles used to execute feeding motion are important for understanding several feeding behaviors and are therefore briefly described. More details regarding cellular and nuclear composition, the structure, electrophysiology, and the molecular components can be found in Avery and You (2012).

The motions of the pharynx are largely regulated by its embedded nervous system. It contains 20 neurons of 14 different types (Albertson and Thomson 1976). Three of these 14 are particularly important for feeding motions: MC, M3, and M4.

MC and M3 control the timing of pumping, a full cycle of contraction and relaxation of the pharyngeal muscle (Avery 1993a): MC controls when a contraction starts (Raizen and Avery 1994, Raizen et al. 1995), and M3, when it ends (Avery 1993b, Raizen and Avery 1994). M4 is necessary for the peristaltic movement within the pharynx to transport trapped bacteria to the grinder, where the bacteria are crushed (Avery and Horvitz 1987). The pumping frequency has been shown to be altered by external cues and the neurons outside the pharynx (Greer et al. 2008). However, the exact connections between extrapharyngeal neurons and the pharynx that control feeding rates or motion are not clearly known.

Pharyngeal neurons contain both neuropeptides and small-molecule neurotransmitters. The most important of the small transmitters are acetylcholine, glutamate, and serotonin. Acetylcholine is released from MC to the pharyngeal muscle to initiate the muscle contraction via a nicotinic channel receptor, EAT-2 (Raizen et al. 1995, McKay et al. 2004). Acetylcholine also regulates a hunger response by controlling pharyngeal muscle responsiveness during starvation via a muscarinic receptor GAR-3 (You et al. 2006). GAR-3 is a *C. elegans* homolog of mammalian M3 muscarinic receptor (Steger and Avery 2004). M3 receptor knockout mice eat less and become skinny, showing conservation in controlling feeding via a similar molecular mechanism (see Section 1.2.1.1). Glutamate is released from M3 to end pharyngeal muscle contraction via an invertebrate-specific glutamate gated chloride channel, AVR-15 (Dent et al. 1997). Serotonin is released from either a neurosecretory-motor neuron (NSM) inside the pharynx or from extrapharyngeal neurons (e.g., ADF) to increase the pumping frequency (Niacaris and Avery 2003, Song et al. 2013). Neuropeptides play important roles, but they are still, for the most part, poorly understood. Recently, Cheong et al. (2015) discovered that one type of neuropeptide homologous to mammalian opioids regulates a hunger response in *C. elegans* (see Section 1.2.1.2).

1.1.2   *C. ELEGANS* AS A MODEL TO STUDY APPETITE CONTROL

Studies from the past 50 years found several fundamental mechanisms of appetite control: specific brain regions integrate signals from the gut, assess the body's nutritional status, and control feeding. Although it has been well known that the hypothalamus in mammals is the executive center for appetite control, it receives input from all over the brain. Because feeding is essential, animals have to use all perceptions to get food. Yet feeding is also dangerous. An animal needs to learn what to eat and what not to eat. Under certain conditions, an animal needs to suppress feeding in order to avoid an immediate danger even if it is still hungry. Indeed, feeding is controlled by input from multiple areas including the reward circuits consisting of the nucleus accumbens and the limbic system including the amygdala. Thus, decoding the circuitry controlling appetite and identifying the neurotransmitters working among the components of the circuit involve the entire brain. This makes the study in animals with a complex brain extremely difficult. Humans are considered to have approximately 100 billion neurons, resulting in as many as 1000 trillion possible synapses (Micheva et al. 2010). Figuring out which connections result in a particular circuit to control appetite and related feeding behaviors is certainly a daunting task.

Luckily, because control of food intake and the related behavior are essential to survival, many aspects of appetite-controlling behavior and the molecular pathways are highly conserved in simpler organisms, including *C. elegans* (You et al. 2008, Valentino et al. 2011, Arshad and Visweswariah 2012, Grimmelikhuijzen and Hauser 2012). This simple model system has contributed to several breakthrough discoveries such as cell death, RNA inference, and use of green fluorescent protein (GFP) as a biomarker. Each of these discoveries led to a Nobel Prize, showing the value and appreciation of the model system.

C. elegans after experiencing starvation and full-refeeding often rests, mimicking the behavioral sequence of satiety and postprandial sleep in rodents (Antin et al. 1975, You et al. 2008, Gallagher et al. 2013a,b, Gallagher and You 2014). For the molecular mechanisms, the satiety quiescence behavior is regulated through transforming growth factor β (TGFβ), insulin and, cyclic guanosine monophosphate (cGMP) pathways that are also conserved in mammals (Valentino et al. 2011).

In addition to conserved behavior and mechanisms, the simplicity of the nervous system of *C. elegans* makes it a great model to study neuronal mechanisms of appetite control. *C. elegans* has only 302 neurons (in a hermaphrodite), each of which is identifiable through differential interference contrast microscopy. The function of each neuron can be studied by selective ablation of that neuron by laser (Bargmann and Avery 1995). In addition, it is the only organism whose entire neural network is mapped by electron microscopy reconstruction, which allows researchers to decode the circuits for simple behaviors such as backward and forward movement as well as for complex learning behaviors such as chemotaxis and thermotaxis (Bargmann 2006, Mori et al. 2007, Zhen and Samuel 2015).

Most importantly, *C. elegans* is a powerful genetic model; they are self-fertilizing hermaphrodites. From egg to adult takes about 3 days. Each worm lays about 300 eggs, which allows large numbers of worms to be bred cheaply, easily, and quickly. The advantage of getting a large number of progeny (easily millions or billions) in a small space within a week is a key feature in genetics; it makes possible large-scale unbiased genetic screens to cover the entire genome. Also the haploid genome size of *C. elegans* is only 100 megabase pairs (Mb) (Coghlan 2005), compared to about 3200 Mb in humans (Morton 1991, International Human Genome Sequence Consortium 2004).

In addition, it is easy to generate transgenic worms that carry a gene of interest (Praitis and Maduro 2011). *C. elegans* researchers have built various transgenic lines where calcium sensors (such as GCaMP) or channel rhodopsin are expressed in the targeted neurons then their neuronal activity is monitored or manipulated in real-time under various conditions. Another beneficial feature is the ease of RNA interference (RNAi) that can be used to knock down gene expression and assess the role of specific genes. Because *C. elegans* feed on bacteria, simply feeding them bacteria that expresses the RNAi of choice can knock down the gene of interest.

It has to be noted that however simple the genome and the nervous system are, studies of metabolism and energy homeostasis in worms reveal conserved fundamental processes and mechanisms, from signaling molecules and receptors to metabolic enzymes (Ashrafi et al. 2003). Insulin signaling plays roles in fat storage, dauer formation, and life span (Kimura et al. 1997). A worm homolog of 5′ adenosine monophosphate-activated protein kinase (AMPK) and a homolog of a nuclear hormone receptor, *nhr-49*, are also engaged in energy homeostasis: mutations in these genes alter fat storage and life span (Apfeld et al. 2004, Van Gilst et al. 2005). Furthermore, neurotransmitters such as serotonin and dopamine, which are known to be important in high-level control of mammalian feeding, are also important in worms, illustrated by the isolation of mutations in biosynthetic enzymes and receptors for these transmitters in screens for mutants with altered fat storage as well as food preference (Sze et al. 2000, Ashrafi et al. 2003, Chase et al. 2004, Song et al. 2013). These findings show that worms and mammals share common mechanisms for signaling, metabolic pathways, and even information processing for energy homeostasis and fat metabolism. Finally, several feeding behaviors and the molecular mechanisms underlying them are also conserved between *C. elegans* and other animals. Through the study of a much simpler model organism such as *C. elegans*, the core molecular basis of appetite-controlling behavior can be unraveled without the complexity that comes with mammalian models.

In this chapter, we describe two main appetite control behaviors, hunger and satiety, in *C. elegans* and discuss the molecular mechanisms underlying them. Then we describe two other food-related behaviors, which show that feeding behavior can be modified by previous experiences and potentially by learning. The integration of molecular mechanisms and learning is summarized in Figure 1.1.

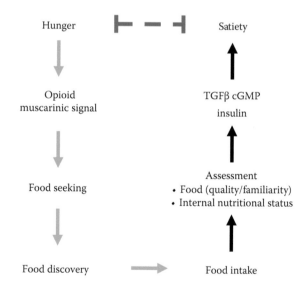

FIGURE 1.1 Appetite control in *C. elegans*. Hunger and satiety are opposite metabolic states potentially antagonizing each other when one state is achieved (shown as the dashed line in dark gray). Hunger evokes signals such as opioid and muscarinic signals to induce food seeking behavior and to prepare the animal for starvation (gray arrows). Upon discovery of food, the animal eats while assessing factors such as the quality and the familiarity of food as well as the animal's internal nutritional status. Eating good food induces signals such as TGFβ, cGMP, and insulin, which in turn promotes satiety (black arrows).

1.2 BEHAVIORS AND MECHANISMS

Satiety and hunger produce opposite behaviors in animals. Hungry animals seek food, increase exploratory behavior, increase alertness, and continue feeding once they encounter food. Satiated animals decrease exploratory behavior, take rest, and stop feeding. This fact suggests that in a broad sense, there are two feeding states: satiated and hungry. If so, two pathways must converge at some point for the animal to make a decision about whether it is hungry or full and whether to continue feeding or to stop. In mammals, the signaling of nutritional status originates in the liver, which monitors the level of both glucose and fatty acids via the hepatic portal vein from the small intestine. The vagus nerve conveys this signal from the liver to the nucleus of the solitary tract (NST) in the medulla. From the NST, nutrient-related information is passed on to the arcuate nucleus of the hypothalamus. Projections from the arcuate nucleus then pass to the paraventricular nucleus of the hypothalamus and the lateral hypothalamic area. Two important neurotransmitters are released from this projection, neuropeptide Y (NPY) and agouti-related peptide (AgRP). In addition to these two neurotransmitters, proopiomelanocortin (POMC) and cocaine and amphetamine-regulated transcripts are released from a group of neurons adjacent to NPY/AgRP neurons. These signals are critical for the delivery of nutritional inputs as well as to integrate and communicate between the nuclei to finally have the animal eat or not. (See reviews by Elmquist et al. 1999 and Schwartz et al. 2000.) The hypothalamus receives input from other brain areas, which could override the energy demands or satisfaction signaled from the gut. These are the general brain areas for motivation and reward such as the nucleus accumbens, ventral tegmental area, dorsal striatum, amygdala, hippocampus, orbitofrontal cortex, cingulate gyrus, and insula. The pleasurable aspect of food is conveyed via cannabinoid and opioid signaling in these areas (Volkow et al. 2011).

In *C. elegans*, the designated area to integrate the signals to regulate appetite has yet to be identified. However, as described in the next section, the relevant feeding behaviors such as satiety or hunger responses and the molecular mechanisms underlying them are conserved.

1.2.1 HUNGER

Hunger is the internal state that results from a lack of nutrients and that motivates the behavioral response. Hungry animals seek food and are eager to eat when they encounter food. Dysregulation of the sensation of hunger often leads to unhealthy conditions; patients with no functional leptin (a fat-derived signal; Masuzaki et al. 1995) feel hungry all the time regardless of their nutritional status, whereas patients with anorexia or cachexia do not feel hungry. In both cases, their brains shut off their bodies' input because of dysregulation of the hunger sensation.

1.2.1.1 Muscarinic Signal

There are only a few molecules known to mediate hunger. The best understood hunger signal in mammals is ghrelin, an endogenous ligand for growth hormone receptor. It is released from the stomach upon fasting and stimulates the orexigenic center in the hypothalamus via the bloodstream and passing through the blood–brain barrier in addition to influencing the tone of the vagus nerve (Date 2012, Scopinho et al. 2012). Subsequently, enhanced NPY release in the hypothalamus motivates the animal to eat (Asakawa et al. 2001, Wren et al. 2001a,b). In *C. elegans*, the muscarinic receptor → MAPK (mitogen-activated protein kinase) pathway is a part of hunger signaling in the pharynx (You et al. 2006). When MPK-1, the *C. elegans* homolog of MAPK-1/2, is activated, its two designated residues (threonine and tyrosine) are phosphorylated. This dual phosphorylation is essential for MAPK activation and thus the marker for MAPK activation (Canagarajah et al. 1997). Specific antibodies for this dual phosphorylation have been used to measure MAPK activation. Endogenous MPK-1 is highly expressed in neurons and muscles including pharyngeal muscles. To measure the phosphorylation of MPK-1 in the pharyngeal muscle specifically, You et al. (2006) targeted the expression of a GFP-tagged MPK-1 to the pharyngeal muscle using a pharynx muscle specific promotor. Starvation and a muscarinic agonist, arecoline, activated pharyngeal muscle MPK-1, but serotonin, also known to act on pharyngeal muscle, did not. Because a Gq-coupled muscarinic receptor, GAR-3, mediates arecoline action in *C. elegans* feeding (Steger and Avery 2004), they tested whether the starvation signal and the muscarinic signal may act on the same GAR-3 and Gq pathway and whether the muscarinic signal could be a starvation signal. Mutations in *gar-3* reduce MPK-1 activation by starvation and by arecoline treatment. In contrast, hyperactivation of Gq (by means of a gain of function mutation of Gq or removal of a negative regulator of Gq) increased MPK-1 activation compared to wild type. If the muscarinic signal mediates a starvation signal, these hyperactive Gq mutants should be more sensitive to starvation than wild type are. Indeed, these mutants are extremely sensitive to starvation, compared with wild type. Inhibiting the pathway either by introducing a mutation in the *gar-3* receptor or by treating the hyperactive Gq mutants with an MAPK inhibitor rescued the sensitivity, showing that the muscarinic signal-Gq-MAPK pathway mediates a starvation response. It has been suggested that the normal muscarinic signal functions to initiate general starvation responses in the pharyngeal muscle, such as to change the pumping rate or pharyngeal muscle responsiveness in preparations for when the animal encounters food later. Overactivation of this pathway for a prolonged time in the hyperactive Gq signaling mutants causes lethality due to a pharyngeal muscle that directly interferes with feeding motion. In fact, wild-type worms initially pump slowly when they are taken off food, but they gradually increase the pumping rate in the first 2 hours of starvation. When the pharyngeal muscle GAR-3 → MPK-1 pathway is blocked with a *gar-3* mutation, the increase in pumping rate is reduced. Conversely, the hyperactive Gq mutants pumping rate increases more in response to starvation. These data suggest that activation of the muscarinic receptor during starvation contributes to the increase in starvation-induced pharyngeal activity. This study also suggests that fine-tuned regulation of this pathway is essential for worm survival during starvation. Subsequently, Kang and Avery (2009) showed that one of the downstream processes that the muscarinic signal initiates as a starvation response is autophagy. Overactivation of the signal leads to excessive autophagy that contributes to early death in the mutants.

1.2.1.2   Opioid Signal

Opioids have been used as analgesics for longer than any other drug. The opioid system is composed of μ-opioid receptors (MORs), δ-opioid receptors, and κ-opioid receptors (KORs) and endogenous ligands for these receptors. Enkephalins, dynorphins, and β-endorphin peptides are produced by proteolytic cleavage of large protein precursors known as preproenkephalin (Penk), preprodynorphin (Pdyn), and POMC, respectively. All opioid peptides share a common N-terminal YGGF signature sequence, which interacts with opioid receptors (Holtzman 1974, Akil et al. 1998).

Many studies have shown that the opioid system modulates food intake; blocking the opioid receptor by naloxone, an opioid receptor blocker, decreases food intake. On the other hand, treating animals with an agonist of the opioid receptor increases food intake (Martin et al. 1963), and β-endorphin stimulates food intake when administered directly into the ventromedial hypothalamus (Grandison and Guidotti 1977). Selective agonists for the μ receptor (DAMGO), the δ receptor (DADLE), and the κ receptor (U50448) also increase food intake (Tepperman and Hirst 1983, Gosnell et al. 1986, Jackson and Cooper 1986). In addition to the homeostatic regulation, opioids also regulate the hedonic food intake, by modulating the palatability of food. Naloxone suppresses intake of sucrose solution and blocks the preference for saccharin solution (Levine et al. 1982, Lynch and Burns 1990). An opioid agonist, DAMGO, increases saccharin intake (Zhang and Kelley 2002).

The opioid system has been observed in invertebrates; biochemical approaches such as immunocytochemistry and radioimmunoassay detected opioids in many invertebrate animals including planarians (Phylum Platyhelminthes) and a parasite trematode, *Schistosoma mansoni* (Venturini et al. 1983, Duvaux-Miret et al. 1990). Treatment with naloxone inhibits a wide range of opioid-mediated responses such as stress-induced analgesia, feeding, mating behavior, and social aggression in invertebrates (Zabala et al. 1984, Kavaliers and Hirst 1986, Kavaliers et al. 1987, Nieto-Fernandez et al. 2009).

Despite all these observations, however, the first invertebrate opioid system with the molecular identities and defined pathway was discovered in *C. elegans*, where it regulates a hunger response (Cheong et al. 2015). This study shows that neuropeptide like proteins (NLP)-24 is a worm opioid and neuropeptide receptor (NPR)-17 is a worm opioid receptor.

C. elegans have 115 neuropeptide genes. Among them, 10 NLPs (*nlp-24, nlp-25, nlp-27, nlp-28, nlp-29, nlp-30, nlp-31, nlp-32, nlp-33,* and *nlp-34*) have an YGGY motif, which is similar to the YGGF motif in the opioid peptides of mammals. The frequency of *C. elegans* pumping is regulated mainly by the firing rate of MC (see Section 1.1.1), a motor neuron embedded in the pharyngeal muscle. MC releases acetylcholine, and its binding to a nicotinic receptor on the pharyngeal muscle initiates an action potential followed by muscle contraction. In the wild-type *C. elegans*, in the presence of food, the usual pumping frequency is over 200 times per minute. This high-frequency pumping absolutely requires MC. Once MC is either genetically or surgically ablated, the frequency decreases to an average of 50 times per minute. Because worms do not pump at a high frequency in the absence of food, it has been assumed that MC fires only when food is present in order for worms to eat as much as possible. Therefore, the MC minus state could represent a hunger state (or absence of food) for the worms. It is also suggested that the residual pumping in the absence of food is probably to survey the environment to increase the chances of taking in food (*C. elegans* are practically blind and they presumably use olfaction to find food). To identify what mediates this MC minus state pumping (or starvation pumping), each of the 115 neuropeptide genes was knocked down by RNAi in MC minus mutants. Cheong found that knocking down *nlp-24* in MC minus worms reduced the pumping rate further. She also found that NPR-17, a G-protein-coupled receptor that shares homology with mammalian opioid receptors and functions in pain suppression (Nieto-Fernandez et al. 2009, Harris et al. 2010), is the functional opioid receptor to mediate this starvation pumping.

The conservation of the signaling system at the molecular level is incredible; morphine induces pumping during starvation, mimicking the NLP-24 role in MC minus worms. The morphine effect on pumping is completely abolished in NPR-17 mutants, strongly suggesting that NPR-17 is the receptor that morphine acts on. Finally, heterologously expressed NPR-17 is activated by specific MOR-1 (loperamide) and KOR-1 (U69593) agonists used in mammals, and this activation is blocked by naloxone (Cheong et al. 2015). This proves that NPR-17 is an opioid receptor and NLP-24 is an endogenous opioid of *C. elegans*.

Based on known opioid roles, we speculate that the opioid during starvation may provide two benefits. First, as the muscarinic signaling does during starvation, opioids stimulate feeding motion to help worms to survey environment and to increase chances of finding food. Second, as a pain reliever, opioids might help the worms feel less stressed during starvation so that they can endure and survive starvation better.

1.2.2 SATIETY

1.2.2.1 Satiety Quiescence

Satiated animals stop eating, decrease exploratory behavior, and often fall asleep, a pattern called the "behavioral sequence of satiety" (Antin et al. 1975). *C. elegans* also display the same behavioral sequence (You et al. 2008). When satiated, they stop eating (measured by pumping rate), stop moving, and become quiescent. The quiescence is the result of satiety because (1) the quiescence is dependent on food quality—worms become quiescent on good food but not on poor food; (2) a decrease in food intake (in feeding mutants) or a decrease in food absorption in the intestine (in absorption mutants) reduces quiescence; and (3) the behavior is dependent on the animal's past experience of starvation—worms that have experienced starvation show enhanced satiety quiescence compared to worms that have not. Satiety quiescence is regulated by neuropeptide signals since *egl-21* mutants, which lack a carboxypeptidase to process neuropeptides, do not produce most peptide signals (Husson et al. 2007), and are completely defective in satiety quiescence. Consistent with the evidence for neuropeptide signaling, insulin and TGFβ signals are also necessary for worms to show satiety quiescence.

Previous studies found that a gain of function mutant of *egl-4*, which encodes a cGMP-dependent protein kinase, shows excessive quiescence under conditions where the wild-type worms do not show quiescence (Avery 1993a, Raizen et al. 2006). You et al. (2008) found that *egl-4* loss of function mutants show no satiety quiescence, whereas the gain of function mutation shows excessive satiety quiescence. This finding suggested a role for cGMP signaling in satiety quiescence, confirmed by the fact that the membrane guanylate cyclase and *C. elegans* homolog of a natriuretic peptide (NP) receptor, DAF-11, and the cGMP-gated cation channel are necessary for satiety quiescence (You et al. 2008). In *C. elegans*, insulin, TGFβ, and cGMP pathways are used in sensing a favorable environment and in making the developmental decision to keep growing and reproducing instead of becoming a dauer, a nonreproductive form specialized for long-term survival (Riddle et al. 1981). In other words, these signals are used to ensure that worms will be in nutritionally favorable conditions. The findings of You et al. imply that these same signals of favorable conditions are used to exhibit satiety quiescence in adults.

1.2.2.2   The Mechanisms: TGFβ and cGMP Pathways in ASI Neurons Regulate Satiety

TGFβ signaling is well studied in cell proliferation, differentiation, and tumor formation (Feng and Derynck 2005). In addition, studies suggest a role of TGFβ in food intake and fat metabolism: (1) Overexpressing a TGFβ family member (MIC-1/GDF-15) in the brain inhibits food intake in wild-type mice and causes weight loss by reducing food intake in leptin-deficient *ob/ob* mice (Johnen et al. 2007). Deficiency of MIC-1, on the other hand, causes an increase in food intake (in females) and induces obesity (in both genders) (Tsai et al. 2013). (2) Exercise activates TGFβ in the brain, and this increase of TGFβ correlates with increased fat mobilization (Shibakusa et al. 2006). (3) Orexin, a neuropeptide that increases appetite, upregulates expression of four sets of signaling genes including TGFβ/SMAD (Sikder and Kodadek 2007). (4) In *C. elegans*, neuronal TGFβ signaling controls fat metabolism (Greer et al. 2008) as well as satiety quiescence (You et al. 2008). These studies suggest that TGFβ signaling regulates food intake and fat metabolism in both mammals and worms. In *C. elegans*, TGFβ is released from a pair of head sensory neurons ASI, which is known to regulate several nutrition-related behaviors such as calorie restriction-dependent longevity (Bishop and Guarente 2007). Gallagher et al. (2013b) found that nutrients directly activate ASI and feeding increases the expression of TGFβ in ASI. These results suggest that nutrients activate ASI and lead to the activation of the TGFβ pathway to induce satiety quiescence.

The cGMP signaling pathway is involved in many essential functions; it regulates phototransduction in the eyes, hypertension, reproduction, attention and hyperactive behavior, vasodilation, circadian rhythms, intestinal homeostasis, and cancer progression (Januszewicz 1995, Oster et al. 2003, Yau and Hardie 2009, Francis et al. 2010, Zhang et al. 2010, Gong et al. 2011, Arshad and Visweswariah 2012, Kim et al. 2013). In addition, it regulates body size, exploratory behavior, stress-induced development, sleep, and feeding in invertebrates (Fujiwara et al. 2002, Raizen et al. 2008, You et al. 2008). Its role in appetite control and obesity was first discovered in *C. elegans* and later in mammals (Valentino et al. 2011). In mammals, a gut peptide, uroguanylin, is released upon feeding and binds to GUCY2C, its receptor in the hypothalamus, to suppress feeding (Valentino et al. 2011). GUCY2C is a membrane guanylyl cyclase (GCY) that produces cGMP upon its activation. Interestingly, there are several previous studies that suggest cGMP functions in obesity. For instance, sildenafil, a medicine that inhibits degradation of cGMP to treat erectile dysfunction, has protective effects in weight gain on a high-fat diet (Ayala et al. 2007, Mitschke et al. 2013). NPs that bind to NP receptors (also GCYs) to produce cGMP are not only important to control blood pressure and heart function (Takei 2001) but also play an important role in lipolysis in adipose tissue via phosphorylation of hormone sensitive lipase by cGMP-dependent protein kinase (PKG) (Sengenes et al. 2000). Furthermore, epidemiological studies show that a certain allele of the NP receptor type C gene is associated with a lean phenotype (Sarzani et al. 2004), suggesting a critical role of NP in fat metabolism.

In *C. elegans*, the cGMP signal is used to perceive most sensations, including temperature, smell, and light (Komatsu et al. 1996, Ward et al. 2008). The cGMP signal is essential for worms to show satiety quiescence; lack of functional PKG led to increased fat storage and a defect in satiety quiescence (You et al. 2008). Together, these findings in mammals and worms highlight an essential role for cGMP signaling in appetite control and metabolism.

How does it regulate appetite and satiety? ASI neurons, whose ablation impairs satiety quiescence and which are activated by nutrients and release TGFβ when the worms are satiated, are also directly activated by 8-Br-cGMP, a membrane permeable form of cGMP. DAF-11, homologous NP receptors, and a GCY expressed in several head neurons including ASI, are necessary for satiety quiescence. Expressing *daf-11* in ASI rescues the defect in satiety quiescence of *daf-11* mutants. All this suggests that ASI is the major neuron to sense nutrients and regulate satiety behavior via TGFβ and cGMP signals.

1.3 FOOD PREFERENCE

1.3.1 QUALITY

Given a choice, *C. elegans* show a preference toward food that supports their growth better. Avery and Shtonda (2003) characterized the quality of food operationally by measuring the growth of *C. elegans*. There is a strong inverse correlation between the quality of food and the size of bacteria; better food is smaller so easier to eat (Avery and Shtonda 2003). The size limitation is one of the most common determinants of food an animal feeds on in nature; when only large seeds were available after drought, the finches with small beak sizes could not feed on them and died. Only the finches with a large beak size survived and were selected (Boag and Grant 1981).

This preference can be modified by experience; using three different quality foods (good, mediocre, and bad), Avery and Shtonda (2003) showed that naïve *C. elegans* L1s that had experienced bad food stayed on the mediocre food and ate it, but the genetically identical naive L1s that had experienced good food from hatching did not stay on the mediocre food. Instead, they left the food a lot more frequently and wandered around, presumably trying to find better food.

Avery and Shtonda (2003) ruled out the possibility that *C. elegans* made the choice based on primary perceptions (such as olfactory cues) by testing several unrelated species of bacteria of similar quality (i.e., similar ability to support *C. elegans* growth). Therefore, their studies strongly suggest that *C. elegans* sense the nutritional value of food to show preference for a better quality of food based on their past experience.

1.3.2 FAMILIARITY

Food can be dangerous for feeders in the wild, mainly because food does not want to be food. Many prey and plants are armed with diverse defense mechanisms such as toxins. Therefore, the feeders would need to make sure what they eat is safe. Familiar food means they are safe so they can eat without experimenting on it. If you have a dog, you should have seen that its responses toward familiar food and nonfamiliar food are as different as day and night. If it is familiar food, the dog is excited from the smell of it. As soon as the food is given, the dog will take a big bite of it without hesitation. On the contrary, if you give the dog a food that it has never experienced before, it hesitates, cautiously tastes it, takes time to eat it.

Song and Avery found that this preference toward familiar food is conserved in *C. elegans*. Using two equally good qualities of bacteria (let us name them A and B for convenience), they showed that *C. elegans* that had fed on bacteria A chose A but the *C. elegans* that had fed on B chose B, when they were given choices between A and B. Song and Avery further discovered that this behavior is mediated by a neuronal serotonin system. Serotonin has been implicated in mimicking food in *C. elegans* (Horvitz et al. 1982, Sze et al. 2000, Niacaris and Avery 2003), exerting several food-related behaviors such as promoting feeding motions and egg-laying and suppressing locomotion. In mammals, serotonin plays a critical role in controlling appetite and food choices by controlling dopamine pathway reward circuits. Song and Avery's work suggests that a conserved reward circuit is used to promote feeding after recognizing familiar food.

1.4 CONCLUSIONS

Although they are simple, *C. elegans* show conserved feeding behavior that enables them to survive an uncertain environment; hunger increases locomotive activity and induces pumping to increase the chances of finding food. Satiation causes them to rest. They can learn what to eat and what not to and change their behavior depending on their past experience of the quality of food. Surprisingly, many of the signals for these behaviors are highly conserved, e.g., a muscarinic acetylcholine signal, opioids, and serotonin. With the simple nervous system, powerful genetics, conserved behavior and genes, and rich resources such as the known connectome of neurons and highly collaborative society of researchers, *C. elegans* proves as an extremely useful model to study fundamental aspects of appetite control behavior and its underlying molecular neuronal mechanisms.

ACKNOWLEDGMENT

We thank Dr. Leon Avery for his invaluable comments. This work is supported by the School of Medicine, Virginia Commonwealth University.

LITERATURE CITED

Akil, H., C. Owens, H. Gutstein, L. Taylor, E. Curran, and S. Watson, 1998. Endogenous opioids: Overview and current issues. *Drug Alcohol Depend* 51 (1–2):127–40.

Albertson, D.G. and J.N. Thomson, 1976. The pharynx of *Caenorhabditis elegans*. *Philos Trans R Soc Lond Series B Biol Sci* 275 (938):299–325.

Antin, J., J. Gibbs, J. Holt, R.C. Young, and G.P. Smith, 1975. Cholecystokinin elicits the complete behavioral sequence of satiety in rats. *J Comp Physiol Psychol* 89 (7):784–90.

Apfeld, J., G. O'Connor, T. McDonagh, P.S. DiStefano, and R. Curtis, 2004. The AMP-activated protein kinase AAK-2 links energy levels and insulin-like signals to lifespan in *C. elegans*. *Genes Dev* 18 (24):3004–9.

Arshad, N. and S.S. Visweswariah, 2012. The multiple and enigmatic roles of guanylyl cyclase C in intestinal homeostasis. *FEBS Lett* 586 (18):2835–40.

Asakawa, A., A. Inui, T. Kaga, H. Yuzuriha, T. Nagata, N. Ueno, S. Makino, M. Fujimiya, A. Niijima, M.A. Fujino, and M. Kasuga, 2001. Ghrelin is an appetite-stimulatory signal from stomach with structural resemblance to motilin. *Gastroenterology* 120 (2):337–45.

Ashrafi, K., F.Y. Chang, J.L. Watts, A.G. Fraser, R.S. Kamath, J. Ahringer, and G. Ruvkun, 2003. Genome-wide RNAi analysis of Caenorhabditis elegans fat regulatory genes. *Nature* 421 (6920):268–72.

Avery, L., 1993a. The genetics of feeding in *Caenorhabditis elegans*. *Genetics* 133 (4):897–917.

Avery, L., 1993b. Motor neuron M3 controls pharyngeal muscle relaxation timing in *Caenorhabditis elegans*. *J Exp Biol* 175:283–97.

Avery, L. and H.R. Horvitz, 1987. A cell that dies during wild-type *C. elegans* development can function as a neuron in a *ced-3* mutant. *Cell* 51 (6):1071–8.

Avery, L. and B.B. Shtonda, 2003. Food transport in the *C. elegans* pharynx. *J Exp Biol* 206 (Pt 14):2441–57.

Avery, L. and Y.Y. You, 2012. *C. elegans* feeding. *WormBook*:1–23.

Ayala, J.E., D.P. Bracy, B.M. Julien, J.N. Rottman, P.T. Fueger, and D.H. Wasserman, 2007. Chronic treatment with sildenafil improves energy balance and insulin action in high fat-fed conscious mice. *Diabetes* 56 (4):1025–33.

Bargmann, C.I., 2006. Chemosensation in *C. elegans*. *WormBook*:1–29.

Bargmann, C.I. and L. Avery, 1995. Laser killing of cells in *Caenorhabditis elegans*. *Methods Cell Biol* 48:225–50.

Bishop, N.A. and L. Guarente, 2007. Two neurons mediate diet-restriction-induced longevity in *C. elegans*. *Nature* 447 (7144):545–9.

Boag, P.T. and P.R. Grant, 1981. Intense natural selection in a population of Darwin's finches (Geospizinae) in the Galapagos. *Science* 214 (4516):82–5.

Canagarajah, B.J., A. Khokhlatchev, M.H. Cobb, and E.J. Goldsmith, 1997. Activation mechanism of the MAP kinase ERK2 by dual phosphorylation. *Cell* 90 (5):859–69.

Chase, D.L., J.S. Pepper, and M.R. Koelle, 2004. Mechanism of extrasynaptic dopamine signaling in *Caenorhabditis elegans*. *Nat Neurosci* 7 (10):1096–103.

Cheong, M.C., A.B. Artyukhin, Y.J. You, and L. Avery, 2015. An opioid-like system regulating feeding behavior in *C. elegans*. *Elife* 4.

Coghlan, A., 2005. Nematode genome evolution. *WormBook*:1–15.

Date, Y., 2012. Ghrelin and the vagus nerve. *Methods Enzymol* 514:261–9.

Dent, J.A., M.W. Davis, and L. Avery, 1997. avr-15 encodes a chloride channel subunit that mediates inhibitory glutamatergic neurotransmission and ivermectin sensitivity in *Caenorhabditis elegans*. *EMBO J* 16 (19):5867–79.

Doncaster, C.C., 1962. Nematode feeding mechanisms. I. Observations on Rhabditis and Pelodera. *Nematologica* 8:313–20.

Duvaux-Miret, O., C. Dissous, J.P. Gautron, E. Pattou, C. Kordon, and A. Capron, 1990. The helminth *Schistosoma mansoni* expresses a peptide similar to human beta-endorphin and possesses a proopiomelanocortin-related gene. *New Biol* 2 (1):93–9.

Elmquist, J.K., C.F. Elias, and C.B. Saper, 1999. From lesions to leptin: Hypothalamic control of food intake and body weight. *Neuron* 22 (2):221–32.

Feng, X.H. and R. Derynck, 2005. Specificity and versatility in tgf-beta signaling through Smads. *Annu Rev Cell Dev Biol* 21:659–93.

Francis, S.H., J.L. Busch, J.D. Corbin, and D. Sibley, 2010. cGMP-dependent protein kinases and cGMP phosphodiesterases in nitric oxide and cGMP action. *Pharmacol Rev* 62 (3):525–63.

Fujiwara, M., P. Sengupta, and S.L. McIntire, 2002. Regulation of body size and behavioral state of *C. elegans* by sensory perception and the EGL-4 cGMP-dependent protein kinase. *Neuron* 36 (6):1091–102.

Gallagher, T., T. Bjorness, R. Greene, Y.J. You, and L. Avery, 2013a. The geometry of locomotive behavioral states in *C. elegans*. *PLoS One* 8 (3):e59865.

Gallagher, T., J. Kim, M. Oldenbroek, R. Kerr, and Y.J. You, 2013b. ASI regulates satiety quiescence in *C. elegans*. *J Neurosci* 33 (23):9716–24.

Gallagher, T. and Y.J. You, 2014. Falling asleep after a big meal: Neuronal regulation of satiety. *Worm* 3:e27938.

Gong, R., C. Ding, J. Hu, Y. Lu, F. Liu, E. Mann, F. Xu, M.B. Cohen, and M. Luo, 2011. Role for the membrane receptor guanylyl cyclase-C in attention deficiency and hyperactive behavior. *Science* 333 (6049):1642–6.

Gosnell, B.A., A.S. Levine, and J.E. Morley, 1986. The stimulation of food intake by selective agonists of mu, kappa and delta opioid receptors. *Life Sci* 38 (12):1081–8.

Grandison, L. and A. Guidotti, 1977. Stimulation of food intake by muscimol and beta endorphin. *Neuropharmacology* 16 (7–8):533–6.

Greer, E.R., C.L. Pérez, M.R. Van Gilst, B.H. Lee, and K. Ashrafi, 2008. Neural and molecular dissection of a *C. elegans* sensory circuit that regulates fat and feeding. *Cell Metab* 8 (2):118–31.

Grimmelikhuijzen, C.J. and F. Hauser, 2012. Mini-review: The evolution of neuropeptide signaling. *Regul Pept* 177(Suppl):S6–9.

Harris, G., H. Mills, R. Wragg, V. Hapiak, M. Castelletto, A. Korchnak, and R.W. Komuniecki, 2010. The monoaminergic modulation of sensory-mediated aversive responses in *Caenorhabditis elegans* requires glutamatergic/peptidergic cotransmission. *J Neurosci* 30 (23):7889–99.

Holtzman, S.G., 1974. Behavioral effects of separate and combined administration of naloxone and D-amphetamine. *J Pharmacol Exp Ther* 189 (1):51–60.

Horvitz, H.R., M. Chalfie, C. Trent, J.E. Sulston, and P.D. Evans, 1982. Serotonin and octopamine in the nematode *Caenorhabditis elegans*. *Science* 216 (4549):1012–4.

Husson, S.J., T. Janssen, G. Baggerman, B. Bogert, A.H. Kahn-Kirby, K. Ashrafi, and L. Schoofs, 2007. Impaired processing of FLP and NLP peptides in carboxypeptidase E (EGL-21)-deficient *Caenorhabditis elegans* as analyzed by mass spectrometry. *J Neurochem* 102 (1):246–60.

International Human Genome Sequence Consortium, 2004. Finishing the euchromatic sequence of the human genome. *Nature* 431 (7011):931–45.

Jackson, A. and S.J. Cooper, 1986. An observational analysis of the effect of the selective kappa opioid agonist, U-50,488H, on feeding and related behaviours in the rat. *Psychopharmacology (Berl)* 90 (2):217–21.

Januszewicz, A., 1995. The natriuretic peptides in hypertension. *Curr Opin Cardiol* 10 (5):495–500.

Johnen, H., S. Lin, T. Kuffner, D.A. Brown, V.W. Tsai, A.R. Bauskin, L. Wu, G. Pankhurst, S. Junankar, M. Hunter, W.D. Fairlie, N.J. Lee, R.F. Enriquez, P.A. Baldock, E. Corey, F.S. Apple, M.M. Murakami, E.J. Lin, C. Wang, M.J. During, A. Sainsbury, H. Herzog, and S.N. Breit, 2007. Tumor-induced anorexia and weight loss are mediated by the TGF-beta superfamily cytokine MIC-1. *Nat Med* 13 (11):1333–40.

Kang, C. and L. Avery, 2009. Systemic regulation of starvation response in *Caenorhabditis elegans*. *Genes Dev* 23 (1):12–7.

Kavaliers, M. and M. Hirst, 1986. Environmental specificity of tolerance to morphine-induced analgesia in a terrestrial snail: Generalization of the behavioral model of tolerance. *Pharmacol Biochem Behav* 25 (6):1201–6.

Kavaliers, M., M.A. Guglick, and M. Hirst, 1987. Opioid involvement in the control of feeding in an insect, the American cockroach. *Life Sci* 40 (7):665–72.

Kim, G.W., J.E. Lin, and S.A. Waldman, 2013. GUCY2C: At the intersection of obesity and cancer. *Trends Endocrinol Metab* 24 (4):165–73.

Kimura, K.D., H.A. Tissenbaum, Y. Liu, and G. Ruvkun, 1997. daf-2, an insulin receptor-like gene that regulates longevity and diapause in *Caenorhabditis elegans*. *Science* 277 (5328):942–6.

Komatsu, H., I. Mori, J.S. Rhee, N. Akaike, and Y. Ohshima, 1996. Mutations in a cyclic nucleotide-gated channel lead to abnormal thermosensation and chemosensation in *C. elegans*. *Neuron* 17 (4):707–18.

Levine, A.S., J.E. Morley, D.M. Brown, and B.S. Handwerger, 1982. Extreme sensitivity of diabetic mice to naloxone-induced suppression of food intake. *Physiol Behav* 28 (6):987–89.

Lynch, W.C. and G. Burns, 1990. Opioid effects on intake of sweet solutions depend both on prior drug experience and on prior ingestive experience. *Appetite* 15 (1):23–32.

Martin, W.R., A. Wickler, C.G. Eades, and F.T. Pescor, 1963. Tolerance to and physical dependence on morphine in rats. *Psychopharmacologia* 4:247–60.

Masuzaki, H., Y. Ogawa, N. Isse, N. Satoh, T. Okazaki, M. Shigemoto, K. Mori, N. Tamura, K. Hosoda, Y. Yoshimasa, H. Jingami, T. Kawada, and K. Nakao, 1995. Human obese gene expression. Adipocyte-specific expression and regional differences in the adipose tissue. *Diabetes* 44 (7):855–8.

McKay, J.P., D.M. Raizen, A. Gottschalk, W.R. Schafer, and L. Avery, 2004. eat-2 and eat-18 are required for nicotinic neurotransmission in the *Caenorhabditis elegans* pharynx. *Genetics* 166 (1):161–9.

Micheva, K.D., B. Busse, N.C. Weiler, N. O'Rourke, and S.J. Smith, 2010. Single-synapse analysis of a diverse synapse population: Proteomic imaging methods and markers. *Neuron* 68 (4):639–53.

Mitschke, M.M., L.S. Hoffmann, T. Gnad, D. Scholz, K. Kruithoff, P. Mayer, B. Haas, A. Sassmann, A. Pfeifer, and A. Kilic, 2013. Increased cGMP promotes healthy expansion and browning of white adipose tissue. *FASEB J* 27 (4):1621–30.

Mori, I., H. Sasakura, and A. Kuhara, 2007. Worm thermotaxis: A model system for analyzing thermosensation and neural plasticity. *Curr Opin Neurobiol* 17 (6):712–9.

Morton, N.E., 1991. Parameters of the human genome. *Proc Natl Acad Sci U S A* 88 (17):7474–6.

Niacaris, T. and L. Avery, 2003. Serotonin regulates repolarization of the *C. elegans* pharyngeal muscle. *J Exp Biol* 206 (Pt 2):223–31.

Nieto-Fernandez, F., S. Andrieux, S. Idrees, C. Bagnall, S.C. Pryor, and R. Sood, 2009. The effect of opioids and their antagonists on the nocifensive response of *Caenorhabditis elegans* to noxious thermal stimuli. *Invert Neurosci* 9 (3–4):195–200.

Oster, H., C. Werner, M.C. Magnone, H. Mayser, R. Feil, M.W. Seeliger, F. Hofmann, and U. Albrecht, 2003. cGMP-dependent protein kinase II modulates mPer1 and mPer2 gene induction and influences phase shifts of the circadian clock. *Curr Biol* 13 (9):725–33.

Praitis, V. and M.F. Maduro, 2011. Transgenesis in *C. elegans*. *Methods Cell Biol* 106:161–85.

Raizen, D.M. and L. Avery, 1994. Electrical activity and behavior in the pharynx of *Caenorhabditis elegans*. *Neuron* 12 (3):483–95.

Raizen, D.M., K.M. Cullison, A.I. Pack, and M.V. Sundaram, 2006. A novel gain-of-function mutant of the cyclic GMP-dependent protein kinase egl-4 affects multiple physiological processes in *Caenorhabditis elegans*. *Genetics* 173 (1):177–87.

Raizen, D.M., R.Y. Lee, and L. Acery, 1995. Interacting genes required for pharyngeal excitation by motor neuron MC in *Caenorhabditis elegans*. *Genetics* 141 (4):1365–82.

Raizen, D.M., J.E. Zimmerman, M.H. Maycock, U.D. Ta, Y.J. You, M.V. Sundaram, and A.I. Pack, 2008. Lethargus is a *Caenorhabditis elegans* sleep-like state. *Nature* 451 (7178):569–72.

Riddle, D.L., M.M. Swanson, and P.S. Albert, 1981. Interacting genes in nematode dauer larva formation. *Nature* 290 (5808):668–71.

Sarzani, R., P. Strazzullo, F. Salvi, R. Iacone, F. Pietrucci, A. Siani, G. Barba, M.C. Gerardi, P. Dessì-Fulgheri, and A. Rappelli, 2004. Natriuretic peptide clearance receptor alleles and susceptibility to abdominal adiposity. *Obes Res* 12 (2):351–6.

Schwartz, M.W., S.C. Woods, D. Porte, R.J. Seeley, and D.G. Baskin, 2000. Central nervous system control of food intake. *Nature* 404 (6778):661–71.

Scopinho, A.A., E.A. Fortaleza, F.M. Corrêa, and L.B. Resstel, 2012. Medial amygdaloid nucleus 5-HT(2)c receptors are involved in the hypophagic effect caused by zimelidine in rats. *Neuropharmacology* 63 (2):301–9.

Sengenes, C., M. Berlan, I. De Glisezinski, M. Lafontan, and J. Galitzky, 2000. Natriuretic peptides: A new lipolytic pathway in human adipocytes. *FASEB J* 14 (10):1345–51.

Seymour, MK, K.A. Wright, and C.C. Doncaster, 1983. The action of the anterior feeding apparatus of *Caenorhabditis elegans* (Nematoda: Rhabditida). *J Zool Soc London* 201:527–39.

Shibakusa, T., Y. Iwaki, W. Mizunoya, S. Matsumura, Y. Nishizawa, K. Inoue, and T. Fushiki, 2006. The physiological and behavioral effects of subchronic intracisternal administration of TGF-beta in rats: Comparison with the effects of CRF. *Biomed Res* 27 (6):297–305.

Sikder, D. and T. Kodadek, 2007. The neurohormone orexin stimulates hypoxia-inducible factor-1 activity. *Genes Dev* 21 (22):2995–3005.

Song, B.M., S. Faumont, S. Lockery, and L. Avery, 2013. Recognition of familiar food activates feeding via an endocrine serotonin signal in *Caenorhabditis elegans*. *Elife* 2:e00329.

Steger, K.A. and L. Avery, 2004. The GAR-3 muscarinic receptor cooperates with calcium signals to regulate muscle contraction in the *Caenorhabditis elegans* pharynx. *Genetics* 167 (2):633–43.

Sze, J.Y., M. Victor, C. Loer, Y. Shi, and G. Ruvkun, 2000. Food and metabolic signalling defects in a *Caenorhabditis elegans* serotonin-synthesis mutant. *Nature* 403 (6769):560–4.

Takei, Y., 2001. Does the natriuretic peptide system exist throughout the animal and plant kingdom? *Comp Biochem Physiol B Biochem Mol Biol* 129 (2–3):559–73.

Tepperman, F.S. and M. Hirst, 1983. Effect of intrahypothalamic injection of [D-Ala2, D-Leu5]enkephalin on feeding and temperature in the rat. *Eur J Pharmacol* 96 (3–4):243–9.

Tsai, V.W., L. Macia, H. Johnen, T. Kuffner, R. Manadhar, S.B. Jørgensen, K.K. Lee-Ng, H.P. Zhang, L. Wu, C.P. Marquis, L. Jiang, Y. Husaini, S. Lin, H. Herzog, D.A. Brown, A. Sainsbury, and S.N. Breit, 2013. TGF-b superfamily cytokine MIC-1/GDF15 is a physiological appetite and body weight regulator. *PLoS One* 8 (2):e55174.

Valentino, M.A., J.E. Lin, A.E. Snook, P. Li, G.W. Kim, G. Marszalowicz, M.S. Magee, T. Hyslop, S. Schulz, and S.A. Waldman, 2011. A uroguanylin-GUCY2C endocrine axis regulates feeding in mice. *J Clin Invest* 121 (9):3578–88.

Van Gilst, M.R., H. Hadjivassiliou, A. Jolly, and K.R. Yamamoto, 2005. Nuclear hormone receptor NHR-49 controls fat consumption and fatty acid composition in *C. elegans*. *PLoS Biol* 3 (2):e53.

Venturini, G., A. Carolei, G. Palladini, V. Margotta, and M.G. Lauro, 1983. Radio-immunological and immunocytochemical demonstration of Met-enkephalin in planaria. *Comp Biochem Physiol C* 74 (1):23–5.

Volkow, N.D., G.J. Wang, and R. Baler, 2011. Reward, dopamine and the control of food intake: Implications for obesity. *Trends Cogn Sci* 15 (1):37–46.

Ward, A., J. Liu, Z. Feng, and X.Z. Xu, 2008. Light-sensitive neurons and channels mediate phototaxis in *C. elegans*. *Nat Neurosci* 11 (8):916–22.

Wren, A.M., L.J. Seal, M.A. Cohen, A.E. Brynes, G.S. Frost, K.G. Murphy, W.S. Dhillo, M.A. Ghatei, and S.R. Bloom, 2001a. Ghrelin enhances appetite and increases food intake in humans. *J Clin Endocrinol Metab* 86 (12):5992.

Wren, A.M., C.J. Small, C.R. Abbott, W.S. Dhillo, L.J. Seal, M.A. Cohen, R.L. Batterham, S. Taheri, S.A. Stanley, M.A. Ghatei, and S.R. Bloom, 2001b. Ghrelin causes hyperphagia and obesity in rats. *Diabetes* 50 (11):2540–7.

Yau, K.W. and R.C. Hardie, 2009. Phototransduction motifs and variations. *Cell* 139 (2):246–64.

You, Y.J., J. Kim, M. Cobb, and L. Avery, 2006. Starvation activates MAP kinase through the muscarinic acetylcholine pathway in *Caenorhabditis elegans* pharynx. *Cell Metab* 3 (4):237–45.

You, Y.J., J. Kim, D.M. Raizen, and L. Avery, 2008. Insulin, cGMP, and TGF-beta signals regulate food intake and quiescence in *C. elegans*: A model for satiety. *Cell Metab* 7 (3):249–57.

Zabala, N.A., A. Miralto, H. Maldonado, J.A. Nuñez, K. Jaffe, and L.D. Calderon, 1984. Opiate receptor in praying mantis: Effect of morphine and naloxone. *Pharmacol Biochem Behav* 20 (5):683–7.

Zhang, M. and A.E. Kelley, 2002. Intake of saccharin, salt, and ethanol solutions is increased by infusion of a mu opioid agonist into the nucleus accumbens. *Psychopharmacology (Berl)* 159 (4):415–23.

Zhang, M., Y.Q. Su, K. Sugiura, G. Xia, and J.J. Eppig, 2010. Granulosa cell ligand NPPC and its receptor NPR2 maintain meiotic arrest in mouse oocytes. *Science* 330 (6002):366–9.

Zhen, M. and A.D. Samuel, 2015. *C. elegans* locomotion: Small circuits, complex functions. *Curr Opin Neurobiol* 33:117–126.

2 Central and Peripheral Regulation of Appetite and Food Intake in *Drosophila*

Audrey Branch and Ping Shen

CONTENTS

2.1 INTRODUCTION

Food intake is a primary behavior executed by all organisms, and the decisions of what, when, and how much to eat have profound consequences on the survival and health of individuals and species. However, characterizing the genetic and neural underpinnings of such complex behavioral decisions is complicated by the inherent difficulties of (1) defining and quantifying related behaviors, (2) the high level of interindividual variation in execution of behavior, and (3) the large number of genes and physiological systems involved (Sokolowski 2001). Given this complexity, invertebrates such as fruit flies (*Drosophila melanogaster*) have emerged as invaluable tools of discovery. Besides its genetic tractability, *D. melanogaster* has a numerically simple nervous system that controls a rich repertoire of robust and quantifiable food-related sensory and motor responses. It is increasingly recognized that the fruit fly represents a powerful complementary animal model for the identification and characterization of general neural principles underlying feeding behavior at the genetic, molecular, cellular, and circuit levels (Lee and Park 2004; Koon et al. 2011; Musselman et al. 2011; Rieder and Larschan 2014; Lushchak et al. 2015).

Flies are homometabolous insects, meaning that their development includes four life stages: embryo, larvae, pupa, and adult (Bainbridge and Bownes 1981). Larvae and adult flies both feed actively, and, like mammals, they modulate their decisions for foraging and food intake in response to changes in environmental stimuli, motivational states, and variation in food quality. These adaptive strategies, either learned or innate, appear to be highly optimized during evolution in order to acquire nutrients for long-term growth and development and to cope with adverse conditions for immediate survival (Brogiolo et al. 2001; Bateson 2002; Kim and Rulifson 2004; Carvalho et al. 2005).

In fruit flies, the availability of nutrients and their absorption and metabolism are also tightly coordinated via central and peripheral signals. Both fly larvae and adults regulate their circulating sugar levels according to food availability and store excess energy in the form of glycogen and lipids, which can be mobilized according to energetic need (Kim and Rulifson 2004; Gutierrez et al. 2007; Rajan and Perrimon 2012). These processes are performed by genetic, molecular, and organ systems that are analogous to those used by vertebrate systems for nutrient uptake, storage, and metabolism (Rulifson et al. 2002; Kim and Rulifson 2004; Gutierrez et al. 2007; Bland et al. 2010; Rajan and Perrimon 2012) and are converted by the CNS into behavioral modifications via neural mechanisms that are genetically and functionally conserved in vertebrates. Thus, like other animals, flies demonstrate adaptive behavioral responses to food, which are dependent on both their internal satiety status and external sensory cues of food quality and nutritional value, allowing discoveries made in the fly to contribute to our understanding of evolutionarily conserved neural and physiological processes.

In the following sections, we will introduce major approaches that are commonly used for studying and quantifying various aspects of fly feeding response. In addition, we will highlight those evolutionarily conserved neural and peripheral substrates and mechanisms that underlie the regulation of these behaviors. A number of excellent reviews are also available on current methodologies for studying food intake in *Drosophila* (Gerber et al. 2013; Itskov and Ribeiro 2013; Deshpande et al. 2014) and the major neural (Nassel and Winther 2010; Pool and Scott 2014), chemosensory (Stocker 1994; Couto et al. 2005; Scott 2005; Hallem et al. 2006; Gerber and Stocker 2007; Vosshall and Stocker 2007; Masse et al. 2009; Montell 2009; Tanimura et al. 2009; Isono and Morita 2010), and cellular mechanisms (Leopold and Perrimon 2007; Nassel and Winther 2010; Itskov and Ribeiro 2013; Rajan and Perrimon 2013; Owusu-Ansah and Perrimon 2014) that regulate these behaviors.

2.2 APPROACHES TO STUDYING APPETITIVE AND CONSUMMATORY BEHAVIORS

The feeding activities of fly larvae and adults are controlled by a series of behavioral subprograms that are unique to their developmental stages. Despite the fact that larvae feed much more frequently than adults do, they do not feed continuously. Rather, the feeding activities of both larvae and adults are subject to regulation by molecular and circuit mechanisms that are highly conserved throughout the fly life cycle. Both larvae and adults will (1) forage for food when driven by physiological needs, (2) cease locomotion when palatable food is detected, (3) initiate a meal, and (4) consume it until postingestive signals trigger cessation of feeding and disengagement from the food (Melcher et al. 2007; Mann et al. 2013; Zhang et al. 2013a). Consequently, studies of feeding behaviors at both of these life stages have and will continue to yield useful insights into the molecular and cellular bases of appetite and feeding controls. Using the fly larva as an example, its central nervous system, along with subsets of neurons producing some of the key signaling molecules for the control of feeding behavior are depicted in Figure 2.1.

2.2.1   FOOD PREFERENCE AND APPETITIVE RESPONSES OF LARVAL AND ADULT FLIES

Both larvae and adults have sophisticated mechanisms for detecting local and long-range cues that guide animals toward food sources they prefer, and many of these systems have been extensively characterized (Vosshall et al. 2000; Scott 2005; Hallem et al. 2006; Benton 2008; Vosshall 2008; Masse et al. 2009; Montell 2009; Tanimura et al. 2009; Yarmolinsky et al. 2009). In general, they both tend to be attracted toward odorants that signal the presence of rotting fruit, including those emitted by the fruit itself or microorganisms that colonize it (Wright 2015). A number of tests have been developed to evaluate the abilities of both larvae and adults to sense volatile and nonvolatile food cues as well as their preferences for foods of various sensory properties and textures (Benton 2008; Gerber et al. 2013). For these experiments, groups of larvae or adult flies are monitored for their movements toward or away from the source(s) containing one or more odorants or tastants, and their distributions around the experimental arena are quantified at defined time points.

Drosophila larvae live on their food source, and they use a diverse array of peripheral sensory neurons located within their body wall to detect various external stimuli, including odorants, tastants, and mechanosensory cues on the surface along which they crawl (Benton 2008). Using these sensory organs, larvae assess environmental conditions, such as the temperature under which they forage, seek potential food sources that emit attractive odors, and evaluate their nutritional values based on appetitive and/or aversive tastes (Thorne et al. 2004; Wang et al. 2004; Wu et al. 2005b; Xu et al. 2010). One type of test for measuring such taste preferences in fly larvae involves monitoring a group of animals that are allowed to move between two nearby feeding substrates for a defined time period. The food preference is quantified using a preference index calculated based on the relative distribution of flies at or near the substrates. Food preference can also be quantified by using one-choice assays, which score and compare the responses of a group of animals to different foods of interest within a defined period of time (Wu et al. 2003). These tests are particularly suited for evaluating the preferences of fly larvae for foods containing various attractive and aversive tastants or of different texture (Fougeron et al. 2011; Masek and Keene 2013; Apostolopoulou et al. 2014). Odortaxis assays are useful for quantifying larval preferences for foods that emit attractive or aversive odors (Fougeron et al. 2011; Gong 2012; Masek and Keene 2013). In most cases, individual or groups of larvae are placed on the middle surface of agarose gel in a Petri dish,

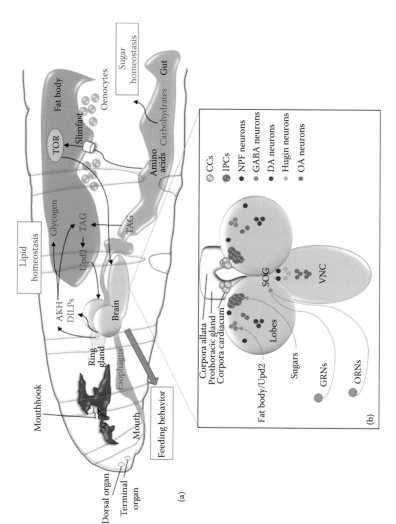

FIGURE 2.1 Overview of larval anatomy and major central and peripheral regulators of feeding behavior. (a) Diagram of the anterior portion of a third instar larva showing the feeding apparatus (mouthhook), chemosensory organs, CNS, and major digestive organs. Circulating signals regulating sugar homeostasis are indicated in blue; those regulating lipid homeostasis are indicated in orange. (b) Diagram of the CNS of a third instar larva displaying the major neurons implicated in the regulation of feeding behavior. Neurotransmitters or neuropeptides produced by each cell type are indicated in the color coded key. Targets of circulating signals and peripheral sensory systems are indicated with blue arrows.

where an odor gradient(s) is established by the foods positioned at opposite sides (Larsson et al. 2004; Fishilevich et al. 2005; Gomez-Marin et al. 2011; Mathew et al. 2013). Again, the movement of the larvae toward the odorant can be tracked and food preference can be calculated either by counting the number of larvae on each side of the dish or by quantifying the distance larvae travel (in terms of X–Y coordinates or in terms of path length). Using a similar assay procedure, groups of larvae can also be tested for their ability to form associative memories in response to the presentation of different types of odorants and tastes (Scherer et al. 2003; Gerber and Stocker 2007; Gerber et al. 2013).

A variation on this approach can be used to assess odor preferences in adult flies (Beshel and Zhong 2013). Adult flies are highly mobile relative to larvae and rely on long-range detection of odors to guide them toward potential foods. Their odor preferences can be assessed using attraction assays in which one or several potential attractants are presented from separate ports in a sealed chamber, and flies are monitored for their movement toward the different odors. When two or more odors are presented simultaneously, the degree of odor-associated attraction can be evaluated as the percentage of flies in each odorized quadrant relative to the total number of flies. As with larvae, such experiments can also be adapted to test the ability of an adult fly to form associative memories (Beck et al. 2000).

Once a fly larva reaches a suitable food, the gustatory detection of palatability causes it to begin ingestive movements in which it uses a pair of external mouth hooks to scoop liquid food or water into its oral cavity. This initial appetitive response of fly larvae to a given food can be quantified by counting the frequency of mouth hook contractions over a period of time (Wu et al. 2005a; Zhang et al. 2013a). Larvae fed ad libitum show a steady baseline contraction rate when placed on liquid sugar media. However, after a brief exposure to appetitive food odors (Wang et al. 2013) or prolonged food deprivation (Wu et al. 2005a), this assay can reliably detect increased appetitive response of individual larvae. For example, fasted larvae display increasingly higher frequencies of mouth hook contraction as food deprivation time is extended (Wu et al. 2005a; Zhang et al. 2013a). In addition, the mouth hook contraction assay is useful for measuring larval appetitive responses to food adulterated by aversive or noxious compounds such as quinine (Wu et al. 2005b) or foods in which the nutrients are difficult to extract (Wu et al. 2005b). For example, under well-nourished conditions, fed larvae decline solid foods; however, fasted larvae display increased use of their mouth hooks to pulverize solid foods in order to extract the embedded nutritious liquid. Thus, this assay can be used to assess the motivation of larvae to work for food (Wu et al. 2003, 2005a,b; Zhang et al. 2013a). While ingestive movements are an indirect readout of intake, the rate of mouth hook contractions of fed, fasted, or appetitive odor-aroused larvae have been shown to positively correlate with the amount of labeled food ingested (Wang et al. 2013; Zhang et al. 2013a), and labels can be added to the feeding media to provide a more quantitative readout. A large number of larvae can be assayed at one time via video recording for later analysis (Zhang et al. 2013a) and individual animals can be exposed to different treatments, making this assay relatively amenable to multiple types of feeding paradigms and treatments that regulate larval appetitive response.

Similarly, in adult flies, appetitive responses are triggered by the gustatory detection of food cues, which cause the fly to extend its proboscis into the food in order to drink. Feeding initiation thresholds and taste preferences can be monitored in adult flies using the proboscis extension response (PER) assay, which is a powerful and widely used method for monitoring preferences and appetitive responses in individual adult flies (Shiraiwa and Carlson 2007). For these experiments, a fly is immobilized (Tompkins et al. 1979; Vargo and Hirsch 1982) and presented with an attractive, sweet solution by application to the mouth (labellum) or tarsi, causing it to extend its proboscis in an all-or-none response and to initiate feeding (Homberg 2004). Conversely, presentation of aversive compounds will inhibit this response (Weiss et al. 2011). Responses are scored as either proboscis extension (positive) or lack of proboscis extension (negative) and can be quantified by measuring the proportion of flies that respond to a given stimulus. While the reflex occurs only when attractive stimuli are given, aversive substances such as bitter or salty compounds can be tested for their ability to inhibit the response when mixed with sugar in a concentration-dependent fashion (Falk and Atidia 1975; Arora et al. 1987; Inagaki et al. 2014). In addition, starvation enhances, while satiety tends to suppress, expression of PER (Edgecomb et al. 1994), making this assay particularly suitable for quantifying hunger-driven appetitive responses to various diets. The response of the proboscis is robust and easily observed, but the requirement for flies to be correctly immobilized and individually observed makes this a relatively low-throughput approach. However, the PER readout can be observed in tandem with live imaging in intact animals, providing an excellent opportunity for identifying basic circuits regulating the execution of this simply but highly adaptable behavior (Cao et al. 2013).

2.2.2 Food Intake of Larval and Adult Flies

Precise quantification of ingestion remains challenging in any organism, and this is also true for flies given the very small mass of food ingested in each feeding bout and meal. While the mass of intake in experimental models is often determined by weighing food before and after each feeding event, the amounts eaten by flies are too small to be accurately weighed. The classic approaches to monitoring fly ingestion therefore rely on the use of food that has been dyed or labeled with traceable molecules. The types of labels, in order of increasing accuracy, are food dyes (Edgecomb et al. 1994; Bross et al. 2005; Min and Tatar 2006), fluorescent molecules (Gasque et al. 2013), and radiolabeled compounds (Brummel et al. 2004; Carvalho et al. 2005, 2006). After flies have been given the labeled food for a period of time, they are assayed for ingestion by either visually scoring the amount of the labeled food in the gut or by grinding up the animals and measuring the amount of dye or label with a spectrophotometer or scintillation counter. Visually scoring flies is less accurate but allows food intake to be repeatedly monitored over time in the same animal. Because tracer methods rely on measuring only the amount of label present in the fly, the results may be influenced by factors other than feeding and may not account for differences in the ingestion ratio, feeding frequency, or retention time of the food or label (Wong et al. 2008, 2009). Fluorescent labels and dyes are accurate reporters of the initial phase of feeding but are not absorbed by the gut and begin to be excreted as feces within roughly 15 minutes of ingestion (Deshpande et al. 2014). For accurate long-term measurement of feeding, radiolabeled feeding substrates must be used, as these are absorbed and continue to accumulate over time (Deshpande et al. 2014). Because these assays determine only the amount of food that is retained in the fly following the assay, supplemental approaches can be used to measure food that is excreted as feces (Edgecomb et al. 1994; Zeng et al. 2011). Despite these limitations, label-based methods can be very powerful for high-throughput screening of a large numbers of flies and are amenable to automation (Gasque et al. 2013). In addition, they are sufficiently quantitative to detect relatively small differences in the mass of food ingested (Zhang et al. 2013a), making them suitable tools for identifying biologically relevant behavioral mechanisms.

Ingestion by adult flies can be dynamically monitored via the Capillary Feeder (CAFÉ) assay, in which flies are allowed to feed from a small capillary tube filled with liquid food and intake is determined by measuring fluid level in the capillary (Ja et al. 2007). This approach allows the experimenter to monitor the temporal aspects of food intake at the level of individual feeding bouts (Ja et al. 2007) with extremely high resolution over long periods of time (Farhadian et al. 2012). In addition, the CAFÉ assay can be adapted to measure food preference (Lee et al. 2008; Sellier et al. 2011). However, this approach does require that flies feed solely on liquid food sources, which may not accurately reflect normal eating patterns (Deshpande et al. 2014), and reduces both egg laying and lifespan (Bass et al. 2007; Lee et al. 2008). Furthermore, this approach is more laborious and fewer animals can be tested at one time (Itskov and Ribeiro 2013). As an alternative, two high-throughput assays have been reported that are designed for quantifying feeding behavior of adult flies. One of them, named the Fly Liquid–Food Interaction Counter (FLIC), detects electrical signals triggered when flies contact liquid food (Ro et al. 2014). One of the unique features of this technique is that it can record transient signals as short as 50 microseconds, and it is possible to distinguish between feeding and taste based on signal characteristics. The second assay is designed to measure the volume of food ingested in single sips by individual flies (Itskov et al. 2014) and is capable of analyzing the microstructure of a meal under different motivational states. Both the CAFÉ and FLIC assays may also detect small but significant changes in food consumption.

2.2.3 Genetic and Neurobiological Manipulation of Feeding Circuits

Perhaps the most valuable aspect of the fly as a model for behavioral neurobiology is the astounding array of genetic tools available for targeting, manipulating, and monitoring neural circuit activity. One particularly important tool set is based on the upstream activation sequence (UAS)/GAL4 system for genetically targeted gene expression, which provides a high level of spatial and temporal control over cell targeting and transgene expression. This system exploits the activity of a yeast transcription factor, GAL4, and it's identified cis-regulatory binding sites (UASs) that, when present upstream of a gene, result in its transcriptional activation by GAL4 (Brand and Perrimon 1993). The GAL4 transcriptional activator can be expressed randomly or in cell types or tissues of interest by placing it under the control of unique gene promotors (Gordon and Scott 2009; Marella et al. 2012). Alternately,

GAL4 expression can be controlled by heat- or drug-inducible promoters for temporal control over transgene expression (Duffy 2002). Variations of this system include the LexA/LexAop and QF/QUAS systems, which can be used alone or in tandem with the UAS/GAL4 system to further refine targeting or to express multiple transgenes (Pfeiffer et al. 2010; del Valle Rodriguez et al. 2012; Riabinina et al. 2015). A wide variety of UAS- and LexAop-based transgenes are available for labeling neurons as well as their nuclear, axonal, and dendritic compartments (Rolls et al. 2007; Nicolai et al. 2010), for monitoring activity (calcium [Akerboom et al. 2013], 3′,5′-cyclic adenosine monophosphate (cAMP) [Shafer et al. 2008], or voltage [Cao et al. 2013]), and for manipulating activity in a temperature- (Pool et al. 2014) or light- (Claridge-Chang et al. 2009; Perisse et al. 2013) dependent fashion. In addition to their use for monitoring the activity of select neuronal populations, these tools can be used to perform exquisitely targeted lesions in individual or small groups of neurons by administration of a targeted laser, allowing for precise loss of function analysis. The body wall of fly larvae is largely transparent, allowing focused laser beams to penetrate the brain and generate lesions in soma and neurites of identifiable central and peripheral neurons labeled with compartment specific markers such as nucleus- or axon-specific GFP (Xu et al. 2010; Wang et al. 2013; Zhang et al. 2013a). This technique has been particularly useful for testing the roles of defined neurons and circuits in feeding regulation in behaving animals. In tandem with the behavioral assays described previously, these genetic tools allow fly researchers a high level of temporal and spatial control and facilitate the characterization of the underlying biology regulating complex behavioral circuits.

2.3 CENTRAL AND PERIPHERAL REGULATION OF FEEDING BEHAVIOR

An extensive body of literature exists on the control of feeding behavior in both larval and adult flies. Like other animals, flies use multiple sensory functions and coordinated motor activities to seek, detect, and ingest food. They also modulate their food intake based on internal energy and nutrient needs and the quality of food sources and environmental conditions under which they forage. A large array of conserved substrates and regulatory systems have been identified that are involved in regulation of these behaviors by central and peripheral pathways, many of which have been extensively characterized (Baker and Thummel 2007; Leopold and Perrimon 2007; Rajan and Perrimon 2011). In this section, we will highlight those that are conserved and prominent. Readers are also referred to other reviews for further information (Baker and Thummel 2007; Leopold and Perrimon 2007; Benton 2008; Masse et al. 2009; Itskov and Ribeiro 2013; Rajan and Perrimon 2013).

2.3.1 MOTIVATIONAL STATE AND UNDERLYING CONTROL MECHANISMS

Like in mammals, feeding motivation in fruit flies is enhanced not only by food deprivation but also by rewarding sensory stimuli. In response to a brief stimulation of appetitive food odor, fed larvae show a significant increase in feeding frequency when presented with sugar-rich food. Two clusters of central dopamine (DA) neurons, one in each brain hemisphere, function as the third-order olfactory neurons. The DA neurons, along with downstream D1-like DA receptor neurons, define a neural circuit that converts diverse odor inputs to brain signals that drive appetitive motivation (Wang et al. 2013). In addition, acute stimulation by food odors triggers a transient increase in circulating glucose in adult flies, although its biological significance remains to be determined (Lushchak et al. 2015). These findings indicate that neural mechanisms underlying reward-driven feeding of palatable food may be conserved across evolution.

The feeding motivation of fruit flies is also altered by energy status and at least two separate neural modulatory systems have been identified that control different aspects of hunger-driven feeding responses in the fly larva. A key neural system that plays a dual role in modulation of larval appetite for sugar-rich food is mediated by octopamine (OA), an invertebrate counterpart of norepinephrine. When one subset of OA neurons in the larval brainstem-like region (named subesophageal ganglia or SOG; Figure 2.1) is ablated using targeted laser beams, fed larvae display increased appetite for sugar food. Conversely, loss of the function of another subset of nearby OA neurons attenuates a hunger-driven hyperphagic response to sugar food (Zhang et al. 2013a). Functional analysis of these OA neurons has led to the discovery of a novel neural activity of the vascular endothelial growth factor receptor (dVEGFR) in hyperphagia. Downregulation of dVEGFR activity in OA neurons attenuates hunger-driven overeating of sugar food, while its upregulation triggers hyperphagia in animals that are well fed (Zhang et al. 2013a), functions that are conserved in rodent feeding behavior models (Branch et al. 2015).

Food-deprived fly larvae are motivated to forage under hostile conditions (e.g., at cold temperatures), to engage in energy-expensive food extraction behaviors, and to accept food of poor quality or taste (Wu et al. 2005a,b). Two conserved neural signaling pathways underlie these hunger-driven feeding motivations. One of the pathways is defined by neuropeptide F (NPF; the fly counterpart of mammalian neuropeptide Y) (Brown et al. 1999; Nassel and Winther 2010; Nassel and Wegener 2011). NPF, whose expression is increased in the brain of hungry larvae, promotes different self-preservative motivations by signaling to neurons that express its receptor NPFR1 as well as the fly insulin-like receptor (dInR). Fly insulin producing cells (IPCs) are located in the median neurosecretory region of the central nervous system (CNS) and act in a fashion similar to the mammalian pancreatic β-cells (Figure 2.1). The release of drosphila insulin-like peptides (dIlps) promotes the storage of circulating sugars and also suppresses foraging motivation and food intake (Oldham and Hafen 2003; Wu et al. 2005a). The dIlps/dInR pathway negatively regulates the activity of the NPFR1 pathway during times of high internal nutrient levels. In fasted flies, the release of at least three of the eight known isoforms (dILP2, 3, and 5) are significantly reduced (Brogiolo et al. 2001; Ikeya et al. 2002). The simultaneous downregulation of dIlp and upregulation of NPF signaling pathways provide a neural control mechanism that drives stress-resistant acquisition and ingestion of food under adverse conditions.

Several studies have analyzed how the fly brain senses the energy state to control food seeking and ingestion (Van der Horst 2003; Kim and Rulifson 2004; Lee and Park 2004; Rajan and Perrimon 2013). The first short-term response to a drop in circulating carbohydrates is activation of corpora cardiac (CC) cells in the neu-roendocrine ring gland, which correspondingly act as pancreatic α-cells (Rajan and Perrimon 2013), releasing a neuropeptide called adipokinetic hormone (AKH) directly into circulation via projections to the aorta (Lee and Park 2004). Decreases in circulating trehalose or glucose are sensed by adenosine triphosphate (ATP)-sensitive potassium channels on CC cells, in a fashion similar to that of pancre-atic α-cells (Kim and Rulifson 2004), resulting in AKH release. AKH acts through a G-protein-coupled receptor, AKHR, located on fat body cells, which mobilizes stored glycogen and fats by increasing lipolysis, glycogenolysis, and production of trehalose (Veelaert et al. 1998; Van der Horst 2003; Kim and Rulifson 2004). This mobilization of energy stores allows starvation-dependent increases in locomotor activity in order to promote food seeking behavior (Kim and Rulifson 2004; Beshel and Zhong 2013; Gruber et al. 2013).

In addition, hunger down-regulates the activity of S6K in IPCs, which reduces insulin release and drives animals to search for and acquire food (Wu et al. 2005a). IPCs are also regulated by several central and peripheral pathways. Centrally, IPCs are targeted by serotonergic and GABAergic neurons, both of which exert an inhibitory influence on their release of dIlps (Enell et al. 2010; Luo et al. 2012). Peripherally, IPC activity is linked to the levels of circulating amino acids, fats, and sugars via signals secreted by the fat body, which acts as a nutrient sensor and secretes growth promoting factors (Davis and Shearn 1977; Britton and Edgar 1998). The fat body expresses an amino acid transporter, Slimfast, which acts as a nonau-tonomous sensor to regulate dIlp signaling based on nutrient levels (Colombani et al. 2003; Geminard et al. 2009) and produces the cytokine Upd2, a Janus kinase (JAK)/ signal transducer and activator of transcription (STAT) pathway ligand function-ally homologous to leptin, in proportion to the circulating levels of fats and sugars (Rajan and Perrimon 2012). Upd2 acts in part by inhibiting GABAergic neurons which synapse on IPCs, resulting in the secretion of dILPs into the circulation to promote systemic growth and fat storage (Rajan and Perrimon 2012). Furthermore, diverse internal sensors for monitoring nutrients are likely present in flies and other animals. For example, taste receptors have been reported in the brain as well as the gastrointestinal tract of flies that function as internal sensors to detect fructose in the body (Miyamoto et al. 2012; Miyamoto and Amrein 2014).

Recent studies have also revealed the roles of two conserved monoamine systems in the central processing of rewarding cues. It has been shown that OA signaling mediates the transient reinforcing properties of the sweet taste of sugar, whereas DA signaling in the fly CNS conveys information regarding rewarding stimuli in a fashion very similar to the reward pathways used by mammals. DA signaling enhances the sensitivity of gustatory receptor neurons (GRNs) to sugar in hungry flies (Inagaki et al. 2012; Marella et al. 2012). It also modulates responses to sucrose (Kim et al. 2007; Krashes et al. 2009; Selcho et al. 2009) and satiety state-dependent appetitive mem-ory formation (Krashes et al. 2009) in the mushroom bodies (MBs), a higher-order brain center important for odor processing and learning (de Belle and Heisenberg 1994; Hitier et al. 1998; Schwaerzel et al. 2003; Margulies et al. 2005; Krashes et al. 2007), via overlapping DA and NPF/NPFR1 signaling mechanisms. The lower appetitive memory performance observed in satiated flies is due to tonic inhibition of subsets of DA neurons in the MB, while stimulation of neurons expressing NPF promotes appetitive memory by suppressing this inhibition and enabling the expression of food-associated conditioned responses. OA-dependent mechanisms also enhance short-term sugar-dependent memory encoding via activation of the OAMB receptor on a subset of DA neurons in the MB (Burke et al. 2012). It therefore appears that subsets of DA neurons in the MB represent short- and long-term reinforcing effects of nutritious sugar in learning and act downstream of OA signals. DA appears to provide a tonic inhibitory signal, which can be modulated by selective NPF/NPFR1 gating mechanisms to promote execution of either appetitive or aversive behavior (Krashes et al. 2009) and also by OA/OAMB gated signaling, which provides gustatory signals regarding food quality (Burke et al. 2012). With this model in mind, DA neurons in the MB can be thought of as a central behavioral subprogram selection circuit, in which subprogram selection is gated by both nutrient detection and satiety state.

2.3.2 Regulatory Systems for Foraging and Food Detection

Foraging behaviors of fruit flies can be enhanced by food deprivation (Yang et al. 2015). The hyperactivity of fasted flies is rapidly suppressed when food is detected through central and peripheral sensory mechanisms, suggesting that such hunger-induced motor activities, mediated by OA signaling, are geared toward searching and acquiring food. A study of motor programs in fly larvae points to a role of a neuropeptide named hugin, which is homologous to mammalian neuromedin U, as a key molecular switch between food intake and locomotion. Furthermore, a pair of interneurons in the spinal cord-like ventral nerve cord has been identified as essential for the inhibition of feeding when an adult fly is walking (Mann et al. 2013). It has also been shown that an OA system in the ventral nerve cord of fly larvae modulates hunger-induced increases in locomotor speed, thereby facilitating larval foraging (Koon et al. 2011). The motor activities of larvae that drive the external mouth hooks to extract nutrients embedded in solid media are also enhanced by food deprivation through the NPF system mentioned earlier (Wu et al. 2003, 2005a).

Both larvae and adult flies have sophisticated sensory systems for detecting volatile and nonvolatile food cues, and many of them have been extensively characterized (Vosshall et al. 2000; Scott 2005; Hallem et al. 2006; Benton 2008; Vosshall 2008; Masse et al. 2009; Montell 2009; Tanimura et al. 2009; Yarmolinsky et al. 2009). Larvae live on their food source. To identify food in their surroundings, they make use of chemosensory neurons that are widely distributed in diverse organs in the head and other parts of the body, including the dorsal organ (DO), which detects odor and taste, and the terminal organ (TO), ventral organ (VO), and pharyngeal sensilla, which are primarily gustatory (Chu and Axtell 1971; Chu-Wang and Axtell 1972a,b; Singh and Singh 1984; Singh 1997). Adult flies are much more mobile and have a more complex chemosensory system to detect long-range cues as well as chemosensory hairs or sensilla located on the antennae, labial and maxillary palps, legs, wings, and mouthparts parts for sensing local gustatory and other sensory cues (Stocker 1994).

The *Drosophila* genome encodes 68 known gustatory receptor genes (Scott et al. 2001) and 61 olfactory receptor genes (Clyne et al. 1999, 2000; Gao and Chess 1999), although their olfactory or gustatory coding capacity has not been fully catalogued

(Scott et al. 2001). In adults, GRNs are found in the DO, TO, VO, and pharyngeal sensilla, while olfactory receptor neurons (ORNs) are located in antennae and maxillary palps (Stocker 1994). For example, gustatory receptor 5a- and 64f- (Gr5a and Gr64f) expressing GRNs have been found to be involved in detection of sugar, salt, fatty acids, and other attractive gustatory cues, while aversive tastes, such as bitter substances and high concentrations of salt, are detected by Gr66-expressing GRNs (Scott et al. 2001; Wang et al. 2004; Dahanukar et al. 2007; Weiss et al. 2011; Marella et al. 2012; Masek and Keene 2013; Zhang et al. 2013b). GRN and ORN expressing neurons located in these chemosensory organs project to the SOG, which is implicated in feeding-related behavioral expression and taste response (Singh and Singh 1984; Singh 1997; Scott et al. 2001; Gendre et al. 2004; Melcher and Pankratz 2005; Melcher et al. 2006), and to protocerebral structures including the lateral horn and MBs, which process and encode this input to guide innate behaviors and form memories (de Belle and Heisenberg 1994; Farris 2008; Claridge-Chang et al. 2009). Large areas of the insect brain are involved in decoding chemosensory signals and transforming them into adaptive commands for motor circuit execution and control (Homberg 2004).

Starvation also enhances a fly's ability to detect and discriminate between different odors and tastes by modifying the activity of ORNs and GRNs. For example, enhancement of odor representations in ORNs and bitter tastes in GRNs is facilitated by short NPF (sNPF) and its receptor sNPFR1 (Root et al. 2011; Inagaki et al. 2014). Starvation decreases insulin signaling pathway regulation of ORNs and increases the fly's expression of sNPFR1, which in turn increases its sensitivity to food-related odors and their foraging behaviors. In addition, increased release of AKH appears to facilitate sNPF-mediated decreases in the sensitivity of GRNs to bitter tastes (Inagaki et al. 2014). Increased responsiveness to taste is largely mediated by overlapping contributions from the OA, DA, and NPF systems, such that sugar sensitivity is increased (Inagaki et al. 2012, 2014; Marella et al. 2012) and bitter sensitivity is decreased (Inagaki et al. 2014). Flies also display taste preference for selected amino acids, and such preferences are greatly enhanced during starvation, possibly due to increased sensitivity of taste cells when flies are deprived of amino acids (Toshima and Tanimura 2012).

2.3.3 REGULATORY SYSTEMS FOR FOOD EVALUATION AND MEAL INITIATION

The decision to initiate a meal is regulated by the detection of nutritive compounds, while detection of noxious stimuli such as aversive taste (Wu et al. 2005b) or temperature (Xu et al. 2010) elicits rejection behaviors. Detection of nutritive compounds involves first taste sensing followed by calorie sensing, and the relative contribution of calorie sensing to feeding choice increases as feeding time progresses (Stafford et al. 2012). While taste sensing is largely performed by peripheral gustatory neurons (Thorne et al. 2004; Wang et al. 2004) and pharyngeal sense organs in the internal mouthparts (LeDue et al. 2015), calorie sensing involves internal sensors located in the brain and other organs (Miyamoto et al. 2012; Dus et al. 2013). For meal initiation to occur, these sensory inputs must override inhibitory thresholds set by central neurons, which gate the activity of feeding motor programs. The precise mechanisms regulating proboscis extension and feeding rate remain under investigation. It has been determined that gustatory neurons (Singh 1997; Thorne et al. 2004; Wang et al. 2004), candidate modulatory neurons (Wu et al. 2003; Wen et al. 2005), and motor neurons that synapse on proboscis muscles (Rajashekhar and Singh 1994) all arborize in the hindbrain-like SOG region of the CNS (Singh and Singh 1984; Singh 1997; Scott et al. 2001; Gendre et al. 2004; Melcher and Pankratz 2005; Melcher et al. 2006; Urbach 2007). The SOG contains several sets of neurons that have been characterized as having direct or indirect roles in feeding behavior expression and quality.

The feeding behavior of adult flies is driven by an organized set of stereotyped motor patterns. It has been reported that a single pair of interneurons is sufficient to command a complete feeding motor program (Flood et al. 2013). In addition, specialized central neurons are required for the execution of the various subprograms involved in feeding, and the activities of such neurons are subject to modification by internal energy status (Gordon and Scott 2009; Flood et al. 2013; Pool et al. 2014). These feeding behavioral subprograms are adaptive, depending on both internal satiety status and external sensory cues of food quality and nutritional value.

It has been reported that fed adult flies wait for a period of at least 30 minutes before feeding on a new food, and this phase of food evaluation can be abolished by food deprivation (Pool et al. 2014). The neuropeptide hugin is essential for establishing this latency to feed (Melcher et al. 2006). Hugin expression is found in roughly 20 neurons located in the larval SOG. Circuit analysis revealed that hugin neurons function as gustatory interneurons that receive input from gustatory sensory neurons and chemosensory neurons of the pharynx and extend axonal processes to the ring glad (a major endocrine organ) and pharyngeal muscles (required for mouth hook movement and ingestion). These observations indicate that hugin controls initiation of meals by suppressing an immediate feeding response.

The activity of hugin is downregulated by starvation and amino acid deprivation (Pool et al. 2014). In contrast to the hugin circuit, which is nutrient responsive and satiety dependent, a novel circuit was recently identified that exerts a tonic inhibitory tone on meal initiation and consumption (Pool et al. 2014) by selectively gating motor neuron output in adult flies. This is mediated by four GABAergic neurons in the ventral region of the SOG, which receive input from GRNs and project to motor neurons regulating food intake. Inactivation of these neurons leads to indiscriminative proboscis extension and consumption of all media tested. This circuit is unique in that it provides a centralized threshold mechanism that a fly can conveniently interact with in order to organize multiple motor programs for ingestive activities regardless of whether they are driven by taste or nutrients (Pool et al. 2014). Recent work has also identified an important role of internal gustatory detection of sweet taste by GRNs in the pharyngeal organs for sustaining feeding after sampling of sweet food (LeDue et al. 2015).

2.3.4 REGULATORY SYSTEMS FOR MEAL SIZE AND FREQUENCY

Once feeding is initiated, the rate of ingestion and duration are dynamically modulated based on internal metabolic status via circulating hormones from neuroendocrine cells and fat tissue. These hormones act as coding mechanisms for the internal availability of carbohydrate and lipid stores (Rajan and Perrimon 2012) and include the *Drosophila* insulin-like peptides (Wu et al. 2005b; Geminard et al. 2009), AKH (Kim and Rulifson 2004), and leptin homolog Unpaired 2. Two fly genes, TfAP2 and Twz, are homologues of mouse AP-2b and Kctd15 implicated in obesity (Williams et al. 2014). They function together to control OA and thereby regulate meal size and frequency. Loss of TfAP2 or Twz in OA neurons leads to larger individual meals, while TfAP2 overexpression reduces the meal size but increases feeding frequency. OA may also play a role in upregulation of drosulfakinin signaling, resulting in inhibition of food consumption (Williams et al. 2014). As noted previously, fly IPCs produce and secrete three of the eight known insulin-like peptide isoforms (dILPs 2, 3, and 5) (Brogiolo et al. 2001) in a nutrient-dependent fashion (Ikeya et al. 2002). In addition, IPCs produce drosulfakinin, a cholecystokinin-like peptide, which acts as a hormonal satiety signal to reduce food intake and heighten discrimination between food choices (Soderberg et al. 2012). Ablation of IPCs or loss of dILP expression in these cells disrupts carbohydrate homeostasis (Geminard et al. 2009), body size regulation (Slaidina et al. 2009; Mirth et al. 2014), and feeding behavior (Wu et al. 2005a). Deletion of the genes for dILP 1–5 results in phenotypes similar to those seen in type I diabetic patients, including elevated circulating sugars, reduced fat storage, and autophagy (Zhang et al. 2009). Further, adult flies develop obesity and insulin resistance when fed high-fat or high-sugar diets (Hull-Thompson et al. 2009; Musselman et al. 2011; Pasco and Leopold 2012), suggesting that mechanisms of insulin resistance are conserved from flies to mammals (Rajan and Perrimon 2013).

Meal termination is regulated by postingestive feedback from the gut, which may inhibit feeding via the recurrent nerve or medial abdominal nerve (Dethier 1976), as well as by the tachykinin-like neuropeptide leucokinin, which acts to signal the amount of food in the foregut (Al-Anzi et al. 2010). Recent work has also identified contributions from posterior enteric neurons in the *Drosophila* digestive system, which innervate the musculature of the gut and may act to convey a stretch-dependent sensation of fullness via pickpocket 1 (PPK1) mechanosensory ion channels (Olds and Xu 2014). Leukokinin mutants increase the amount of food consumed per meal and increase the intermeal interval, suggesting that leukokinin mediates the decision to stop feeding. An additional source of postingestive feedback comes from specialized neurons in the central nervous system, which directly monitor circulating energy levels and alter feeding probability based on internal need. For example, some central neurons express receptors that respond to specific nutrients such as fructose (Miyamoto et al. 2012) and amino acids (Bjordal et al. 2014) and modify feeding and other behaviors accordingly (Burke and Waddell 2011; Dus et al. 2011; Fujita and Tanimura 2011; Stafford et al. 2012).

2.4 CONCLUSION AND FUTURE DIRECTIONS

Drosophila larvae and adults have been proven to be useful models for characterization of conserved molecular and neural bases of feeding behaviors. A broad array of conserved neural substrates including monoamines, neuropeptides, and other regulatory genes and pathways have been identified and characterized in flies for their roles in regulation of foraging activities, food detection and evaluation, feeding decisions, feeding motivation, and execution of ingestive motor activities. These studies have generated a substantial body of novel and complementary knowledge that demonstrates that fruit flies and vertebrate animals share conserved neural substrates and mechanisms for the control of diverse aspects of feeding behavior.

In the next decade, we are likely to see more rapid progresses in several areas of fly feeding research, partly due to promising new technical advances. For example, more efficient knock-in and knock-out technologies will enable researchers to modulate the activity of individual neurons or gene activity in neurons of interest in transgenic flies. Emerging tools for high-resolution mapping of neural circuits in the fly brain will also make it possible to analyze how a network of interacting pathways coordinately mediates feeding control. At present, much remains to be studied about the hierarchy or independence of the neural circuits, their neural plasticity, and temporal dynamics of their regulation. This information is needed to piece together how feeding is dynamically regulated over short and long time periods. In addition, our knowledge about cognitive functions related to feeding decisions remains rudimentary. Feeding behavior is influenced by a multitude of environmental and physiological factors, and future work will lead to a deeper understanding of the integrated effects of these factors on the feeding response, especially on a long-term basis.

LITERATURE CITED

Akerboom, J. et al. 2013 Genetically encoded calcium indicators for multi-color neural activity imaging and combination with optogenetics. *Front Mol Neurosci* 6:2.

Al-Anzi, B., Armand, E., Nagamei, P., Olszewski, M., Sapin, V., Waters, C., Zinn, K., Wyman, R.J., and Benzer, S. 2010 The leucokinin pathway and its neurons regulate meal size in *Drosophila*. *Curr Biol* 20(11):969–978.

Apostolopoulou, A.A., Mazija, L., Wust, A., and Thum, A.S. 2014 The neuronal and molecular basis of quinine-dependent bitter taste signaling in *Drosophila* larvae. *Front Behav Neurosci* 8:6.

Arora, K., Rodrigues, V., Joshi, S., Shanbhag, S., and Siddiqi, O. 1987 A gene affecting the specificity of the chemosensory neurons of *Drosophila*. *Nature* 330(6143):62–63.

Bainbridge, S.P. and Bownes, M. 1981 Staging the metamorphosis of *Drosophila melanogaster*. *J Embryol Exp Morphol* 66:57–80.

Baker, K.D. and Thummel, C.S. 2007 Diabetic larvae and obese flies—Emerging studies of metabolism in *Drosophila*. *Cell Metab* 6(4):257–266.

Bass, T.M., Grandison, R.C., Wong, R., Martinez, P., Partridge, L., and Piper, M.D. 2007 Optimization of dietary restriction protocols in *Drosophila*. *J Gerontol A Biol Sci Med Sci* 62(10):1071–1081.

Bateson, M. 2002 Recent advances in our understanding of risk-sensitive foraging preferences. *Proc Nutr Soc* 61(4):509–516.

Beck, C.D., Schroeder, B., and Davis, R.L. 2000 Learning performance of normal and mutant *Drosophila* after repeated conditioning trials with discrete stimuli. *J Neurosci* 20(8):2944–2953.

Benton, R. 2008 Chemical sensing in *Drosophila*. *Curr Opin Neurobiol* 18(4):357–363.

Beshel, J. and Zhong, Y. 2013 Graded encoding of food odor value in the *Drosophila* brain. *J Neurosci* 33(40):15693–15704.

Bjordal, M., Arquier, N., Kniazeff, J., Pin, J.P., and Leopold, P. 2014 Sensing of amino acids in a dopaminergic circuitry promotes rejection of an incomplete diet in *Drosophila*. *Cell* 156(3):510–521.

Bland, M.L., Lee, R.J., Magallanes, J.M., Foskett, J.K., and Birnbaum, M.J. 2010 AMPK supports growth in *Drosophila* by regulating muscle activity and nutrient uptake in the gut. *Develop Biol* 344(1):293–303.

Branch, A., Bobilev, A., Negrao, N.W., Cai, H., and Shen, P. 2015 Prevention of palatable diet-induced hyperphagia in rats by central injection of a VEGFR kinase inhibitor. *Behav Brain Res* 278:506–513.

Brand, A.H. and Perrimon, N. 1993 Targeted gene expression as a means of altering cell fates and generating dominant phenotypes. *Development* 118(2):401–415.

Britton, J.S. and Edgar, B.A. 1998 Environmental control of the cell cycle in *Drosophila*: Nutrition activates mitotic and endoreplicative cells by distinct mechanisms. *Development* 125(11):2149–2158.

Brogiolo, W., Stocker, H., Ikeya, T., Rintelen, F., Fernandez, R., and Hafen, E. 2001 An evolutionarily conserved function of the *Drosophila* insulin receptor and insulin-like peptides in growth control. *Curr Biol* 11(4):213–221.

Bross, T.G., Rogina, B., and Helfand, S.L. 2005 Behavioral, physical, and demographic changes in *Drosophila* populations through dietary restriction. *Aging Cell* 4(6):309–317.

Brown, M.R., Crim, J.W., Arata, R.C., Cai, H.N., Chun, C., and Shen, P. 1999 Identification of a *Drosophila* brain-gut peptide related to the neuropeptide Y family. *Peptides* 20(9):1035–1042.

Brummel, T., Ching, A., Seroude, L., Simon, A.F., and Benzer, S. 2004 *Drosophila* lifespan enhancement by exogenous bacteria. *Proc Natl Acad Sci U S A* 101(35):12974–12979.

Burke, C.J. and Waddell, S. 2011 Remembering nutrient quality of sugar in *Drosophila*. *Curr Biol* 21(9):746–750.

Burke, C.J., Huetteroth W., Owald, D., Perisse, E., Krashes, M.J., Das, G., Gohl, D., Silies, M., Certel, S., and Waddell, S. 2012 Layered reward signalling through octopamine and dopamine in *Drosophila*. *Nature* 492(7429):433–437.

Cao, G., Platisa, J., Pieribone, V.A., Raccuglia, D., Kunst, M., and Nitabach, M.N. 2013 Genetically targeted optical electrophysiology in intact neural circuits. *Cell* 154(4):904–913.

Carvalho, G.B., Kapahi, P., and Benzer, S. 2005 Compensatory ingestion upon dietary restriction in *Drosophila melanogaster*. *Nat Methods* 2(11):813–815.

Carvalho, G.B., Kapahi, P., Anderson, D.J., and Benzer, S. 2006 Allocrine modulation of feeding behavior by the sex peptide of *Drosophila*. *Curr Biol* 16(7):692–696.

Chu, I.W. and Axtell, R.C. 1971 Fine structure of the dorsal organ of the house fly larva, *Musca domestica* L. *Z Zellforsch Mikrosk Anat* 117(1):17–34.

Chu-Wang, I.W. and Axtell, R.C. 1972a Fine structure of the terminal organ of the house fly larva, *Musca domestica* L. *Z Zellforsch Mikrosk Anat* 127(3):287–305.

Chu-Wang, I.W. and Axtell, R.C. 1972b Fine structure of the ventral organ of the house fly larva, *Musca domestica* L. *Z Zellforsch Mikrosk Anat* 130(4):489–495.

Claridge-Chang, A., Roorda, R.D., Vrontou, E., Sjulson, L., Li, H., Hirsh, J., and Miesenböck, G. 2009 Writing memories with light-addressable reinforcement circuitry. *Cell* 139(2): 405–415.

Clyne, P.J., Warr, C.G., and Carlson, J.R. 2000 Candidate taste receptors in *Drosophila*. *Science* 287(5459):1830–1834.

Clyne, P.J., Warr, C.G., Freeman, M.R., Lessing, D., Kim, J., and Carlson, J.R. 1999 A novel family of divergent seven-transmembrane proteins: Candidate odorant receptors in *Drosophila*. *Neuron* 22(2):327–338.

Colombani, J., Raisin, S., Pantalacci, S., Radimerski, T., Montagne, J., and Léopold, P. 2003 A nutrient sensor mechanism controls *Drosophila* growth. *Cell* 114(6):739–749.

Couto, A., Alenius, M., and Dickson, B.J. 2005 Molecular, anatomical, and functional organization of the *Drosophila* olfactory system. *Curr Biol* 15(17):1535–1547.

Dahanukar, A., Lei, Y.T., Kwon, J.Y., and Carlson, J.R. 2007 Two Gr genes underlie sugar reception in *Drosophila*. *Neuron* 56(3):503–516.

Davis, K.T. and Shearn, A. 1977 In vitro growth of imaginal disks from *Drosophila melanogaster*. *Science* 196(4288):438–440.

de Belle, J.S. and Heisenberg, M. 1994 Associative odor learning in *Drosophila* abolished by chemical ablation of mushroom bodies. *Science* 263(5147):692–695.

del Valle Rodriguez, A., Didiano, D., and Desplan, C. 2012 Power tools for gene expression and clonal analysis in *Drosophila*. *Nat Methods* 9(1):47–55.

Deshpande, S.A., Carvalho, G.B., Amador, A., Phillips, A.M., Hoxha, S., Lizotte, K.J., Ja, W.W. 2014 Quantifying *Drosophila* food intake: Comparative analysis of current methodology. *Nat Methods* 11(5):535–540.

Dethier, V.G. 1976 *The Hungry Fly* (Harvard University Press, Cambridge, MA).

Duffy, J.B. 2002 GAL4 system in *Drosophila*: A fly geneticist's Swiss army knife. *Genesis* 34(1–2):1–15.

Dus, M., Ai, M., and Suh, G.S. 2013 Taste-independent nutrient selection is mediated by a brain-specific Na+/solute co-transporter in *Drosophila*. *Nat Neurosci* 16(5):526–528.

Dus, M., Min, S., Keene, A.C., Lee, G.Y., and Suh, G.S. 2011 Taste-independent detection of the caloric content of sugar in *Drosophila*. *Proc Natl Acad Sci U S A* 108(28):11644–11649.

Edgecomb, R.S., Harth, C.E., and Schneiderman, A.M. 1994 Regulation of feeding behavior in adult *Drosophila melanogaster* varies with feeding regime and nutritional state. *J Exp Biol* 197:215–235.

Enell, L.E., Kapan, N., Soderberg, J.A., Kahsai, L., and Nassel, D.R. 2010 Insulin signaling, lifespan and stress resistance are modulated by metabotropic GABA receptors on insulin producing cells in the brain of *Drosophila*. *PloS One* 5(12):e15780.

Falk, R. and Atidia, J. 1975 Mutation affecting taste perception in *Drosophila melanogaster*. *Nature* 254(5498):325–326.

Farhadian, S.F., Suarez-Farinas, M., Cho, C.E., Pellegrino, M., and Vosshall, L.B. 2012 Post-fasting olfactory, transcriptional, and feeding responses in *Drosophila*. *Physiol Behav* 105(2):544–553.

Farris, S.M. 2008 Structural, functional and developmental convergence of the insect mushroom bodies with higher brain centers of vertebrates. *Brain Behav Evol* 72(1):1–15.

Fishilevich, E., Domingos, A.I., Asahina, K., Naef, F., Vosshall, L.B., Louis, M. 2005 Chemotaxis behavior mediated by single larval olfactory neurons in *Drosophila*. *Curr Biol* 15(23):2086–2096.

Flood, T.F., Iguchi, S., Gorczyca, M., White, B., Ito, K., and Yoshihara, M. 2013 A single pair of interneurons commands the *Drosophila* feeding motor program. *Nature* 499(7456):83–87.

Fougeron, A.S., Farine, J.P., Flaven-Pouchon, J., Everaerts, C., and Ferveur, J.F. 2011 Fatty-acid preference changes during development in *Drosophila melanogaster*. *PloS One* 6(10):e26899.

Fujita, M. and Tanimura, T. 2011 *Drosophila* evaluates and learns the nutritional value of sugars. *Curr Biol* 21(9):751–755.

Gao, Q. and Chess, A. 1999 Identification of candidate *Drosophila* olfactory receptors from genomic DNA sequence. *Genomics* 60(1):31–39.

Gasque, G., Conway, S., Huang, J., Rao, Y., and Vosshall, L.B. 2013 Small molecule drug screening in *Drosophila* identifies the 5HT2A receptor as a feeding modulation target. *Sci Rep* 3:srep02120.

Geminard, C., Rulifson, E.J., and Leopold, P. 2009 Remote control of insulin secretion by fat cells in *Drosophila*. *Cell Metab* 10(3):199–207.

Gendre, N., Lüer, K., Friche, S., Grillenzoni, N., Ramaekers, A., Technau, G.M., and Stocker, R.F. 2004 Integration of complex larval chemosensory organs into the adult nervous system of *Drosophila*. *Development* 131(1):83–92.

Gerber, B. and Stocker, R.F. 2007 The *Drosophila* larva as a model for studying chemosensation and chemosensory learning: A review. *Chem Senses* 32(1):65–89.

Gerber, B., Biernacki, R., Thrum, J. 2013 Odor-taste learning assays in *Drosophila* larvae. *Cold Spring Harb Protoc.* Mar 1;2013(3).

Gomez-Marin, A., Stephens, G.J., and Louis, M. 2011 Active sampling and decision making in *Drosophila* chemotaxis. *Nat Commun* 2:441.

Gong, Z. 2012 Innate preference in *Drosophila melanogaster*. *Sci China Life Sci* 55(1):8–14.

Gordon, M.D. and Scott, K. 2009 Motor control in a *Drosophila* taste circuit. *Neuron* 61(3): 373–384.

Gruber, F., Knapek, S., Fujita, M., Matsuo, K., Bräcker, L., Shinzato, N., Siwanowicz, I., Tanimura, T., and Tanimoto, H. 2013 Suppression of conditioned odor approach by feeding is independent of taste and nutritional value in *Drosophila*. *Curr Biol* 23(6):507–514.

Gutierrez, E., Wiggins, D., Fielding, B., and Gould, A.P. 2007 Specialized hepatocytelike cells regulate *Drosophila* lipid metabolism. *Nature* 445(7125):275–280.

Hallem, E.A., Dahanukar, A., and Carlson, J.R. 2006 Insect odor and taste receptors. *Ann Rev Entomol* 51:113–135.

Hitier, R., Heisenberg, M., and Preat, T. 1998 Abnormal mushroom body plasticity in the *Drosophila* memory mutant amnesiac. *Neuroreport* 9(12):2717–2719.

Homberg, U. 2004 *Multisensory Processing in the Insect Brain: Methods in Insect Sensory Neuroscience* (CRC Press, Boca Raton, London, New York, Washington, DC).

Hull-Thompson, J., Muffat, J., Sanchez, D., Walker, D.W., Benzer, S., Ganfornina, M.D., and Jasper, H. 2009 Control of metabolic homeostasis by stress signaling is mediated by the lipocalin NLaz. *PLoS Genet* 5(4):e1000460.

Ikeya, T., Galic, M., Belawat, P., Nairz, K., and Hafen, E. 2002 Nutrient-dependent expression of insulin-like peptides from neuroendocrine cells in the CNS contributes to growth regulation in *Drosophila*. *Curr Biol* 12(15):1293–1300.

Inagaki, H.K., Ben-Tabou de-Leon, S., Wong, A.M., Jagadish, S., Ishimoto, H., Barnea, G., Kitamoto, T., Axel, R., and Anderson, D.J. 2012 Visualizing neuromodulation in vivo: TANGO-mapping of dopamine signaling reveals appetite control of sugar sensing. *Cell* 148(3):583–595.

Inagaki, H.K., Panse, K.M., and Anderson, D. 2014 Independent, reciprocal neuromodulatory control of sweet and bitter taste sensitivity during starvation in *Drosophila*. *Neuron* 19;84(4):806–820.

Isono, K. and Morita, H. 2010 Molecular and cellular designs of insect taste receptor system. *Front Cell Neurosci* 4:20.

Itskov, P.M. and Ribeiro, C. 2013 The dilemmas of the gourmet fly: The molecular and neuronal mechanisms of feeding and nutrient decision making in *Drosophila*. *Front Neurosci* 7:12.

Itskov, P.M., Moreira, J.M., Vinnik, E., Lopes, G., Safarik, S., Dickinson, M.H., and Ribeiro, C. 2014 Automated monitoring and quantitative analysis of feeding behavior in *Drosophila*. *Nat Commun* 5:4560.

Ja, W.W., Carvalho, G.B., Mak, E.M., de la Rosa, N.N., Fang, A.Y., Liong, J.C., Brummel, T., and Benzer, S. 2007 Prandiology of *Drosophila* and the CAFE assay. *Proc Natl Acad Sci U S A* 104(20):8253–8256.

Kim, S.K. and Rulifson, E.J. 2004 Conserved mechanisms of glucose sensing and regulation by *Drosophila* corpora cardiaca cells. *Nature* 431(7006):316–320.

Kim, Y.C., Lee, H.G., and Han, K.A. 2007 D1 dopamine receptor dDA1 is required in the mushroom body neurons for aversive and appetitive learning in *Drosophila*. *The J Neurosci* 27(29):7640–7647

Koon, A.C. et al. 2011 Autoregulatory and paracrine control of synaptic and behavioral plasticity by octopaminergic signaling. *Nat Neurosci* 14(2):190–199.

Krashes, M.J., DasGupta, S., Vreede, A., White, B., Armstrong, J.D., and Waddell, S. 2009 A neural circuit mechanism integrating motivational state with memory expression in *Drosophila*. *Cell* 139(2):416–427.

Krashes, M.J., Keene, A.C., Leung, B., Armstrong, J.D., and Waddell, S. 2007 Sequential use of mushroom body neuron subsets during *Drosophila* odor memory processing. *Neuron* 53(1):103–115.

Larsson, M.C., Domingos, A.I., Jones, W.D., Chiappe, M.E., Amrein, H., Vosshall, L.B. 2004 Or83b encodes a broadly expressed odorant receptor essential for *Drosophila* olfaction. *Neuron* 43(5):703–714.

LeDue, E.E., Chen, Y.C., Jung, A.Y., Dahanukar, A., and Gordon, M.D. 2015 Pharyngeal sense organs drive robust sugar consumption in *Drosophila*. *Nat Commun* 6:6667.

Lee, G. and Park, J.H. 2004 Hemolymph sugar homeostasis and starvation-induced hyperactivity affected by genetic manipulations of the adipokinetic hormone-encoding gene in *Drosophila melanogaster*. *Genetics* 167(1):311–323.

Lee, K.P., Simpson, S.J., Clissold, F.J., Brooks, R., Ballard, J.W., Taylor, P.W., Soran, N., and Raubenheimer, D. 2008 Lifespan and reproduction in *Drosophila*: New insights from nutritional geometry. *Proc Natl Acad Sci U S A* 105(7):2498–2503.

Leopold, P. and Perrimon, N. 2007 *Drosophila* and the genetics of the internal milieu. *Nature* 450(7167):186–188.

Luo, J., Becnel, J., Nichols, C.D., and Nassel, D.R. 2012 Insulin-producing cells in the brain of adult *Drosophila* are regulated by the serotonin 5-HT1A receptor. *Cell Mol Life Sci* 69(3):471–484.

Lushchak, O.V., Carlsson, M.A., and Nassel, D.R. 2015 Food odors trigger an endocrine response that affects food ingestion and metabolism. *Cell Mol Life Sci* 72(16):3143–3155.

Mann, K., Gordon, M.D., and Scott, K. 2013 A pair of interneurons influences the choice between feeding and locomotion in *Drosophila*. *Neuron* 79(4):754–765.

Marella, S., Mann, K., and Scott, K. 2012 Dopaminergic modulation of sucrose acceptance behavior in *Drosophila*. *Neuron* 73(5):941–950.

Margulies, C., Tully, T., and Dubnau, J. 2005 Deconstructing memory in *Drosophila*. *Curr Biol* 15(17):R700–R713.

Masek, P. and Keene, A.C. 2013 *Drosophila* fatty acid taste signals through the PLC pathway in sugar-sensing neurons. *PLoS Genetics* 9(9):e1003710.

Masse, N.Y., Turner, G.C., and Jefferis, G.S. 2009 Olfactory information processing in *Drosophila*. *Curr Biol* 19(16):R700–R713.

Mathew, D., Martelli, C., Kelley-Swift, E., Brusalis, C., Gershow, M., Samuel, A.D., Emonet, T., Carlson, J.R. 2013 Functional diversity among sensory receptors in a *Drosophila* olfactory circuit. *Proc Natl Acad Sci U S A* 110(23):E2134–E2143.

Melcher, C. and Pankratz, M.J. 2005 Candidate gustatory interneurons modulating feeding behavior in the *Drosophila* brain. *PLoS Biol* 3(9):e305.

Melcher, C., Bader R., Walther, S., Simakov, O., and Pankratz, M.J. 2006 Neuromedin U and its putative *Drosophila* homolog hugin. *PLoS Biol* 4(3):e68.

Melcher, C., Bader, R., and Pankratz, M.J. 2007 Amino acids, taste circuits, and feeding behavior in *Drosophila*: Towards understanding the psychology of feeding in flies and man. *J Endocrinol* 192(3):467–472.

Min, K.J. and Tatar, M. 2006 *Drosophila* diet restriction in practice: Do flies consume fewer nutrients? *Mech Ageing Dev* 127(1):93–96.

Mirth, C.K., Tang, H.Y., Makohon-Moore, S.C., Salhadar, S., Gokhale, R.H., Warner, R.D., Koyama, T., Riddiford, L.M., and Shingleton, A.W. 2014 Juvenile hormone regulates body size and perturbs insulin signaling in *Drosophila*. *Proc Natl Acad Sci U S A* 111(19):7018–7023.

Miyamoto, T. and Amrein, H. 2014 Diverse roles for the *Drosophila* fructose sensor Gr43a. *Fly (Austin)* 8(1):19–25.

Miyamoto, T., Slone, J., Song, X., and Amrein, H. 2012 A fructose receptor functions as a nutrient sensor in the *Drosophila* brain. *Cell* 151(5):1113–1125.

Montell, C. 2009 A taste of the *Drosophila* gustatory receptors. *Curr Opin Neurobiol* 19(4):345–353.

Musselman, L.P. et al. 2011 A high-sugar diet produces obesity and insulin resistance in wild-type *Drosophila*. *Dis Model Mech* 4(6):842–849.

Nassel, D.R. and Wegener, C. 2011 A comparative review of short and long neuropeptide F signaling in invertebrates: Any similarities to vertebrate neuropeptide Y signaling? *Peptides* 32(6):1335–1355.

Nassel, D.R. and Winther, A.M. 2010 *Drosophila* neuropeptides in regulation of physiology and behavior. *Prog Neurobiol* 92(1):42–104.

Nicolai, L.J., Ramaekers, A., Raemaekers, T., Drozdzecki, A., Mauss, A.S., Yan, J., Landgraf, M., Annaert, W., and Hassan, B.A. 2010 Genetically encoded dendritic marker sheds light on neuronal connectivity in *Drosophila*. *Proc Natl Acad Sci U S A* 107(47):20553–20558.

Oldham, S. and Hafen, E. 2003 Insulin/IGF and target of rapamycin signaling: A TOR de force in growth control. *Trends Cell Biol* 13(2):79–85.

Olds, W.H. and Xu, T. 2014 Regulation of food intake by mechanosensory ion channels in enteric neurons. *Elife* 3.

Owusu-Ansah, E. and Perrimon, N. 2014 Modeling metabolic homeostasis and nutrient sensing in *Drosophila*: Implications for aging and metabolic diseases. *Dis Model Mech* 7(3):343–350.

Pasco, M.Y. and Leopold, P. 2012 High sugar-induced insulin resistance in *Drosophila* relies on the lipocalin Neural Lazarillo. *PloS One* 7(5):e36583.

Perisse, E., Burke, C., Huetteroth, W., and Waddell, S. 2013 Shocking revelations and saccharin sweetness in the study of *Drosophila* olfactory memory. *Current Biol* 23(17):R752–R763.

Pfeiffer, B.D., Ngo, T.T., Hibbard, K.L., Murphy, C., Jenett, A., Truman, J.W., and Rubin, G.M. 2010 Refinement of tools for targeted gene expression in *Drosophila*. *Genetics* 186(2):735–755.

Pool, A.H. and Scott, K. 2014 Feeding regulation in *Drosophila*. *Curr Opin Neurobiol* 29:57–63.

Pool, A.H., Kim, D.J., Dunbar-Yaffe, R., Nikolaev, V.O., Lohse, M.J., and Taghert, P.H. 2014 Four GABAergic interneurons impose feeding restraint in *Drosophila*. *Neuron* 83(1):164–177.

Rajan, A. and Perrimon, N. 2011 *Drosophila* as a model for interorgan communication: Lessons from studies on energy homeostasis. *Develop Cell* 21(1):29–31.

Rajan, A. and Perrimon, N. 2012 *Drosophila* cytokine unpaired 2 regulates physiological homeostasis by remotely controlling insulin secretion. *Cell* 151(1):123–137.

Rajan, A. and Perrimon, N. 2013 Of flies and men: Insights on organismal metabolism from fruit flies. *BMC Biol* 11:38.

Rajashekhar, K.P. and Singh, R.N. 1994 Organization of motor neurons innervating the proboscis musculature in *Drosophila melanogaster* Meigen (Diptera: Drosophilidae). *Int J Insect Morphol. Embryol.* 23:225–242.

Riabinina, O., Luginbuhl, D., Marr, E., Liu, S., Wu, M.N., Luo, L., and Potter, C.J. 2015 Improved and expanded Q-system reagents for genetic manipulations. *Nat Methods* 12(3):219–222, 215 p following 222.

Rieder, L.E. and Larschan, E.N. 2014 Wisdom from the fly. *Trends Genet* 30(11):479–481.

Ro, J., Harvanek, Z.M., and Pletcher, S.D. 2014 FLIC: High-throughput, continuous analysis of feeding behaviors in *Drosophila*. *PloS One* 9(6):e101107.

Rolls, M.M., Satoh, D., Clyne, P.J., Henner, A.L., Uemura, T., and Doe, C.Q. 2007 Polarity and intracellular compartmentalization of *Drosophila* neurons. *Neural Dev* 2:7.

Root, C.M., Ko, K.I., Jafari, A., and Wang J.W. 2011 Presynaptic facilitation by neuropeptide signaling mediates odor-driven food search. *Cell* 145(1):133–144.

Rulifson, E.J., Kim, S.K., and Nusse, R. 2002 Ablation of insulin-producing neurons in flies: Growth and diabetic phenotypes. *Science* 296(5570):1118–1120.

Scherer, S., Stocker, R.F., and Gerber, B. 2003 Olfactory learning in individually assayed *Drosophila* larvae. *Learn Mem* 10(3):217–225.

Schwaerzel, M., Monastirioti, M., Scholz, H., Friggi-Grelin, F., Birman, S., and Heisenberg, M. 2003 Dopamine and octopamine differentiate between aversive and appetitive olfactory memories in *Drosophila*. *J Neurosci* 23(33):10495–10502.

Scott, K. 2005 Taste recognition: Food for thought. *Neuron* 48(3):455–464.

Scott, K., Brady, R., Cravchik, A., Morozov, P., Rzhetsky, A., Zuker, C., and Axel, R. 2001 A chemosensory gene family encoding candidate gustatory and olfactory receptors in *Drosophila*. *Cell* 104(5):661–673.

Selcho, M., Pauls, D., Han, K.A., Stocker, R.F., and Thum, A.S. 2009 The role of dopamine in *Drosophila* larval classical olfactory conditioning. *PloS One* 4(6):e5897.

Sellier, M.J., Reeb, P., and Marion-Poll, F. 2011 Consumption of bitter alkaloids in *Drosophila melanogaster* in multiple-choice test conditions. *Chem Senses* 36(4):323–334.

Shafer O.T. et al. 2008 Widespread receptivity to neuropeptide PDF throughout the neuronal circadian clock network of *Drosophila* revealed by real-time cyclic AMP imaging. *Neuron* 58(2):223–237.

Shiraiwa, T. and Carlson, J.R. 2007 Proboscis extension response (PER) assay in *Drosophila*. *J Vis Exp* (3):193.

Singh, R.N. 1997 Neurobiology of the gustatory systems of *Drosophila* and some terrestrial insects. *Microsc Res Tech* 39(6):547–563.

Singh, R.N. and Singh, K. 1984 Fine structure of the sensory organs of *Drosophila melanogaster* Meigen larva (Diptera: Drosophilidae). *Int J Insect Morphol Embryol* 13:255–273.

Slaidina, M., Delanoue, R., Gronke, S., Partridge, L., and Leopold, P. 2009 A *Drosophila* insulin-like peptide promotes growth during nonfeeding states. *Develop Cell* 17(6):874–884.

Soderberg, J.A., Carlsson, M.A., and Nassel, D.R. 2012 Insulin-producing cells in the *Drosophila* brain also express satiety-inducing cholecystokinin-like peptide, drosulfakinin. *Front Endocrinol (Lausanne)* 3:109.

Sokolowski, M.B. 2001 *Drosophila*: Genetics meets behaviour. *Nat Rev Genet* 2(11):879–890.

Stafford, J.W., Lynd, K.M., Jung, A.Y., and Gordon, M.D. 2012 Integration of taste and calorie sensing in *Drosophila*. *J Neurosci* 32(42):14767–14774.

Stocker, R.F. 1994 The organization of the chemosensory system in *Drosophila melanogaster*: A review. *Cell Tiss Res* 275(1):3–26.

Tanimura, T., Hiroi, M., Inoshita, T., and Marion-Poll, F. 2009 Neurophysiology of gustatory receptor neurones in *Drosophila*. *SEB Exp Biol Ser* 63:59–76.

Thorne, N., Chromey, C., Bray, S., and Amrein, H. 2004 Taste perception and coding in *Drosophila*. *Curr Biol* 14(12):1065–1079.

Tompkins, L., Cardosa, M.J., White, F.V., and Sanders, T.G. 1979 Isolation and analysis of chemosensory behavior mutants in *Drosophila melanogaster*. *Proc Natl Acad Sci U S A* 76(2):884–887.

Toshima, N. and Tanimura, T. 2012 Taste preference for amino acids is dependent on internal nutritional state in *Drosophila melanogaster*. *J Exp Biol* 215(Pt 16):2827–2832.

Urbach, R. 2007 A procephalic territory in *Drosophila* exhibiting similarities and dissimilarities compared to the vertebrate midbrain/hindbrain boundary region. *Neural Dev* 2:23.

Van der Horst, D.J. 2003 Insect adipokinetic hormones: Release and integration of flight energy metabolism. *Comp Biochem Physiol B Biochem Mol Biol* 136(2):217–226.

Vargo, M. and Hirsch, J. 1982 Central excitation in the fruit fly (*Drosophila melanogaster*). *J Comp Physiol Psychol* 96(3):452–459.

Veelaert, D., Schoofs, L., and De Loof, A. 1998 Peptidergic control of the corpus cardiacum-corpora allata complex of locusts. *Int Rev Cytol* 182:249–302.

Vosshall, L.B. 2008 Scent of a fly. *Neuron* 59(5):685–689.

Vosshall, L.B. and Stocker, R.F. 2007 Molecular architecture of smell and taste in *Drosophila*. *Annu Rev Neurosci* 30:505–533.

Vosshall, L.B., Wong, A.M., and Axel, R. 2000 An olfactory sensory map in the fly brain. *Cell* 102(2):147–159.

Wang, Y., Pu, Y., and Shen, P. 2013 Neuropeptide-gated perception of appetitive olfactory inputs in *Drosophila* larvae. *Cell Rep* 3(3):820–830.

Wang, Z., Singhvi, A., Kong, P., and Scott, K. 2004 Taste representations in the *Drosophila* brain. *Cell* 117(7):981–991.

Weiss, L.A., Dahanukar, A., Kwon, J.Y., Banerjee, D., and Carlson, J.R. 2011 The molecular and cellular basis of bitter taste in *Drosophila*. *Neuron* 69(2):258–272.

Wen, T., Parrish, C.A., Xu, D., Wu, Q., and Shen, P. 2005 *Drosophila* neuropeptide F and its receptor, NPFR1, define a signaling pathway that acutely modulates alcohol sensitivity. *Proc Natl Acad Sci U S A* 102(6):2141–2146.

Williams, M.J., Goergen, P., Rajendran, J., Zheleznyakova, G., Hägglund, M.G., Perland, E., Bagchi, S., Kalogeropoulou, A., Khan, Z., Fredriksson, R., and Schiöth, H.B. 2014 Obesity-linked homologues TfAP-2 and Twz establish meal frequency in *Drosophila melanogaster*. *PLoS Genet* 10(9):e1004499.

Wong, R., Piper, M.D., Blanc, E., and Partridge, L. 2008 Pitfalls of measuring feeding rate in the fruit fly *Drosophila melanogaster*. *Nat Methods* 5(3):214–215.

Wong, R., Piper, M.D., Wertheim, B., and Partridge L. 2009 Quantification of food intake in *Drosophila*. *PloS One* 4(6):e6063.

Wright, G.A. 2015 Olfaction: Smells like fly food. *Curr Biol* 25(4):R144–R146.

Wu, Q., Wen, T., Lee, G., Park, J.H., Cai, H.N., and Shen, P. 2003 Developmental control of foraging and social behavior by the *Drosophila* neuropeptide Y-like system. *Neuron* 39(1):147–161.

Wu, Q., Zhang, Y., Xu, J., and Shen, P. 2005a Regulation of hunger-driven behaviors by neural ribosomal S6 kinase in *Drosophila*. *Proc Natl Acad Sci U S A* 102(37):13289–13294.

Wu, Q., Zhao, Z., and Shen, P. 2005b Regulation of aversion to noxious food by *Drosophila* neuropeptide Y- and insulin-like systems. *Nat Neurosci* 8(10):1350–1355.

Xu, J., Li, M., and Shen, P. 2010 A G-protein-coupled neuropeptide Y-like receptor suppresses behavioral and sensory response to multiple stressful stimuli in *Drosophila*. *J Neurosci* 30(7):2504–2512.

Yang, Z., Yu, Y., Zhang, V., Tian, Y., Qi, W., and Wang, L. 2015 Octopamine mediates starvation-induced hyperactivity in adult *Drosophila*. *Proc Natl Acad Sci U S A* 112(16):5219–5224.

Yarmolinsky, D.A., Zuker, C.S., and Ryba, N.J. 2009 Common sense about taste: From mammals to insects. *Cell* 139(2):234–244.

Zeng, C., Du, Y., Alberico, T., Seeberger, J., Sun, X., and Zou, S. 2011 Gender-specific prandial response to dietary restriction and oxidative stress in *Drosophila melanogaster*. *Fly (Austin)* 5(3):174–180.

Zhang, H., Liu, J., Li, C.R., Momen, B., Kohanski, R.A., and Pick L. 2009 Deletion of *Drosophila* insulin-like peptides causes growth defects and metabolic abnormalities. *Proc Natl Acad Sci U S A* 106(46):19617–19622.

Zhang, T., Branch, A., and Shen, P. 2013a Octopamine-mediated circuit mechanism underlying controlled appetite for palatable food in *Drosophila*. *Proc Natl Acad Sci U S A* 110(38):15431–15436.

Zhang, Y.V., Ni, J., and Montell, C. 2013b The molecular basis for attractive salt-taste coding in *Drosophila*. *Science* 340(6138):1334–1338.

3 The Hamster as a
Model for Human
Ingestive Behavior

Ruth B.S. Harris

CONTENTS

3.1   INTRODUCTION

Hamsters are one of the less common rodent models used for the study of ingestive behavior. These animals can be a valuable tool for investigating certain aspects of human behavior and metabolism that cannot be replicated in rats and mice. This chapter will focus on two of those aspects: (i) the appetitive behaviors of food foraging and hoarding and (ii) stress-induced weight gain.

There are many species of hamsters, but laboratory-based studies on ingestive behavior have been almost exclusively limited to Syrian/Golden hamsters (*Mesocricetus auratus*) and Siberian/Djungarian hamsters (*Phodopus sungorus*). In a natural setting, hamster physiology and behavior adjust according to seasonal changes in the environment and photoperiod, with duration of nocturnal melatonin release and activity in the suprachiasmatic nucleus acting as the signal that coordinates changes in physiology and behavior (Bartness et al. 1993). Winter-like short day length suppresses reproductive function, causing gonadal regression in both Syrian and Siberian hamsters. Siberian hamsters also change their coat color from agouti to white, lose body fat, and use temporary, daily torpor to improve energy efficiency in cold environments. Body temperature and metabolic rate are decreased for several hours during the daylight hours to conserve energy that is needed for nocturnal foraging in subzero ambient temperatures (Ruf and Heldmaier 1992; Ruf et al. 1993). The capacity for nonshivering thermogenesis is increased (Heldmaier, Steinlechner, and Rafael 1982) and may facilitate the recovery of normothermia at the end of daily torpor. By contrast, Syrian hamsters housed in short photoperiod days gain body fat (Campbell, Tabor, and Davis 1983; McElroy and Wade 1986) primarily by reducing energy expenditure (Wade 1983). Gonadal involution, change in coat color, inhibition of food intake (Hoffman 1973), changes in body fat mass (Wade and Bartness 1984a; Bartness 1996), and 55% of the change in thermogenic capacity (Heldmaier, Steinlechner, and Rafael 1982) can be replicated in the laboratory by reducing the photoperiod to a short day length.

3.2   APPETITIVE VERSUS CONSUMMATORY INGESTIVE BEHAVIOR

Craig (1931) described instinctive behaviors as consisting of two phases: appetitive, which is a state of agitation that drives the animal to search for a stimulus that is absent, and consummatory, during which the stimulus is received and is followed by a state of rest. In the context of food intake, appetite drives an animal to find and obtain food. The second, consummatory phase during which food is eaten is dependent upon successful completion of the appetitive phase. A majority of laboratory research on the control of food intake investigates hormonal, neurological, and physiological factors that impact the amount of food consumed, meal size, meal frequency, and food choice. These studies are conducted in animals housed either individually or in groups in a cage with controlled (usually constant) access to an excess of food and water. The amount of food consumed is assumed to be determined by mechanisms that control hunger and satiety because food is freely available and very little effort has to be made to obtain that food. The experimental animals tend to remain lean despite few opportunities for activity but will gain weight if offered a calorically dense (Lemonnier 1972), palatable (Kanarek and Orthen-Gambill 1982), or varied (Rothwell and Stock 1979) diet. These studies have identified factors that drive food intake in humans but are limited to evaluation of the consummatory phase of eating (Berthoud 2004). By contrast, in order to eat either inside or outside the home, humans and other animals living in their natural habitat have to exert some effort on leaving the home environment to look for food that is then brought back and stored in a safe location for future consumption.

Although we do not always consider ourselves to be foragers or food hoarders, there are few individuals who, by choice, fail to have some food stored in their living area. The majority of US consumers live within a mile of their local grocery store (US Department of Agriculture 2009; Liu, Han, and Cohen 2015) and visit the store an average of 2.2 times a week (Food Marketing Institute 2012) but are willing to travel further (i.e., work harder) for a better selection of foods or for price discounts (Food Marketing Institute 2012). These infrequent visits to the store each week require people to anticipate their future energy requirements and to bring home adequate supplies to feed the family for a number of days following each foraging expedition.

There are a limited number of studies focused on appetitive behavior in humans, but it has been shown that food purchases and storage are influenced by physiological state. People who go to the grocery store hungry buy more than those who are not hungry when they shop (Dodd, Stalling, and Bedell 1977; Mela, Aaron, and Gatenby 1996; Nederkoorn et al. 2009; Bevelander, Anschutz, and Engels 2011). Both hungry and obese individuals increase the number of calorically dense items purchased (Ransley et al. 2003; Nederkoorn et al. 2009) and the number of unplanned food purchases made (Tom 1983). Obese people store more perishable food at home by maintaining a greater number of refrigerators and freezers and store food in more locations outside the kitchen than do nonobese individuals (Emery et al. 2015).

Understanding the underlying mechanisms involved in human foraging and food storage (hoarding) behaviors has the potential to identify novel factors contributing to the currently high rates of overweight and obesity. Although the amount of food eaten outside of the home has doubled in the past 30 years, food prepared at home still accounts for 68% of daily caloric intake (Lin and Guthrie 2012). If obese people tend to purchase more calorically dense foods and store them in multiple locations around the home (Emery et al. 2015), then this raises the potential for the appetitive behavior of the primary food shopper to influence not only their own adiposity but also that of other members of the household. Consistent with this, it has been shown that early exposure to unhealthy food influences a child's food preferences (Nepper and Chai 2016) and children with a preference for high-fat foods have parents who are fatter than parents of children who prefer low fat foods (Fisher and Birch 1995).

3.3 RODENT MODELS OF FOOD HOARDING

Rodents and all other species tested (Collier, Johnson, and Mathis 2002) will work to obtain food. In the laboratory, the effort required to obtain food can be increased by linking the delivery of food pellets to rotations of a running wheel (Perrigo and Bronson 1983), the torque on the wheel (Collier, Johnson, and Mathis 2002), the number of lever presses (Kanoski et al. 2014), or distance travelled in a tunnel or maze (Cabanac and Swiergiel 1989). In these situations, the amount of work performed to obtain food reaches a plateau, at which point intake starts to decline if the work requirement continues to increase. For example, young female mice increase their running activity in proportion to the number of revolutions required for each pellet up to 135 revolutions per pellet, after which running activity plateaus and food intake decreases (Perrigo and Bronson 1983). If work has to be done to initiate access to food that is then freely available, meal size increases and meal frequency decreases as the effort required to initiate the meal is increased (Collier, Johnson, and Mathis 2002). An elegant series of studies by the Collier laboratory suggest that this may be because the time required to obtain food is a critical aspect of procurement cost (Collier, Johnson, and Mathis 2002).

3.3.1 FOOD HOARDING BY RATS

Animals that hoard food can be divided into two general categories of scatter hoarders, which bury small amounts of food in multiple, widely distributed sites, and larder hoarders, which hoard food at one site that can be easily defended. Rats do not normally hoard food, although they may move it around (Deacon 2009), but they can be induced to hoard if they have been food restricted to lose weight. For example, rats exposed to the cold and given a choice of hoarding food or insulating material will hoard insulating material if they are fed but hoard food if they are food deprived (Fantino and Cabanac 1984). These data imply that food hoarding in rats is limited to conditions of negative energy balance, and food deprivation studies show that the amount of food hoarded by rats is proportional to the amount of weight that has been lost (Fantino and Cabanac 1980; Cabanac and Swiergiel 1989) and is inversely proportional to the amount of work associated with foraging (Cabanac and Swiergiel 1989). The degree of weight loss required for initiation of hoarding does not, however, change with the cost associated with foraging (Cabanac and Swiergiel 1989; Charron and Cabanac 2004). Hoarding studies with rats follow a protocol that allows access to food for only a few hours a day during which the rats forage, hoard, and consume food. At the end of this period, the hoarded food is removed. Under these experimental conditions, the size of the food hoard changes, but the amount of food consumed during the experimental period is the same for all conditions (Cabanac and Swiergiel 1989), indicating the presence of separate control systems for the different behaviors and leading to the suggestion that hunger is a stronger drive for appetitive than consummatory behavior (Borker and Gogate 1981).

3.3.2 FOOD HOARDING BY HAMSTERS

Unlike rats, many rodents, including hamsters (Humphries, Thomas, and Kramer 2003), hoard food as an integral part of an innate ingestive behavior that is fully developed by 21 days of age (Etienne, Emmanuelli, and Zinder 1982). Hamsters are larder hoarders and food transport is facilitated by large cheek pouches that allow the animals to carry multiple pieces of food, unlike rats that transport one pellet at a time (Charron and Cabanac 2004). Foraging and hoarding are achieved through an organized series of events that involve leaving the nest to look for food, filling the pouch with food, returning to the nest, and emptying the pouch (Etienne, Emmanuelli, and Zinder 1982). In this chapter, foraging refers to the total amount of food obtained (eaten and stored), whereas hoarding refers to the amount of food taken back to the burrow and stored. Hamsters are nocturnal and in free-feeding conditions hoard 5 to 10 times more food at night than during the day (Waddell 1951). Laboratory-based studies of foraging and hoarding use a housing system consisting of two cages connected by a length of vertical tubing that acts as a tunnel. The cage at the bottom of the tubing is dark and contains bedding, representing the animals' "burrow." The top cage is the foraging area that is lit, open to the external environment, and stocked with food and water. This food may be freely available or the cage may be fitted with a running wheel that allows a food pellet to be delivered when the animal runs a prescribed number of revolutions. The running wheel allows foraging effort to be increased beyond that required for the hamster to climb up the tunnel and the number of revolutions required for each pellet can be varied. Control conditions include cages in which a wheel is available, but pellets are freely available to account for increases in activity that are unrelated to foraging and cages in which the wheel is locked to account for changes in foraging and hoarding caused by the energy used for locomotor activity in the wheel (Day and Bartness 2001). Diagrams of experimental foraging-hoarding systems have been published elsewhere (Bartness and Clein 1994; Garretson et al. 2015).

Experimental animals hoard 10%–20% of the food that they earn through foraging (Day and Bartness 2001; Garretson and Bartness 2014) and approximately one-third of their daily food intake is taken from the hoard (Wood and Bartness 1996b). Although it has been suggested that the activity of transporting food and hoarding, rather than food accumulation, is a rewarding experience for hamsters, there is ample data to show that hoarding responds to energy demand and likely represents a behavior that optimizes survival (Waddell 1951). Female hamsters that have a choice of reproductive behavior or feeding, foraging, and hoarding will spend more time with their mates when food is freely available but transfer their preference to feeding, foraging, and hoarding following a period of food deprivation (Schneider et al. 2007). Similar types of behavior have been reported for human populations experiencing chronic food shortages. When the food supply is limited, a high level of anxiety related to building up food reserves (hoarding) develops, and individuals become more selfish as they protect the limited amount of food they have available. If famine ensues, then all activity is focused on procuring food (Keys et al. 1950).

3.3.2.1 Energy Deficit and Food Hoarding

Both Syrian and Siberian hamsters increase foraging and hoarding following food deprivation (Bartness and Clein 1994; Buckley and Schneider 2003) irrespective of day length (Wood and Bartness 1996b). A 32-hour period of food deprivation increases foraging by approximately 30%, but may cause a 3-fold increase in food hoarding (Day and Bartness 2003). This effect is greatest in animals that hoard large quantities of food in baseline conditions (Buckley and Schneider 2003), and if there is a choice of diets, then food-restricted hamsters show an exaggerated preference for high-calorie food (Day, Mintz, and Bartness 1999). In contrast to the increase in hoarding, it is well documented that, unlike rats and mice that overeat when food becomes available ad libitum (Harris and Martin 1984; Harris, Kasser, and Martin 1986; Trayhurn and Jennings 1988), hamsters do not increase their food intake during refeeding and may die due to a failure to compensate for an extended period of food deprivation (Silverman and Zucker 1976; Bartness and Clein 1994; Buckley and Schneider 2003). In fact, Syrian hamsters that hoard the most eat the least amount of food during refeeding (Buckley and Schneider 2003; Garretson and Bartness 2014). Despite the failure to overeat, the food-deprived animals slowly regain body weight (Bartness and Clein 1994), presumably due to a decrease in energy expenditure, and the size of the food hoard comes back down to control levels as body weight is regained (Bartness and Clein 1994). In Siberian hamsters, the severity of food deprivation does not change the size of the hoard but increases the number of days that an enlarged hoard is maintained (Bartness and Clein 1994). The size of the hoard is monitored because if pellets are removed from a hoard, then hamsters respond by bringing more pellets back to the burrow, whereas if pellets are added to the hoard, then fewer pellets are brought back to the burrow (Garretson and Bartness 2014). Similarly, if the caloric density of the diet is changed, then hamsters will adjust the size of their food hoard in an attempt to control the total amount of energy present in the hoard (Wood and Bartness 1996a). Although the size of a food hoard is controlled, it may be limited if foraging effort is excessive (Day and Bartness 2001), in which case the food-deprived animals take longer to recover to baseline body weight.

Increased food hoarding also is apparent in hamsters that experience other energetically demanding situations, such as pregnancy and lactation. Unlike rats or mice, Syrian hamsters do not increase food intake or reduce activity during pregnancy but deplete body fat stores by as much as 40% (Bhatia and Wade 1993). Siberian hamsters do increase food intake (Schneider and Wade 1987; Bartness 1997) but also lose a substantial amount of body fat despite a decrease in thermogenic capacity (Schneider and Wade 1987). Both species exhibit a substantial increase in hoarding during pregnancy and lactation (Miceli and Malsbury 1982; Bartness 1997). Because the increase in hoarding following food deprivation and pregnancy is associated with a reduced body weight and loss of body fat (Bartness 1997; Day, Mintz, and Bartness 1999), the possibility that a signal related to fat mass could initiate the increase in food hoarding has been explored.

3.3.2.2   Lipectomy and Food Hoarding

Partial lipectomy is the surgical removal of individual fat depots that results in a reduction in total body energy stores but differs from fat loss caused by an energy deficit because the size of the fat cells in the remaining fat depots do not change. Over time, the animals correct for the loss of fat by enlargement of remaining depots (Hausman et al. 2004). Removal of two major fat depots (inguinal and epididymal) from Siberian hamsters (Wood and Bartness 1997) has been shown to increase hoarding but not change food intake in the lipectomized animals. Hoarding returns to control levels as body fat and body weight are restored. There is no relation between the amount of fat removed and hoard size, but loss of gonadal fat (epididymal) results in a greater increase in hoarding than removal of subcutaneous fat when the cost of foraging is increased (Dailey and Bartness 2008), suggesting that fat required for support of essential physiological functions such as reproduction may have a greater impact on appetitive behavior.

3.3.2.3   Leptin and Food Hoarding

The link between body fat mass and hoarding has also been explored in experiments in which hamsters are treated with leptin, an adipose-derived hormone proposed to be a feedback signal in the control of energy balance (Zhang et al. 1994). In normal-weight animals, circulating concentrations of leptin reflect body fat mass (Considine et al. 1996) and administration of exogenous leptin inhibits food intake of mice that have been food deprived for 24 hours (Rentsch, Levens, and Chiesi 1995).

Food deprivation causes a substantial drop in circulating concentrations of leptin in Siberian hamsters, and if this is prevented by peripheral injection of leptin, then the increase in food intake and hoarding of both Siberian and Syrian hamsters during refeeding also is prevented if foraging requires little effort (Buckley and Schneider 2003, Keen-Rhinehart and Bartness 2008). If work (10 wheel revolutions/pellet) is required for foraging, then the inhibitory effect of leptin on food intake and hoarding is attenuated. This may be due in part to the increased energy cost of foraging and also because hoarding has already been suppressed by the requirement for wheel running (Keen-Rhinehart and Bartness 2008).

Despite the evidence from lipectomy and leptin studies implying a link between adiposity and appetitive behavior, the natural reduction in body fat mass of Siberian hamsters housed in short day length is not associated with a significant increase in foraging or hoarding compared with that of naturally fatter animals housed in long photoperiod days (Teubner and Bartness 2009a). Thus, the increase in hoarding by food-deprived hamsters may be due to a combination of stimuli associated with a state of negative energy balance, rather than a specific response to reduced fat mass. Alternatively, the response may be initiated by the hamsters being forced to reduce body fat mass to a level that is less than would be appropriate for the current environment, and in this situation, the hamsters evaluate energy stored in the food hoard as an integral part of the available energy substrate.

Although rats and mice overeat until body weight is restored to control levels when food becomes freely available following a period of food deprivation (Harris and Martin 1984; Harris, Kasser, and Martin 1986; Trayhurn and Jennings 1988), 32-hour food-deprived Siberian hamsters increase their food intake for only a few hours but increase the size of their food hoard until body weight returns to baseline levels (Day and Bartness 2003). Similarly, severe food deprivation is followed by hyperphagia in humans (Keys et al. 1950), but a short fast of 36 hours or less does not induce overeating when food becomes available (Johnstone et al. 2002; Levitsky and DeRosimo 2010). There is, however, some evidence that people buy more food and more calorically dense food if they shop when they are hungry (Dodd, Stalling, and Bedell 1977; Mela, Aaron, and Gatenby 1996; Nederkoorn et al. 2009; Bevelander, Anschutz, and Engels 2011). These data suggest that in both humans and hamsters, food intake and foraging and hoarding are controlled independently of one another.

3.3.2.4 Metabolic Signals and Food Hoarding

The Bartness laboratory has taken advantage of the hamster model to investigate metabolic factors that influence hoarding and to test the importance of neuropeptides known to influence consummatory behavior on this appetitive behavior. This work was most recently reviewed in depth in 2011 (Bartness et al. 2011) and will be summarized here.

Because hoarding is increased following periods of negative energy balance (see Section 3.3.2.1), several studies have tested whether limiting cellular energy metabolism stimulates appetitive behavior. Glucoprivation, achieved by blocking glycolysis with the nonmetabolizable glucose analog 2-deoxyglucose (2DG), produces a robust increase in food intake of rats (Ritter and Slusser 1980) and laboratory mice (Rowland, Bellush, and Carlton 1985). The increase in intake lasts for approximately

6 hours, is dose dependent, and is accompanied by hyperglycemia (Ritter and Slusser 1980). Methyl palmoxirate (MP), which inhibits mitochondrial fatty acid oxidation, also stimulates food intake of rats for at least 8 hours (Horn and Friedman 1998). By contrast, although 2DG does induce hyperglycemia and MP increases circulating levels of free fatty acids and decreases ketones (Lazzarini, Schneider, and Wade 1988), neither 2DG nor MP stimulates food intake in Syrian hamsters (Slusser and Ritter 1980; Rowland, Bellush, and Carlton 1985; Lazzarini, Schneider, and Wade 1988), irrespective of whether they are offered chow or a preferred high-fat diet (Sclafani and Eisenstadt 1980, Schneider et al. 1988). Similarly, neither 2DG nor MP affects either food intake or hoarding in Siberian hamsters when administered alone or in combination (Bartness and Clein 1994). High doses of insulin, which cause hypoglycemia by promoting glucose uptake in insulin sensitive tissues but glucoprivation in insulin-insensitive tissue, stimulate food intake in rats (Booth 1968) and Syrian hamsters (Ritter and Balch 1978) but do not affect food intake or hoarding in Siberian hamsters (Bartness and Clein 1994). These data do not necessarily eliminate substrate availability as a factor that influences hoarding but do indicate that these metabolic signals of limited glucose or fatty acid utilization do not activate the same control mechanisms in hamsters as they do in rats.

3.3.2.5   Central Control of Food Hoarding

Food intake and energy balance are controlled by a complex interaction between multiple hormones and neuropeptides. Ingestive behavior refers to food acquisition and consumption of defined meals, the initiation and duration of which are determined by "short-term" signals that monitor factors such as gastric distension, blood glucose, and other indices of immediate energy flux. By contrast, energy intake and expenditure are rarely matched on a daily basis, but energy balance is achieved when intake and expenditure are considered over a period of days. These two systems interact so that disruption of energy balance influences sensitivity toward satiety signals that determine meal size (Maniscalco and Rinaman 2013) and a sustained disruption of the normal feeding pattern can result in a shift in energy balance (Stanley et al. 1989). The experiments described earlier examine hoarding in conditions of energy deficit and address the issue of whether signals associated with energy balance influence foraging and hoarding behaviors. By contrast, the investigation of peripheral hormones and central neuropeptides that influence hoarding have, by necessity, focused on factors known to influence consummatory behavior and can generally be categorized as "short-term" signals. Although the control of food intake involves an integrated response to peripheral signals and multiple areas of the brain (Grill and Kaplan 2002; Grill 2006), the role played by hypothalamic nuclei has received the most attention (e.g., Schwartz et al. 2000). Therefore, it is not surprising that studies investigating appetitive behavior have initially focused on hypothalamic neuropeptides known to contribute to the control of food intake.

Neuropeptide Y (NPY) is a 36-amino-acid peptide that is widely distributed in the brain (Adrian et al. 1983; Allen et al. 1983) and periphery (Thomas, Ryu, and Bartness 2016). NPY influences multiple physiologic systems (Herring 2015; Reichmann and Holzer 2016; Tilan and Kitlinska 2016), one of which is the control of ingestive behavior. The arcuate nucleus of the hypothalamus contains a set of orexigenic neurons that coexpress NPY and agouti-related protein (AgRP) and a second set of anorexigenic neurons that coexpress propiomelanocortin (POMC) and cocaine and amphetamine regulated peptide (CART). The NPY/AgRP neurons project to the paraventricular nucleus of the hypothalamus (PVN) and the perifornical (PFH) hypothalamus and also inhibit activity of POMC/CART neurons. Injection of NPY into the PVN or the PFH of fed rats increases food intake in a dose-dependent manner (Clark et al. 1984; Stanley and Leibowitz 1985; Stanley et al. 1993). A single injection will stimulate food intake for several hours (Stanley and Leibowitz 1985), whereas repeated administration in rats leads to weight gain (Stanley et al. 1989). The pattern of food intake following NPY injection into the PFH replicates that produced by food deprivation and involves an increase in both meal size and meal frequency (Marin Bivens; Thomas, and Stanley 1998). There are five subtypes of NPY receptors, and Y1 and Y5 appear to play a critical role in NPY-induced feeding (Kamiji and Inui 2007).

Seeley, Payne, and Woods (1995) were the first to report that central administration of NPY increased food intake in animals that had to perform a minimal level of appetitive behavior, such as moving toward a food hopper or licking a spout for sucrose solution, but did not stimulate intake of rats that had sucrose solution delivered directly into the oral cavity, which did not require any appetitive behavior. These observations led to the conclusion that NPY has its primary effect on the appetitive and not the consummatory phase of food intake. In addition, Ammar et al. (2000) performed a series of studies examining appetitive versus consummatory behavior in rats receiving central injections of NPY. They report that rats receiving intraoral delivery of sucrose do not consume more sucrose but do visit a bottle from which they expect to obtain sucrose more frequently when they are treated with NPY, even if the bottle is empty. In addition, NPY injection changes the preference of male rats away from a sexually receptive female toward to a bottle of sucrose. These observations lead to the conclusion that NPY is not an orexigenic peptide, but one that directs attention toward food.

The potential effects of NPY on appetitive behavior in rats (Seeley, Payne, and Woods 1995; Ammar et al. 2000), together with evidence that NPY meets all of the criteria required for an endogenous orexigenic signal (Kalra et al. 1999), made it an obvious candidate for testing in hamster foraging and hoarding experiments. Central injection of NPY increases short-term food intake in both Syrian (Kulkosky et al. 1988) and Siberian hamsters (Boss-Williams and Bartness 1996). The response is independent of photoperiod length and is short-lived (approximately 30 minutes) as with other species, but Siberian hamsters are more sensitive to low-dose NPY compared with rats (Boss-Williams and Bartness 1996). Injection of NPY into the third ventricle of Siberian hamsters produces robust increases in foraging, food intake, and hoarding (Day, Keen-Rhinehart, and Bartness 2005). Foraging is increased about 5-fold during the first hour after injection when the work required to obtain a pellet is moderate (10 revolutions), but only by 50% when the work required is increased (50 revolutions/pellet). Food intake is increased 7- to 10-fold for 2 to 4 hours after injection and only in animals for which pellets are contingent on running. Food hoarding is increased 10- to 20-fold in animals that do not have to work for food and the effect lasts for up to 24 hours. All three behaviors are also stimulated by injection of a Y1 or a Y5 receptor agonist although the magnitude of response is less than that produced by NPY (Day, Keen-Rhinehart, and Bartness 2005). In addition, NPY stimulates hoarding more than food intake, whereas the Y1 receptor agonist increases hoarding but has a minimal effect on food intake, and the Y5 receptor agonist primarily affects food intake, supporting the notion of different control systems for appetitive and consummatory behaviors.

The relative importance of the PVN and PFH in mediating the changes in foraging and hoarding has also been investigated (Dailey and Bartness 2009). NPY in the PVN inhibits foraging independent of whether pellets have to be earned by wheel running; by contrast, NPY in the PFA stimulates foraging with a greater effect in animals for which pellets are contingent on wheel running. NPY in either nuclei increases hoarding about 5-fold for at least 24 hours and the effect is greatest in animals that have free access to pellets. Stimulation of food intake lasts for about 4 hours and is greater when NPY is injected into the PFH than when it is injected into the PVN. Antagonism of the Y1 receptor in the PVN prevents an increase in hoarding by food-deprived hamsters, whereas antagonism of receptors in the PFH prevents both foraging and hoarding. These results demonstrate that the effects of NPY on appetitive and feeding behavior are mediated by a distributed network and that specific behaviors may be controlled through specific sites and by specific receptor subtypes.

As noted previously, AgRP, a melanocortin receptor (MCR) antagonist, is an orexigenic agent that is coexpressed with NPY in neurons of the arcuate nucleus of the hypothalamus. There are two MCRs that influence food intake and energy balance. MCR3 is expressed at relatively high levels in the arcuate and dorsomedial ventromedial nuclei of the hypothalamus (Roselli-Rehfuss et al. 1993). MCR4 expression is widely distributed throughout the forebrain and hindbrain (Mountjoy et al. 1994). Deletion of either MCR3 or MCR4 results in an increase in body fat mass in mice (Zhang et al. 2005), although MCR4 appears to be more important in mediating energy expenditure whereas MCR3 may influence food intake.

AgRP expression is modestly increased in the hypothalamus of Siberian hamsters housed in a short day photoperiod, compared with long-day photoperiod (Mercer et al. 2000), with a much more robust increase in expression in animals that have been food deprived for 24 hours. This contrasts with NPY expression, which is not changed by photoperiod or food deprivation (Mercer et al. 2000). In fed hamsters housed in long photoperiod days, third ventricle injection of AgRP increases food intake but has a much greater impact on foraging and hoarding (Day and Bartness 2004). The greatest effect is achieved with a low dose of AgRP (0.1 nmol). Food intake is doubled for several hours after injection. Foraging is also doubled, but for 24 hours, and hoarding is increased 10- or 12-fold during the hours after injection and remains above control levels for up to 7 days after a single injection in animals that have free access to food (Day and Bartness 2004). NPY and AgRP are coexpressed in neurons in the arcuate nucleus and expression of both increases in food deprived hamsters. Therefore, it is not too surprising that they have additive effects on food intake, foraging, and hoarding. Injection of a mixture of subthreshold doses of NPY and AgRP into the third ventricle causes a significant increase in food intake for 1 hour in hamsters with free access to food and increases hoarding for 48 hours with the greatest effect in animals having to run to obtain food pellets (Teubner, Keen-Rhinehart, and Bartness 2012).

Peroxisome proliferator-activated receptor γ (PPARγ) is a nuclear receptor that is expressed in both peripheral and central tissues, including hypothalamic nuclei and AgRP/POMC neurons in the arcuate nucleus (Sarruf et al. 2009). In the periphery, PPARγ plays a role in the control of lipid synthesis and adipogenesis (Medina-Gomez et al. 2007). In the brain, this receptor may function as an intermediary between hunger signals and activation of central orexigenic mechanisms. Acute activation of hypothalamic PPARγ in rats stimulates food intake and exaggerates weight gain, whereas antagonism of the receptor inhibits food intake of food-deprived but not fed rats and inhibits consumption of a high-fat diet (Ryan et al. 2011). In fed hamsters, a single third ventricle injection of rosiglitazone, a PPARγ receptor agonist, increases arcuate nucleus expression of AgRP and NPY and increases wheel running, food intake, and food hoarding for at least 7 days. Expression of PPARγ in AgRP-expressing cells is increased in food-deprived hamsters, and infusion of the receptor antagonist attenuates the increase in AgRP and NPY expression, food intake, and hoarding but does not affect foraging (Garretson et al. 2015). The natural ligands for PPARγ are fatty acids and prostaglandins (Kliewer et al. 1997) and it has yet to be determined how they may influence centrally expressed receptor activation.

3.3.2.6 Gut-Derived Hormones and Food Hoarding

Cholecystokinin (CCK), a hormone present in the brain (Schneider, Monahan, and Hirsch 1979) and released from the duodenum and jejunum in response to the presence of fat and protein (Liddle et al. 1985), stimulates meal termination (Muurahainen et al. 1988) and initiates a sequence of behaviors that are typical of satiety (Gibbs and Smith 1982). CCK also initiates changes in the gastrointestinal function that promote digestion of food in the small intestine (Bragado, Tashiro, and Williams 2000) and inhibit gastric emptying (Shillabeer and Davison 1987). CCK has multiple biologically active forms, with CCK-8 and CCK-33 being the most frequently used to investigate satiation. More recently CCK-58, which is the most abundant in the circulation, has been shown to have significant effects on both meal size and intermeal interval (Overduin et al. 2014). There are two CCK receptor subtypes: CCK_A/CCK_1 and CCK_B/CCK_2. CCK_A receptors located on gastrointestinal vagal afferents that project to the hindbrain (Campos et al. 2012) are essential for the satiating effects of CCK (Moran 2000). Peripheral injections of CCK acutely inhibit food intake of Syrian (Campos et al. 2012) and Siberian (Teubner and Bartness 2009b) hamsters. CCK-33 also significantly inhibits food hoarding but has no effect on foraging in Siberian hamsters (Teubner and Bartness 2009b). This lack of effect on foraging that is contingent on wheel running demonstrates the specificity of response to hoarding, which is significantly inhibited by a lower dose of CCK than is needed to inhibit food intake. In addition, the percentage inhibition of hoarding is greater than the inhibition of feeding for any dose of CCK tested (Teubner and Bartness 2009b). The inhibition of both appetitive and consummatory behavior is apparent in both fed and food-deprived animals but is limited to the first hour after an intraperitonal injection of CCK. These results show that appetitive behaviors respond not only to energy deficits but also to "short-term" signals of current energy sufficiency, consistent with observations that people buy more food when they shop before eating their evening meal than if they shop after their evening meal (Dodd, Stalling, and Bedell 1977).

In direct contrast to CCK, ghrelin, a peptide hormone secreted primarily by the stomach (Kojima et al. 1999), has multiple physiologic functions that include stimulating food intake and insulin release and down-regulating thermogenesis (see Muller et al. 2015 for review). Ghrelin release increases with fasting or food restriction and peripheral administration of ghrelin increases appetite (Wren et al. 2001), the hedonic response to food (Malik et al. 2008; Goldstone et al. 2014) and food intake (Wren et al. 2001). The central response to ghrelin is widely distributed and includes multiple areas known to influence food intake, including the dorsal vagal complex (Faulconbridge et al. 2003), ventral tegmental area (Naleid et al. 2005), arcuate, paraventricular, lateral and dorsomedial nuclei of the hypothalamus (Lawrence et al. 2002; Faulconbridge, Grill, and Kaplan 2005). Central activity of ghrelin appears to be necessary for stimulation of food intake because vagal deafferentation does not block the response to an intraperitoneal injection of ghrelin (Arnold et al. 2006). Because ghrelin-induced increases in food intake can be blocked by preadministration of NPY receptor antagonists (Lawrence et al. 2002) or antagonists of MCRs (MCR3, MCR4) (Keen-Rhinehart and Bartness 2007), it appears that the origexigenic neuropeptides expressed in the arcuate nucleus of the hypothalamus (see Section 3.3.2.5) are intermediaries in the feeding response.

Ghrelin production is lower in hamsters than in mice or rats (Yabuki et al. 2004) and does not change with the photoperiod (Tups et al. 2004) but is increased following 48 hours of food deprivation, as is hypothalamic expression of ghrelin's receptor: growth hormone secretagogue receptor. Ghrelin release does not, however, change with chronic food restriction (Tups et al. 2004), suggesting that it plays a more important role in the short-term control of food intake than long-term control of energy balance. Peripheral injections of ghrelin that raise circulating concentrations of ghrelin in fed hamsters to the same levels as those found in 48-hour food-deprived hamsters stimulate foraging for 24 hours, food intake for 1 hour, and hoarding for 5 days (Keen-Rhinehart and Bartness 2005). These ghrelin-induced increases in appetitive and feeding behavior are smaller than the 10- to 20-fold increases produced by 48 hours of food deprivation (Keen-Rhinehart and Bartness 2007). Consistent with the data from rats (Arnold et al. 2006), centrally administered ghrelin produces larger increases in food intake and hoarding than do peripheral injections, and blockade of central ghrelin receptors prevents the response to peripheral injections of ghrelin. Blockade of central ghrelin receptors also transiently inhibits food intake and hoarding in food-deprived animals (Thomas, Ryu, and Bartness 2016), confirming the biological relevance of this hormone in the initiation of hoarding behavior in hungry animals. Hamsters housed in a short-day photoperiod are less sensitive to ghrelin than those housed in a long-day photoperiod (Bradley et al. 2010), and the reduced sensitivity is associated with a reduction in activation of NPY-expressing neurons in the arcuate nucleus (Bradley et al. 2010). These data suggest that ghrelin is likely to contribute to the control of appetitive behavior and that the short-day change in sensitivity represents adaptation to limited food supplies and hostile foraging conditions for animals living in the wild during the winter months.

3.3.3 SUMMARY OF HAMSTERS AS A MODEL FOR APPETITIVE INGESTIVE BEHAVIOR

The hamster provides a unique model for investigating appetitive behavior that is typical of that reported for humans. The studies described previously show that hormones and neuropeptides known to influence consummatory behavior and energy balance also have a significant effect on appetitive behaviors, which have to be successful in order for an animal to eat. Conditions in which body energy stores have been depleted, such as food deprivation and pregnancy and lactation, have a greater effect on food hoarding than food intake in hamsters, suggesting that the primary response to an energy deficit is to prepare for a future repetition of the energy insufficiency rather than an immediate replenishment of body energy stores. Observations that hamsters hoard according to the energy density of food pellets and also compensate for external manipulation of their food hoard also lends credence to the idea that the hamsters are monitoring energy sufficiency by integrating the amount of energy stored in the hoard with that in body energy stores.

Studies completed to date examining gut-derived hormones that promote or terminate meals and orexigenic neuropeptides have started to delineate potential pathways through which hoarding is controlled. Although many of the same hormones and neuropeptides appear to be involved in the control of appetitive and consummatory behaviors, they seem to be functioning to produce independent outcomes on food intake and hoarding, possibly by activation of different receptor subtypes or by activation of neurons with different projection patterns. The results from experiments with NPY also illustrate that behaviors measured in rats and mice that do not have to work to obtain food may erroneously interpret the results in relation to food intake, when they are really driven by appetitive behavior. A majority of the studies conducted so far have investigated the effects of "short-term" signals that modulate hoarding for a period of hours (e.g., CCK) separately from those related to shifts in energy balance and body fat that have sustained effects on hoarding (e.g., leptin). Several investigators have shown that leptin, a signal that is present in proportion to the size of body fat stores, extends and exaggerates the inhibitory effect of CCK on food intake and this represents some of the first evidence for mechanisms that allow energy balance to be maintained through modulation of short-term signals. It would be of interest to determine whether a similar integration of response occurs with appetitive behavior.

3.4 HAMSTERS AS A MODEL FOR STRESS-INDUCED WEIGHT GAIN

Stress has been defined as a state of threatened homeostasis (Stratakis, Gold, and Chrousos 1995) that can be physical or psychological (Armario et al. 1996), and its severity is determined not only by the nature of the threat itself but also by the past experience of the individual and by their perception of the threat. The physiological, endocrine, and neurological systems that facilitate the appropriate whole animal response to a threat have been reviewed in detail elsewhere (Richard, Lin, and Timofeeva 2002; Kovacs 2013; Stengel and Tache 2014) and will be mentioned only briefly here. Exposure to a stressor activates the sympathetic nervous system

(SNS), which releases epinephrine from the adrenal medulla and acts on peripheral systems to initiate a coordinated "fight or flight" response. At the same time, the hypothalamic–pituitary–adrenal (HPA) axis stimulates release of glucocorticoids (GC) from the adrenal cortex (Raber 1998). Hamsters secrete both cortisol and corticosterone, but cortisol appears to be the GC that has the greatest impact on metabolism and energy balance (Solomon et al. 2011). GC receptors are widely distributed in the periphery and change metabolism to mobilize energy stores. In the brain, multiple systems are activated and GCs contribute to the integrated response to a specific stress (Ulrich-Lai and Herman 2009).

Although activation of the SNS and HPA axis initiates the appropriate response to an acute psychological or physical challenge, chronic stress can eventually become life-threatening (Seyle 1976). GCs have the potential to remodel neuronal structures to produce sustained changes in physiology and behavior (McEwen 2012). If these changes are appropriate, then the individual will adapt to a constantly challenging environment; however, if the changes are inappropriate, they can lead to the development of chronic disease (McEwen 1998, McEwen and Wingfield 2003). In recent years, there has also been a growing acceptance that the chronic stress associated with work and home life contributes to the current high incidence of obesity (Spencer and Tilbrook 2011; Wardle et al. 2011) and metabolic syndrome (Bergmann, Gyntelberg, and Faber 2014).

3.4.1 STRESS-INDUCED WEIGHT GAIN IN HUMANS

It has long been recognized that there is a direct association between stress responsiveness and incidence of binge eating in both men and women (Wolf and Crowther 1983; Schaumberg and Earleywine 2013), but it is clear from the literature that only subgroups of the population are susceptible to stress-induced weight gain. In particular, female restrained eaters (Weinstein, Shide, and Rolls 1997; Greeno and Wing 1994) are more likely to overeat in response to stress than are unrestrained eaters (Heatherton, Herman, and Polivy 1991; Zellner et al. 2006). Restrained eaters make conscious decisions about food that are unrelated to hunger but are driven by cues associated with certain food choices and their potential impact on control of body weight. This approach to food selection may not result in a reduced energy intake because extended periods of self-imposed food restriction (van Strien et al. 2006) may be mixed with intermittent periods of disinhibition and overeating (Herman and Polivy 1984). Self-reported restrained eating has been identified as a risk factor for development of obesity in adolescent girls (Stice et al. 2005), but in order for stress to increase food intake, an individual has to be both a restrained eater and someone who is easily disinhibited and experiences frequent bouts of overeating (Westenhoefer et al. 1994). Not all restrained eaters are easily disinhibited, and those who are not may in fact lose weight in response to stress (Yeomans and Coughlan 2009). By contrast, those who are easily disinhibited will choose more calorically dense foods when they are placed in a stressful situation (Rutters et al. 2009; Roberts, Campbell, and Troop 2014).

The effects of stress on energy balance in different animal models has been reviewed in depth elsewhere (Harris 2015), and in contrast to humans, a majority of chronically stressed experimental animals lose weight. This is true for rats and mice subjected to restraint stress (Harris et al. 2002; Chotiwat, Kelso, and Harris 2010), chronic unpredictable mild stress (Michel et al. 2005; Farhan et al. 2014), or social defeat (Keeney and Hogg 1999; Buwalda et al. 2001). Two exceptions are hamsters subjected to social defeat and nonhuman primates housed in social groups. The studies with cymologous monkeys have been reported exclusively by the Wilson laboratory at Emory University and are discussed in detail in Chapter 4 of this book. In these experiments, female monkeys that are group housed develop a social hierarchy that results in the subordinates being chronically stressed (Wilson et al. 2014). Subordinate monkeys consistently eat more than the dominant females regardless of dietary composition (Arce et al. 2010).

3.4.2 SOCIAL DEFEAT AS AN EXPERIMENTAL CHRONIC STRESSOR

It has been suggested that chronic social stress may be typical of an animal's natural habitat (Koolhaas et al. 1997, Blanchard, McKittrick, and Blanchard 2001), in which dominance is established and animals are exposed to predators when they leave the burrow to forage for food. Chronic social defeat is a combined physical and psychological stressor that has been used extensively in the laboratory as a mouse model of depression (Krishnan and Nestler 2011). These experiments are limited to males because females do not establish social dominance. The social defeat paradigm involves placing a subordinate male in the home cage of a dominant male for 4–10 minutes each day. Because the aggressive male attacks the intruder, the duration of direct exposure is limited to the first day and physical contact is prevented on subsequent days by placing mesh between the resident and intruder animals. In a majority of studies, repeatedly placing a subordinate mouse in close proximity to an aggressive male causes weight loss and depression-like behavior (Kudryavtseva, Bakshtanovskaya, and Koryakina 1991; Avgustinovich, Kovalenko, and Kudryavtseva 2005). There are some recent studies in which social defeat results in reversible weight gain in the subordinate mouse. Continuous visual, olfactory, and auditory contact with a dominant male for 8 days with intermittent physical contact causes weight gain in some strains of mice (Moles et al. 2006) but not others (Bartolomucci et al. 2004; Sanghez et al. 2013). Mice also gain weight on a protocol in which the subordinate is subjected to progressively shorter durations of exposure to different dominant resident mice each day (Goto et al. 2014), but in this situation, the weight gain is due to increased water retention and no change in body fat mass.

3.4.3 STRESS-INDUCED WEIGHT GAIN IN HAMSTERS

Although there are very few reports on the effects of chronic stress in hamsters, it appears that weight gain is a consistent response in both male and female Syrian hamsters. Borer et al. (1988) group or single housed adult female Syrian hamsters for 100 days. The group-housed animals grew faster and gained 50% more body fat than the single-housed controls irrespective of whether they were housed in long or short photoperiods. There was a nonsignificant increase in food intake that could account for approximately half of the increase in body energy stores and a reduction in resting metabolic rate, facilitated by huddling, accounted for the remaining weight gain. In a subsequent experiment, Meisel et al. (1990) found the same effect on body weight, with group-housed animals gaining three times more weight during the experiment than single-housed controls did. For this study, in addition to growing faster and increasing body fat mass, the group-housed animals were found to have enlarged adrenals. Both male and female hamster live in isolation and defend their territory in the wild (Staffend and Meisel 2012); therefore, group housing is experienced as a chronic social stress (Meisel et al. 1990).

No further studies have been reported on group-housed hamsters, but the work was followed up using a different social stress in male hamsters. Young (9-week-old) male Syrian hamsters were housed in long photoperiod conditions and subjected to 7-minute sessions of social defeat before being returned to their individual home cages (Foster et al. 2006; Solomon et al. 2007). The animals were stressed intermittently for a total of 15 times during a 34-day period. Excess weight gain was apparent after about 10 days, when the hamsters had been stressed three times but did not become significant until day 24, by which time they had been stressed nine times. Both the subordinate and aggressive males gained weight, but the increase in food intake was greater in the subordinates and an increase in body fat was apparent only in the subordinates because the aggressive males gained lean tissue (Solomon et al. 2007). There was a small but significant increase in food intake, but a doubling of feed efficiency in the stressed animals compared with their controls. Animals defeated only once did not increase food intake, feed efficiency, or weight gain; therefore, repeated or chronic stress was essential to initiate the changes in energy utilization that resulted in increased body fat, but it did not matter whether the defeat occurred on consecutive days or at random intervals (Foster et al. 2006). There were no changes in circulating testosterone or cortisol in the subordinate hamsters at the end of the study, nor were their adrenal glands enlarged. This difference between the female group-housed and the socially defeated animals may have been due to the difference in severity of the stress because the defeated males returned to their home cages every day whereas the group housed animals were in a constant state of stress for the duration of the study.

Although the initiation of weight gain requires activation of stress-related systems, they are not required for the sustained shift in efficiency of energy utilization and overeating. This was confirmed by a failure of chronic infusions of GC into adrenal-intact animals to replicate stress-induced weight gain (Solomon et al. 2011). By contrast, a similar weight gain, caused entirely by an increase in efficiency of energy utilization, can be achieved with four daily sessions of footshock (Solomon et al. 2007). Although this suggests that weight gain would be generalized to any repeated stress, repeated restraint stress decreases food intake and causes weight loss in Syrian hamsters (King-Herbert et al. 1997), just as it does in rats and mice.

3.4.4 SUMMARY OF THE HAMSTER AS A MODEL FOR STRESS-INDUCED WEIGHT GAIN

In addition to the need to identify the mechanistic basis of weight gain, which is highly dependent upon increased energy efficiency, there are a number of other aspects of this model that still need to be investigated. One is whether chronic social stress causes weight gain in Siberian hamsters as it does in Syrian hamsters. Only one paper has been published on social defeat in Siberian hamsters, and this focused on immune function but had no information on body weight (Chester, Bonu, and Demas 2010). If the response is initiated by release of GC, or modulation of SNS activity, then one would expect a similar response in Siberian and Syrian hamsters. There are, however, species differences in body fat accumulation during a short photoperiod, where Syrian hamsters gain body fat (Wade and Bartness 1984b), but Siberian hamsters reduce their fat mass (Bartness 1996). Similarly, Siberian hamsters exposed to a long photoperiod and offered a high-fat diet increase food intake, but do not gain weight possibly because of a significant increase in brown fat thermogenesis (McElroy et al. 1986). By contrast, Syrian hamsters do not overeat a high-fat diet but become obese due to a reduction in energy expenditure despite an increase in brown fat thermogenic capacity (Wade 1983). Therefore, it is quite possible that whatever underlying mechanisms cause opposing shifts in body fat mass in response to seasonal changes and diet could also influence the gain in body fat caused by chronic stress. Second, all of the studies with chronic stress have the animals housed in cages with free access to food, and it would be of interest to determine whether the effects on consummatory behavior are accompanied by changes in appetitive behavior.

ACKNOWLEDGMENT

Timothy J. Bartness, PhD, was the intended author of this chapter but was unable to complete the task. This chapter is written in acknowledgment of his unique contribution to the understanding of ingestive behavior through investigation of the foraging and hoarding behavior of Siberian hamsters.

LITERATURE CITED

Adrian, T. E., J. M. Allen, S. R. Bloom, M. A. Ghatei, M. N. Rossor, G. W. Roberts, T. J. Crow, K. Tatemoto, and J. M. Polak. 1983. Neuropeptide Y distribution in human brain. *Nature* 306:584–6.

Allen, Y. S., T. E. Adrian, J. M. Allen, K. Tatemoto, T. J. Crow, S. R. Bloom, and J. M. Polak. 1983. Neuropeptide Y distribution in the rat brain. *Science* 221:877–9.

Ammar, A. A., F. Sederholm, T. R. Saito, A. J. Scheurink, A. E. Johnson, and P. Sodersten. 2000. NPY-leptin: Opposing effects on appetitive and consummatory ingestive behavior and sexual behavior. *Am J Physiol Regul Integr Comp Physiol* 278:R1627–33.

Arce, M., V. Michopoulos, K. N. Shepard, Q. C. Ha, and M. E. Wilson. 2010. Diet choice, cortisol reactivity, and emotional feeding in socially housed rhesus monkeys. *Physiol Behav* 101:446–55.

Armario, A., O. Marti, T. Molina, J. de Pablo, and M. Valdes. 1996. Acute stress markers in humans: Response of plasma glucose, cortisol and prolactin to two examinations differing in the anxiety they provoke. *Psychoneuroendocrinology* 21:17–24.

Arnold, M., A. Mura, W. Langhans, and N. Geary. 2006. Gut vagal afferents are not necessary for the eating-stimulatory effect of intraperitoneally injected ghrelin in the rat. *J Neurosci* 26:11052–60.

Avgustinovich, D. F., I. L. Kovalenko, and N. N. Kudryavtseva. 2005. A model of anxious depression: Persistence of behavioral pathology. *Neurosci Behav Physiol* 35:917–24.

Bartness, T. J. 1996. Photoperiod, sex, gonadal steroids, and housing density affect body fat in hamsters. *Physiol Behav* 60:517–29.

Bartness, T. J. 1997. Food hoarding is increased by pregnancy, lactation, and food deprivation in Siberian hamsters. *Am J Physiol* 272:R118–25.

Bartness, T. J., and M. R. Clein. 1994. Effects of food deprivation and restriction, and metabolic blockers on food hoarding in Siberian hamsters. *Am J Physiol* 266:R1111–7.

Bartness, T. J., E. Keen-Rhinehart, M. J. Dailey, and B. J. Teubner. 2011. Neural and hormonal control of food hoarding. *Am J Physiol Regul Integr Comp Physiol* 301:R641–55.

Bartness, T. J., J. B. Powers, M. H. Hastings, E. L. Bittman, and B. D. Goldman. 1993. The timed infusion paradigm for melatonin delivery: What has it taught us about the melatonin signal, its reception, and the photoperiodic control of seasonal responses? *J Pineal Res* 15:161–90.

Bartolomucci, A., T. Pederzani, P. Sacerdote, A. E. Panerai, S. Parmigiani, and P. Palanza. 2004. Behavioral and physiological characterization of male mice under chronic psychosocial stress. *Psychoneuroendocrinology* 29:899–910.

Bergmann, N., F. Gyntelberg, and J. Faber. 2014. The appraisal of chronic stress and the development of the metabolic syndrome: A systematic review of prospective cohort studies. *Endocr Connect* 3:R55–80.

Berthoud, H. R. 2004. Mind versus metabolism in the control of food intake and energy balance. *Physiol Behav* 81:781–93.

Bevelander, K. E., D. J. Anschutz, and R. C. Engels. 2011. Social modeling of food purchases at supermarkets in teenage girls. *Appetite* 57:99–104.

Bhatia, A. J., and G. N. Wade. 1993. Energy balance in pregnant hamsters: A role for voluntary exercise? *Am J Physiol* 265:R563–7.

Blanchard, R. J., C. R. McKittrick, and D. C. Blanchard. 2001. Animal models of social stress: Effects on behavior and brain neurochemical systems. *Physiol Behav* 73:261–71.

Booth, D. A. 1968. Effects of intrahypothalamic glucose injection on eating and drinking elicited by insulin. *J Comp Physiol Psychol* 65:13–6.

Borer, K. T., A. Pryor, C. A. Conn, R. Bonna, and M. Kielb. 1988. Group housing accelerates growth and induces obesity in adult hamsters. *Am J Physiol* 255:R128–33.

Borker, A. S., and M. G. Gogate. 1981. Hunger versus hoarding and body weight in rats. *Indian J Physiol Pharmacol* 25:365–8.

Boss-Williams, K. A., and T. J. Bartness. 1996. NPY stimulation of food intake in Siberian hamsters is not photoperiod dependent. *Physiol Behav* 59:157–64.

Bradley, S. P., L. M. Pattullo, P. N. Patel, and B. J. Prendergast. 2010. Photoperiodic regulation of the orexigenic effects of ghrelin in Siberian hamsters. *Horm Behav* 58:647–52.

Bragado, M. J., M. Tashiro, and J. A. Williams. 2000. Regulation of the initiation of pancreatic digestive enzyme protein synthesis by cholecystokinin in rat pancreas in vivo. *Gastroenterology* 119:1731–9.

Buckley, C. A., and J. E. Schneider. 2003. Food hoarding is increased by food deprivation and decreased by leptin treatment in Syrian hamsters. *Am J Physiol Regul Integr Comp Physiol* 285:R1021–9.

Buwalda, B., W. A. Blom, J. M. Koolhaas, and G. van Dijk. 2001. Behavioral and physiological responses to stress are affected by high-fat feeding in male rats. *Physiol Behav* 73:371–7.

Cabanac, M., and A. H. Swiergiel. 1989. Rats eating and hoarding as a function of body weight and cost of foraging. *Am J Physiol* 257:R952–7.

Campbell, C. S., J. Tabor, and J. D. Davis. 1983. Small effect of brown adipose tissue and major effect of photoperiod on body weight in hamsters (*Mesocricetus auratus*). *Physiol Behav* 30:349–52.

Campos, C. A., J. S. Wright, K. Czaja, and R. C. Ritter. 2012. CCK-induced reduction of food intake and hindbrain MAPK signaling are mediated by NMDA receptor activation. *Endocrinology* 153:2633–46.

Charron, I., and M. Cabanac. 2004. Influence of pellet size on rat's hoarding behavior. *Physiol Behav* 82:447–51.

Chester, E. M., T. Bonu, and G. E. Demas. 2010. Social defeat differentially affects immune responses in Siberian hamsters (*Phodopus sungorus*). *Physiol Behav* 101:53–8.

Chotiwat, C., E. W. Kelso, and R. B. Harris. 2010. The effects of repeated restraint stress on energy balance and behavior of mice with selective deletion of CRF receptors. *Stress* 13:203–13.

Clark, J. T., P. S. Kalra, W. R. Crowley, and S. P. Kalra. 1984. Neuropeptide Y and human pancreatic polypeptide stimulate feeding behavior in rats. *Endocrinology* 115:427–9.

Collier, G., D. F. Johnson, and C. Mathis. 2002. The currency of procurement cost. *J Exp Anal Behav* 78:31–61.

Considine, R. V., M. K. Sinha, M. L. Heiman, A. Kriauciunas, T. W. Stephens, M. R. Nyce, J. P. Ohannesian, C. C. Marco, L. J. McKee, T. L. Bauer, and J. F. Caro. 1996. Serum immunoreactive-leptin concentrations in normal-weight and obese humans. *N Engl J Med* 334:292–5.

Craig, W. 1931. Appetites and aversions as constituents of instincts. *The Biological Bulletin* 34:91–107.

Dailey, M. E., and T. J. Bartness. 2008. Fat pad-specific effects of lipectomy on foraging, food hoarding, and food intake. *Am J Physiol Regul Integr Comp Physiol* 294:R321–8.

Dailey, M. J., and T. J. Bartness. 2009. Appetitive and consummatory ingestive behaviors stimulated by PVH and perifornical area NPY injections. *Am J Physiol Regul Integr Comp Physiol* 296:R877–92.

Day, D. E., and T. J. Bartness. 2001. Effects of foraging effort on body fat and food hoarding in Siberian hamsters. *J Exp Zool* 289:162–71.

Day, D. E., and T. J. Bartness. 2003. Fasting-induced increases in food hoarding are dependent on the foraging-effort level. *Physiol Behav* 78:655–68.

Day, D. E., and T. J. Bartness. 2004. Agouti-related protein increases food hoarding more than food intake in Siberian hamsters. *Am J Physiol Regul Integr Comp Physiol* 286:R38–45.

Day, D. E., E. Keen-Rinehart, and T. J. Bartness. 2005. Role of NPY and its receptor subtypes in foraging, food hoarding, and food intake by Siberian hamsters. *Am J Physiol Regul Integr Comp Physiol* 289:R29–36.

Day, D. E., E. M. Mintz, and T. J. Bartness. 1999. Diet self-selection and food hoarding after food deprivation by Siberian hamsters. *Physiol Behav* 68:187–94.

Deacon, R. M. 2009. Burrowing: A sensitive behavioural assay, tested in five species of laboratory rodents. *Behav Brain Res* 200:128–33.

Dodd, D. K., R. B. Stalling, and J. Bedell. 1977. Grocery purchases as a function of obesity and assumed food deprivation. *Int J Obes* 1:43–7.

Emery, C. F., K. L. Olson, V. S. Lee, D. L. Habash, J. L. Nasar, and A. Bodine. 2015. Home environment and psychosocial predictors of obesity status among community-residing men and women. *Int J Obes (Lond)* 39:1401–7.

Etienne, A. S., E. Emmanuelli, and M. Zinder. 1982. Ontogeny of hoarding in the golden hamster: The development of motor patterns and their sequential coordination. *Dev Psychobiol* 15:33–45.

Fantino, M., and M. Cabanac. 1980. Body weight regulation with a proportional hoarding response in the rat. *Physiol Behav* 24:939–42.

Fantino, M., and M. Cabanac. 1984. Effect of a cold ambient temperature on the rat's food hoarding behavior. *Physiol Behav* 32:183–90.

Farhan, M., H. Ikram, S. Kanwal, and D. J. Haleem. 2014. Unpredictable chronic mild stress induced behavioral deficits: A comparative study in male and female rats. *Pak J Pharm Sci* 27:879–84.

Faulconbridge, L. F., D. E. Cummings, J. M. Kaplan, and H. J. Grill. 2003. Hyperphagic effects of brainstem ghrelin administration. *Diabetes* 52:2260–5.

Faulconbridge, L. F., H. J. Grill, and J. M. Kaplan. 2005. Distinct forebrain and caudal brainstem contributions to the neuropeptide Y mediation of ghrelin hyperphagia. *Diabetes* 54:1985–93.

Fisher, J. O., and L. L. Birch. 1995. Fat preferences and fat consumption of 3- to 5-year-old children are related to parental adiposity. *J Am Diet Assoc* 95:759–64.

Food Marketing Institute. 2012. *U.S. grocery shopper trends.* Arlington, VA: Food Marketing Institute.

Foster, M. T., M. B. Solomon, K. L. Huhman, and T. J. Bartness. 2006. Social defeat increases food intake, body mass, and adiposity in Syrian hamsters. *Am J Physiol Regul Integr Comp Physiol* 290:R1284–93.

Garretson, J. T., and T. J. Bartness. 2014. Dynamic modification of hoarding in response to hoard size manipulation. *Physiol Behav* 127:8–12.

Garretson, J. T., B. J. Teubner, K. L. Grove, A. Vazdarjanova, V. Ryu, and T. J. Bartness. 2015. Peroxisome proliferator-activated receptor gamma controls ingestive behavior, agouti-related protein, and neuropeptide Y mRNA in the arcuate hypothalamus. *J Neurosci* 35:4571–81.

Gibbs, J., and G. P. Smith. 1982. Gut peptides and food in the gut produce similar satiety effects. *Peptides* 3:553–7.

Goldstone, A. P., C. G. Prechtl, S. Scholtz, A. D. Miras, N. Chhina, G. Durighel, S. S. Deliran, C. Beckmann, M. A. Ghatei, D. R. Ashby, A. D. Waldman, B. D. Gaylinn, M. O. Thorner, G. S. Frost, S. R. Bloom, and J. D. Bell. 2014. Ghrelin mimics fasting to enhance human hedonic, orbitofrontal cortex, and hippocampal responses to food. *Am J Clin Nutr* 99:1319–30.

Goto, T., Y. Kubota, Y. Tanaka, W. Iio, N. Moriya, and A. Toyoda. 2014. Subchronic and mild social defeat stress accelerates food intake and body weight gain with polydipsia-like features in mice. *Behav Brain Res* 270:339–48.

Greeno, C. G., and R. R. Wing. 1994. Stress-induced eating. *Psychol Bull* 115:444–64.

Grill, H. J. 2006. Distributed neural control of energy balance: Contributions from hindbrain and hypothalamus. *Obesity (Silver Spring)* 14 Suppl 5:216S–221S.

Grill, H. J., and J. M. Kaplan. 2002. The neuroanatomical axis for control of energy balance. *Front Neuroendocrinol* 23:2–40.

Harris, R. B. 2015. Chronic and acute effects of stress on energy balance: Are there appropriate animal models? *Am J Physiol Regul Integr Comp Physiol* 308:R250–65.

Harris, R. B., and R. J. Martin. 1984. Recovery of body weight from below "set point" in mature female rats. *J Nutr* 114:1143–50.

Harris, R. B., T. R. Kasser, and R. J. Martin. 1986. Dynamics of recovery of body composition after overfeeding, food restriction or starvation of mature female rats. *J Nutr* 116:2536–46.

Harris, R. B., T. D. Mitchell, J. Simpson, S. M. Redmann, Jr., B. D. Youngblood, and D. H. Ryan. 2002. Weight loss in rats exposed to repeated acute restraint stress is independent of energy or leptin status. *Am J Physiol Regul Integr Comp Physiol* 282:R77–88.

Hausman, D. B., J. Lu, D. H. Ryan, W. P. Flatt, and R. B. Harris. 2004. Compensatory growth of adipose tissue after partial lipectomy: Involvement of serum factors. *Exp Biol Med (Maywood)* 229:512–20.

Heatherton, T. F., C. P. Herman, and J. Polivy. 1991. Effects of physical threat and ego threat on eating behavior. *J Pers Soc Psychol* 60:138–43.

Heldmaier, G., S. Steinlechner, and J. Rafael. 1982. Nonshivering thermogenesis and cold resistance during seasonal acclimatization in the DJungarian hamster. *J Comp Physiol* 149:1–9.

Herman, C. P., and J. Polivy. 1984. A boundary model for the regulation of eating. *Res Publ Assoc Res Nerv Ment Dis* 62:141–56.

Herring, N. 2015. Autonomic control of the heart: Going beyond the classical neurotransmitters. *Exp Physiol* 100:354–8.

Hoffman, K. 1973. The influence of photoperiod and melatonin on testis size, body weight and pelage color in the Djungarian hamster (*Phodopus sungorus*). *J Comp Physiol* 85:267–82.

Horn, C. C., and M. I. Friedman. 1998. Methyl palmoxirate increases eating behavior and brain Fos-like immunoreactivity in rats. *Brain Res* 781:8–14.

Humphries, M. M., D. W. Thomas, and D. L. Kramer. 2003. The role of energy availability in mammalian hibernation: A cost–benefit approach. *Physiol Biochem Zool* 76:165–79.

Johnstone, A. M., P. Faber, E. R. Gibney, M. Elia, G. Horgan, B. E. Golden, and R. J. Stubbs. 2002. Effect of an acute fast on energy compensation and feeding behaviour in lean men and women. *Int J Obes Relat Metab Disord* 26:1623–8.

Kalra, S. P., M. G. Dube, S. Pu, B. Xu, T. L. Horvath, and P. S. Kalra. 1999. Interacting appetite-regulating pathways in the hypothalamic regulation of body weight. *Endocr Rev* 20:68–100.

Kamiji, M. M., and A. Inui. 2007. Neuropeptide y receptor selective ligands in the treatment of obesity. *Endocr Rev* 28:664–84.

Kanarek, R. B., and N. Orthen-Gambill. 1982. Differential effects of sucrose, fructose and glucose on carbohydrate-induced obesity in rats. *J Nutr* 112:1546–54.

Kanoski, S. E., A. L. Alhadeff, S. M. Fortin, J. R. Gilbert, and H. J. Grill. 2014. Leptin signaling in the medial nucleus tractus solitarius reduces food seeking and willingness to work for food. *Neuropsychopharmacology* 39:605–13.

Keen-Rinehart, E., and T. J. Bartness. 2005. Peripheral ghrelin injections stimulate food intake, foraging, and food hoarding in Siberian hamsters. *Am J Physiol Regul Integr Comp Physiol* 288:R716–22.

Keen-Rinehart, E., and T. J. Bartness. 2007. MTII attenuates ghrelin- and food deprivation-induced increases in food hoarding and food intake. *Horm Behav* 52:612–20.

Keen-Rinehart, E., and T. J. Bartness. 2008. Leptin inhibits food-deprivation-induced increases in food intake and food hoarding. *Am J Physiol Regul Integr Comp Physiol* 295:R1737–46.

Keeney, A. J., and S. Hogg. 1999. Behavioural consequences of repeated social defeat in the mouse: Preliminary evaluation of a potential animal model of depression. *Behav Pharmacol* 10:753–64.

Keys, A., J. Brozek, A. Henschel, O. Mickelson, and H. L. Taylor. 1950. *The biology of human starvation*. 2 vols. Minneapolis, MN: The University of Minnesota Press.

King-Herbert, A. P., T. W. Hesterburg, P. P. Thevenaz, T. E. Hamm, Jr., O. R. Moss, D. B. Janszen, and J. I. Everitt. 1997. Effects of immobilization restraint on Syrian golden hamsters. *Lab Anim Sci* 47:362–6.

Kliewer, S. A., S. S. Sundseth, S. A. Jones, P. J. Brown, G. B. Wisely, C. S. Koble, P. Devchand, W. Wahli, T. M. Willson, J. M. Lenhard, and J. M. Lehmann. 1997. Fatty acids and eicosanoids regulate gene expression through direct interactions with peroxisome proliferator-activated receptors alpha and gamma. *Proc Natl Acad Sci U S A* 94:4318–23.

Kojima, M., H. Hosoda, Y. Date, M. Nakazato, H. Matsuo, and K. Kangawa. 1999. Ghrelin is a growth-hormone-releasing acylated peptide from stomach. *Nature* 402:656–60.

Koolhaas, J. M., P. Meerlo, S. F. De Boer, J. H. Strubbe, and B. Bohus. 1997. The temporal dynamics of the stress response. *Neurosci Biobehav Rev* 21:775–82.

Kovacs, K. J. 2013. CRH: The link between hormonal-, metabolic- and behavioral responses to stress. *J Chem Neuroanat* 54:25–33.

Krishnan, V., and E. J. Nestler. 2011. Animal models of depression: Molecular perspectives. *Curr Top Behav Neurosci* 7:121–47.

Kudryavtseva, N. N., I. V. Bakshtanovskaya, and L. A. Koryakina. 1991. Social model of depression in mice of C57BL/6J strain. *Pharmacol Biochem Behav* 38:315–20.

Kulkosky, P. J., G. W. Glazner, H. D. Moore, C. A. Low, and S. C. Woods. 1988. Neuropeptide Y: Behavioral effects in the golden hamster. *Peptides* 9:1389–93.

Lawrence, C. B., A. C. Snape, F. M. Baudoin, and S. M. Luckman. 2002. Acute central ghrelin and GH secretagogues induce feeding and activate brain appetite centers. *Endocrinology* 143:155–62.

Lazzarini, S. J., J. E. Schneider, and G. N. Wade. 1988. Inhibition of fatty acid oxidation and glucose metabolism does not affect food intake or hunger motivation in Syrian hamsters. *Physiol Behav* 44:209–13.

Lemonnier, D. 1972. Effect of age, sex, and sites on the cellularity of the adipose tissue in mice and rats rendered obese by a high-fat diet. *J Clin Invest* 51:2907–15.

Levitsky, D. A., and L. DeRosimo. 2010. One day of food restriction does not result in an increase in subsequent daily food intake in humans. *Physiol Behav* 99:495–9.

Liddle, R. A., I. D. Goldfine, M. S. Rosen, R. A. Taplitz, and J. A. Williams. 1985. Cholecystokinin bioactivity in human plasma. Molecular forms, responses to feeding, and relationship to gallbladder contraction. *J Clin Invest* 75:1144–52.

Lin, B. H., and J. Guthrie. 2012. Nutritional quality of food prepared at home and away from home. www.ers.usda.gov: Economic Research Service.

Liu, J. L., B. Han, and D. A. Cohen. 2015. Beyond neighborhood food environments: Distance traveled to food establishments in 5 US cities, 2009–2011. *Prev Chronic Dis* 12:E126.

Malik, S., F. McGlone, D. Bedrossian, and A. Dagher. 2008. Ghrelin modulates brain activity in areas that control appetitive behavior. *Cell Metab* 7:400–9.

Maniscalco, J. W., and L. Rinaman. 2013. Overnight food deprivation markedly attenuates hindbrain noradrenergic, glucagon-like peptide-1, and hypothalamic neural responses to exogenous cholecystokinin in male rats. *Physiol Behav* 121:35–42.

Marin Bivens, C. L., W. J. Thomas, and B. G. Stanley. 1998. Similar feeding patterns are induced by perifornical neuropeptide Y injection and by food deprivation. *Brain Res* 782:271–80.

McElroy, J. F., and G. N. Wade. 1986. Short photoperiod stimulates brown adipose tissue growth and thermogenesis but not norepinephrine turnover in Syrian hamsters. *Physiol Behav* 37:307–11.

McElroy, J. F., P. W. Mason, J. M. Hamilton, and G. N. Wade. 1986. Effects of diet and photoperiod on NE turnover and GDP binding in Siberian hamster brown adipose tissue. *Am J Physiol* 250:R383–8.

McEwen, B. S. 1998. Stress, adaptation, and disease. Allostasis and allostatic load. *Ann N Y Acad Sci* 840:33–44.

McEwen, B. S. 2012. The ever-changing brain: Cellular and molecular mechanisms for the effects of stressful experiences. *Dev Neurobiol* 72:878–90.

McEwen, B. S., and J. C. Wingfield. 2003. The concept of allostasis in biology and biomedicine. *Horm Behav* 43:2–15.

Medina-Gomez, G., S. L. Gray, L. Yetukuri, K. Shimomura, S. Virtue, M. Campbell, R. K. Curtis, M. Jimenez-Linan, M. Blount, G. S. Yeo, M. Lopez, T. Seppanen-Laakso, F. M. Ashcroft, M. Oresic, and A. Vidal-Puig. 2007. PPAR gamma 2 prevents lipotoxicity by controlling adipose tissue expandability and peripheral lipid metabolism. *PLoS Genet* 3:e64.

Meisel, R. L., T. C. Hays, S. N. Del Paine, and V. R. Luttrell. 1990. Induction of obesity by group housing in female Syrian hamsters. *Physiol Behav* 47:815–7.

Mela, D. J., J. I. Aaron, and S. J. Gatenby. 1996. Relationships of consumer characteristics and food deprivation to food purchasing behavior. *Physiol Behav* 60:1331–5.

Mercer, J. G., K. M. Moar, A. W. Ross, N. Hoggard, and P. J. Morgan. 2000. Photoperiod regulates arcuate nucleus POMC, AGRP, and leptin receptor mRNA in Siberian hamster hypothalamus. *Am J Physiol Regul Integr Comp Physiol* 278:R271–81.

Miceli, M. O., and C. W. Malsbury. 1982. Sagittal knife cuts in the near and far lateral preoptic area-hypothalamus disrupt maternal behaviour in female hamsters. *Physiol Behav* 28:856–67.

Michel, C., M. Duclos, M. Cabanac, and D. Richard. 2005. Chronic stress reduces body fat content in both obesity-prone and obesity-resistant strains of mice. *Horm Behav* 48:172–9.

Moles, A., A. Bartolomucci, L. Garbugino, R. Conti, A. Caprioli, R. Coccurello, R. Rizzi, B. Ciani, and F. R. D'Amato. 2006. Psychosocial stress affects energy balance in mice: Modulation by social status. *Psychoneuroendocrinology* 31:623–33.

Moran, T. H. 2000. Cholecystokinin and satiety: Current perspectives. *Nutrition* 16:858–65.

Mountjoy, K. G., M. T. Mortrud, M. J. Low, R. B. Simerly, and R. D. Cone. 1994. Localization of the melanocortin-4 receptor (MC4-R) in neuroendocrine and autonomic control circuits in the brain. *Molecular Endocrinology* 8:1298–308.

Muller, T. D., R. Nogueiras, M. L. Andermann, Z. B. Andrews, S. D. Anker, J. Argente, R. L. Batterham, S. C. Benoit, C. Y. Bowers, F. Broglio, F. F. Casanueva, D. D'Alessio, I. Depoortere, A. Geliebter, E. Ghigo, P. A. Cole, M. Cowley, D. E. Cummings, A. Dagher, S. Diano, S. L. Dickson, C. Dieguez, R. Granata, H. J. Grill, K. Grove, K. M. Habegger, K. Heppner, M. L. Heiman, L. Holsen, B. Holst, A. Inui, J. O. Jansson, H. Kirchner, M. Korbonits, B. Laferrere, C. W. LeRoux, M. Lopez, S. Morin, M. Nakazato, R. Nass, D. Perez-Tilve, P. T. Pfluger, T. W. Schwartz, R. J. Seeley, M. Sleeman, Y. Sun, L. Sussel, J. Tong, M. O. Thorner, A. J. van der Lely, L. H. van der Ploeg, J. M. Zigman, M. Kojima, K. Kangawa, R. G. Smith, T. Horvath, and M. H. Tschop. 2015. Ghrelin. *Mol Metab* 4:437–60.

Muurahainen, N., H. R. Kissileff, A. J. Derogatis, and F. X. Pi-Sunyer. 1988. Effects of cholecystokinin-octapeptide (CCK-8) on food intake and gastric emptying in man. *Physiol Behav* 44:645–9.

Naleid, A. M., M. K. Grace, D. E. Cummings, and A. S. Levine. 2005. Ghrelin induces feeding in the mesolimbic reward pathway between the ventral tegmental area and the nucleus accumbens. *Peptides* 26:2274–9.

Nederkoorn, C., R. Guerrieri, R. C. Havermans, A. Roefs, and A. Jansen. 2009. The interactive effect of hunger and impulsivity on food intake and purchase in a virtual supermarket. *Int J Obes (Lond)* 33:905–12.

Nepper, M. J., and W. Chai. 2016. Parents' barriers and strategies to promote healthy eating among school-age children. *Appetite* 103:157–64.

Overduin, J., J. Gibbs, D. E. Cummings, and J. R. Reeve, Jr. 2014. CCK-58 elicits both satiety and satiation in rats while CCK-8 elicits only satiation. *Peptides* 54:71–80.

Perrigo, G., and F. H. Bronson. 1983. Foraging effort, food intake, fat deposition and puberty in female mice. *Biol Reprod* 29:455–63.

Raber, J. 1998. Detrimental effects of chronic hypothalamic–pituitary–adrenal axis activation. From obesity to memory deficits. *Mol Neurobiol* 18:1–22.

Ransley, J. K., J. K. Donnelly, H. Botham, T. N. Khara, D. C. Greenwood, and J. E. Cade. 2003. Use of supermarket receipts to estimate energy and fat content of food purchased by lean and overweight families. *Appetite* 41:141–8.

Reichmann, F., and P. Holzer. 2016. Neuropeptide Y: A stressful review. *Neuropeptides* 55:99–109.

Rentsch, J., N. Levens, and M. Chiesi. 1995. Recombinant ob-gene product reduces food intake in fasted mice. *Biochem Biophys Res Commun* 214:131–6.

Richard, D., Q. Lin, and E. Timofeeva. 2002. The corticotropin-releasing factor family of peptides and CRF receptors: Their roles in the regulation of energy balance. *Eur J Pharmacol* 440:189–97.

Ritter, R. C., and O. K. Balch. 1978. Feeding in response to insulin but not to 2-deoxy-D-glucose in the hamster. *Am J Physiol* 234:E20–4.

Ritter, R. C., and P. Slusser. 1980. 5-Thio-D-glucose causes increased feeding and hyperglycemia in the rat. *Am J Physiol* 238:E141–4.

Roberts, C. J., I. C. Campbell, and N. Troop. 2014. Increases in weight during chronic stress are partially associated with a switch in food choice towards increased carbohydrate and saturated fat intake. *Eur Eat Disord Rev* 22:77–82.

Roselli-Rehfuss, L., K. G. Mountjoy, L. S. Robbins, M. T. Mortrud, M. J. Low, J. B. Tatro, M. L. Entwistle, R. B. Simerly, and R. D. Cone. 1993. Identification of a receptor for gamma melanotropin and other proopiomelanocortin peptides in the hypothalamus and limbic system. *Proc Natl Acad Sci U S A* 90:8856–60.

Rothwell, N. J., and M. J. Stock. 1979. Regulation of energy balance in two models of reversible obesity in the rat. *J Comp Physiol Psychol* 93:1024–34.

Rowland, N. E., L. L. Bellush, and J. Carlton. 1985. Metabolic and neurochemical correlates of glucoprivic feeding. *Brain Res Bull* 14:617–24.

Ruf, T., and G. Heldmaier. 1992. The impact of daily torpor on energy requirements in the Djungarian hamster, Phodopus sungorus. *Physiol Zool* 65:994–1010.

Ruf, T., A. Stieglitz, S. Steinlechner, J. L. Blank, and G. Heldmaier. 1993. Cold exposure and food restriction facilitate physiological responses to short photoperiod in Djungarian hamsters (*Phodopus sungorus*). *J Exp Zool* 267:104–12.

Rutters, F., A. G. Nieuwenhuizen, S. G. Lemmens, J. M. Born, and M. S. Westerterp-Plantenga. 2009. Acute stress-related changes in eating in the absence of hunger. *Obesity (Silver Spring)* 17:72–7.

Ryan, K. K., B. Li, B. E. Grayson, E. K. Matter, S. C. Woods, and R. J. Seeley. 2011. A role for central nervous system PPAR-gamma in the regulation of energy balance. *Nat Med* 17:623–6.

Sanghez, V., M. Razzoli, S. Carobbio, M. Campbell, J. McCallum, C. Cero, G. Ceresini, A. Cabassi, P. Govoni, P. Franceschini, V. de Santis, A. Gurney, I. Ninkovic, S. Parmigiani, P. Palanza, A. Vidal-Puig, and A. Bartolomucci. 2013. Psychosocial stress induces hyperphagia and exacerbates diet-induced insulin resistance and the manifestations of the metabolic syndrome. *Psychoneuroendocrinology* 38:2933–42.

Sarruf, D. A., F. Yu, H. T. Nguyen, D. L. Williams, R. L. Printz, K. D. Niswender, and M. W. Schwartz. 2009. Expression of peroxisome proliferator-activated receptor-gamma in key neuronal subsets regulating glucose metabolism and energy homeostasis. *Endocrinology* 150:707–12.

Schaumberg, K., and M. Earleywine. 2013. Evaluating the acquired preparedness model for bulimic symptoms and problem drinking in male and female college students. *Eat Behav* 14:47–52.

Schneider, J. E., and G. N. Wade. 1987. Body composition, food intake, and brown fat thermogenesis in pregnant Djungarian hamsters. *Am J Physiol* 253:R314–20.

Schneider, B. S., J. W. Monahan, and J. Hirsch. 1979. Brain cholecystokinin and nutritional status in rats and mice. *J Clin Invest* 64:1348–56.

Schneider, J. E., J. F. Casper, A. Barisich, C. Schoengold, S. Cherry, J. Surico, A. DeBarba, F. Fabris, and E. Rabold. 2007. Food deprivation and leptin prioritize ingestive and sex behavior without affecting estrous cycles in Syrian hamsters. *Horm Behav* 51:413–27.

Schneider, J. E., S. J. Lazzarini, M. I. Friedman, and G. N. Wade. 1988. Role of fatty acid oxidation in food intake and hunger motivation in Syrian hamsters. *Physiol Behav* 43:617–23.

Schwartz, M. W., S. C. Woods, D. Porte, Jr., R. J. Seeley, and D. G. Baskin. 2000. Central nervous system control of food intake. *Nature* 404:661–71.

Sclafani, A., and D. Eisenstadt. 1980. 2-Deoxy-D-glucose fails to induce feeding in hamsters fed a preferred diet. *Physiol Behav* 24:641–3.

Seeley, R. J., C. J. Payne, and S. C. Woods. 1995. Neuropeptide Y fails to increase intraoral intake in rats. *Am J Physiol* 268:R423–7.

Seyle, H. 1976. *The stress of life*. Revised ed. New York: McGraw-Hill Book Co.

Shillabeer, G., and J. S. Davison. 1987. Proglumide, a cholecystokinin antagonist, increases gastric emptying in rats. *Am J Physiol* 252:R353–60.

Silverman, H. J., and I. Zucker. 1976. Absence of post-fast food compensation in the golden hamster (*Mesocricetus auratus*). *Physiol Behav* 17:271–85.

Slusser, P. G., and R. C. Ritter. 1980. Increased feeding and hyperglycemia elicited by intracerebroventricular 5-thioglucose. *Brain Res* 202:474–8.

Solomon, M. B., M. T. Foster, T. J. Bartness, and K. L. Huhman. 2007. Social defeat and footshock increase body mass and adiposity in male Syrian hamsters. *Am J Physiol Regul Integr Comp Physiol* 292:R283–90.

Solomon, M. B., R. R. Sakai, S. C. Woods, and M. T. Foster. 2011. Differential effects of glucocorticoids on energy homeostasis in Syrian hamsters. *Am J Physiol Endocrinol Metab* 301:E307–16.

Spencer, S. J., and A. Tilbrook. 2011. The glucocorticoid contribution to obesity. *Stress* 14:233–46.

Staffend, N. A., and R. L. Meisel. 2012. Aggressive experience increases dendritic spine density within the nucleus accumbens core in female Syrian hamsters. *Neuroscience* 227:163–9.

Stanley, B. G., and S. F. Leibowitz. 1985. Neuropeptide Y injected in the paraventricular hypothalamus: A powerful stimulant of feeding behavior. *Proc Natl Acad Sci U S A* 82:3940–3.

Stanley, B. G., K. C. Anderson, M. H. Grayson, and S. F. Leibowitz. 1989. Repeated hypothalamic stimulation with neuropeptide Y increases daily carbohydrate and fat intake and body weight gain in female rats. *Physiol Behav* 46:173–7.

Stanley, B. G., W. Magdalin, A. Seirafi, W. J. Thomas, and S. F. Leibowitz. 1993. The perifornical area: The major focus of (a) patchily distributed hypothalamic neuropeptide Y-sensitive feeding system(s). *Brain Res* 604:304–17.

Stengel, A., and Y. Tache. 2014. CRF and urocortin peptides as modulators of energy balance and feeding behavior during stress. *Front Neurosci* 8:52.

Stice, E., K. Presnell, H. Shaw, and P. Rohde. 2005. Psychological and behavioral risk factors for obesity onset in adolescent girls: A prospective study. *J Consult Clin Psychol* 73:195–202.

Stratakis, C. A., P. W. Gold, and G. P. Chrousos. 1995. Neuroendocrinology of stress: Implications for growth and development. *Horm Res* 43:162–7.

Teubner, B. J., and T. J. Bartness. 2009a. Body mass loss during adaptation to short winterlike days increases food foraging, but not food hoarding. *Physiol Behav* 97:135–40.

Teubner, B. J., and T. J. Bartness. 2009b. Cholecystokinin-33 acutely attenuates food foraging, hoarding and intake in Siberian hamsters. *Peptides* 2010 31:618–24.

Teubner, B. J., E. Keen-Rhinehart, and T. J. Bartness. 2012. Third ventricular coinjection of subthreshold doses of NPY and AgRP stimulate food hoarding and intake and neural activation. *Am J Physiol Regul Integr Comp Physiol* 302:R37–48.

Thomas, M. A., V. Ryu, and T. J. Bartness. 2016. Central ghrelin increases food foraging/hoarding that is blocked by GHSR antagonism and attenuates hypothalamic paraventricular nucleus neuronal activation. *Am J Physiol Regul Integr Comp Physiol* 310:R275–85.

Tilan, J., and J. Kitlinska. 2016. Neuropeptide Y (NPY) in tumor growth and progression: Lessons learned from pediatric oncology. *Neuropeptides* 55:55–66.

Tom, G. 1983. Effect of deprivation on the grocery shopping behavior of obese and nonobese consumers. *Int J Obes* 7:307–11.

Trayhurn, P., and G. Jennings. 1988. Nonshivering thermogenesis and the thermogenic capacity of brown fat in fasted and/or refed mice. *Am J Physiol* 254:R11–6.

Tups, A., M. Helwig, R. M. Khorooshi, Z. A. Archer, M. Klingenspor, and J. G. Mercer. 2004. Circulating ghrelin levels and central ghrelin receptor expression are elevated in response to food deprivation in a seasonal mammal (*Phodopus sungorus*). *J Neuroendocrinol* 16:922–8.

Ulrich-Lai, Y. M., and J. P. Herman. 2009. Neural regulation of endocrine and autonomic stress responses. *Nat Rev Neurosci* 10:397–409.

US Department of Agriculture. 2009. Access to affordable and Nutritious food: Measuring and understanding food deserts and their consequences. Report to Congress. Washington, DC: US Department of Agriculture Economic Research Service.

van Strien, T., R. C. Engels, W. van Staveren, and C. P. Herman. 2006. The validity of dietary restraint scales: Comment on Stice et al. (2004). *Psychol Assess* 18:89–94; discussion 95–9.

Waddell, D. 1951. Hoarding behavior in the golden hamster. *J Comp Physiol Psychol* 44:383–8.

Wade, G. N. 1983. Dietary obesity in golden hamsters: Reversibility and effects of sex and photoperiod. *Physiol Behav* 30:131–7.

Wade, G. N., and T. J. Bartness. 1984a. Effects of photoperiod and gonadectomy on food intake, body weight, and body composition in Siberian hamsters. *Am J Physiol* 246:R26–30.

Wade, G. N., and T. J. Bartness. 1984b. Seasonal obesity in Syrian hamsters: Effects of age, diet, photoperiod, and melatonin. *Am J Physiol* 247:R328–34.

Wardle, J., Y. Chida, E. L. Gibson, K. L. Whitaker, and A. Steptoe. 2011. Stress and adiposity: A meta-analysis of longitudinal studies. *Obesity (Silver Spring)* 19:771–8.

Weinstein, S. E., D. J. Shide, and B. J. Rolls. 1997. Changes in food intake in response to stress in men and women: Psychological factors. *Appetite* 28:7–18.

Westenhoefer, J., P. Broeckmann, A. K. Munch, and V. Pudel. 1994. Cognitive control of eating behaviour and the disinhibition effect. *Appetite* 23:27–41.

Wilson, M. E., C. J. Moore, K. F. Ethun, and Z. P. Johnson. 2014. Understanding the control of ingestive behavior in primates. *Horm Behav* 66:86–94.

Wolf, E. M., and J. H. Crowther. 1983. Personality and eating habit variables as predictors of severity of binge eating and weight. *Addict Behav* 8:335–44.

Wood, A. D., and T. J. Bartness. 1996a. Caloric density affects food hoarding and intake by Siberian hamsters. *Physiol Behav* 59:897–903.

Wood, A. D., and T. J. Bartness. 1996b. Food deprivation-induced increases in hoarding by Siberian hamsters are not photoperiod-dependent. *Physiol Behav* 60:1137–45.

Wood, A. D., and T. J. Bartness. 1997. Partial lipectomy, but not PVN lesions, increases food hoarding by Siberian hamsters. *Am J Physiol* 272:R783–92.

Wren, A. M., L. J. Seal, M. A. Cohen, A. E. Brynes, G. S. Frost, K. G. Murphy, W. S. Dhillo, M. A. Ghatei, and S. R. Bloom. 2001. Ghrelin enhances appetite and increases food intake in humans. *J Clin Endocrinol Metab* 86:5992.

Yabuki, A., T. Ojima, M. Kojima, Y. Nishi, H. Mifune, M. Matsumoto, R. Kamimura, T. Masuyama, and S. Suzuki. 2004. Characterization and species differences in gastric ghrelin cells from mice, rats and hamsters. *J Anat* 205:239–46.

Yeomans, M. R., and E. Coughlan. 2009. Mood-induced eating. Interactive effects of restraint and tendency to overeat. *Appetite* 52:290–8.

Zellner, D. A., S. Loaiza, Z. Gonzalez, J. Pita, J. Morales, D. Pecora, and A. Wolf. 2006. Food selection changes under stress. *Physiol Behav* 87:789–93.

Zhang, Y., G. E. Kilroy, T. M. Henagan, V. Prpic-Uhing, W. G. Richards, A. W. Bannon, R. L. Mynatt, and T. W. Gettys. 2005. Targeted deletion of melanocortin receptor subtypes 3 and 4, but not CART, alters nutrient partitioning and compromises behavioral and metabolic responses to leptin. *FASEB J* 19:1482–91.

Zhang, Y., R. Proenca, M. Maffei, M. Barone, L. Leopold, and J. M. Friedman. 1994. Positional cloning of the mouse obese gene and its human homologue. *Nature* 372:425–32.

4 Beyond Homeostasis
Understanding the Impact of Psychosocial Factors on Appetite Using Nonhuman Primate Models

Mark E. Wilson and Vasiliki Michopoulos

CONTENTS

4.1 INTRODUCTION

Animal models have proven to be exceptionally informative in defining neuropeptide regulation of appetite and energy homeostasis (Gao and Horvath 2007, Berthoud 2012, Williams and Elmquist 2012). More recent studies using a range of animal models and molecular tools are elucidating how epigenetic changes resulting from specific prenatal and postnatal dietary environments or experiences affect metabolic processes and appetite regulation (Levin 2008, Zambrano and Nathanielsz 2013, Burdge and Lillycrop 2014). Taken together, these approaches are helping to define possible treatment interventions for eating disorders in people (Casper, Sullivan, and Tecott 2008, Foltin 2012, van Gestel et al. 2014, Lutter, Croghan, and Cui 2016). The choice of animal used is best dictated by the question being addressed. Because of similarities in physiology and neurobiology, studies of captive nonhuman primates have begun to contribute significantly to our understanding of appetite regulation (see Wilson et al. 2014 for a review). Importantly, the use of nonhuman primate models provides the unique opportunity to extend analyses beyond a focus on the homeostatic regulation of appetite. This is particularly relevant given the well-established notion that a number of psychosocial factors influence food intake in people (Bruce and Ricciardelli 2015), including chronic stressor exposure (Tsenkova, Boylan, and Ryff 2013), even in children (Nguyen-Rodriguez, Unger, and Spruijt-Metz 2009). While the importance of psychosocial factors can be modeled in nonprimate animals (Tamashiro, Hegeman, and Sakai 2006), socially housed nonhuman primates share many characteristics in addition to physiology and neurobiology, with humans increasing the translational value of these pre-clinical studies.

4.2 LIVING IN AN OBESOGENIC ENVIRONMENT

Diet-induced obesity (DIO) has been a well-established strategy in animal models, including nonhuman primates, to study the susceptibility to and consequences of obesity (e.g., Hariri and Thibault 2010, Bremer et al. 2011, Panchal and Brown 2011, Rosini, Silva, and Moraes 2012, Hansen et al. 2013, Pound, Kievit, and Grove 2014). The DIO approach is modeled after the fact that people generally live in an obesogenic environment where highly palatable, calorically dense foods are readily available. An obvious difference between the DIO approach and what occurs naturally in human societies is that people typically have dietary choices, with some individuals exercising cognitive restraint of consuming calorically dense food, an outcome that likely plays a role in the variation in rates of obesity. Despite the fact that nearly all studies of DIO feed only an obesogenic diet and do not give animals a dietary choice, some animals nonetheless show a range of susceptibility to developing obesity (Levin et al. 1997, Archer and Mercer 2007). The DIO model assumes that animals will consume the same number of calories such that differences in obesity-related phenotypes are due to differences in metabolic responses to the diet (Levin et al. 1997, Blundell and Cooling 2000, Woods et al. 2004), perhaps due to differences in genetics (Levin 2000, Yazbek et al. 2010). However, it is unclear whether equivalent amounts of caloric intake occur consistently in research subjects in a DIO paradigm. While differences in energy expenditure could also account for differential metabolic responses to an obesogenic diet (Assaad et al. 2014, Blundell and Cooling 2000, Thivel et al. 2014, Sullivan, Koegler, and Cameron 2006), differences in feeding behavior and calories consumed are likely important.

Despite the increasing appreciation of how gut hormones and neuropeptides regulate appetite, social context and cognitive processes also have a significant impact on food intake and resulting alterations in body composition. Indeed, the field has a limited understanding of how these social and cognitive factors interact with the satiety and orexigenic signals to shape feeding behavior. In the present-day dietary environment, energy intake in humans may largely be unrelated to maintaining homeostasis but due to signals that thwart the action of canonical satiety hormones (Thivel et al. 2013). Indeed, it is becoming well accepted that the dietary variety (Cohen 2008, Cohen and Babey 2012, Feinle-Bisset 2014) as well as the cognitive salience and reward value of food (Zheng and Berthoud 2007, Berridge 2009) can facilitate food intake beyond satiety, likely contributing to differences in body composition in human populations (Van Vugt 2010, Booth and Booth 2011, Berthoud

2012). Given similarities to humans in cortical structures and mesolimbic circuits that govern executive control of appetitive behaviors (Kolb 1984, Reep 1984, Preuss 1995, Van Eden and Buijs 2000, Heidbreder and Groenewegen 2003, Haber and Knutson 2010, Petrides et al. 2012, Yeterian et al. 2012), nonhuman primates provide a unique opportunity to model the nonhomeostatic regulation of feeding behavior in people. This is highlighted in studies using rhesus monkeys that show that the orbitofrontal cortex (OFC) and amygdala are important regions for assessing food salience that likely interact with satiety-inducing neuropeptides to influence the timing of meal termination (Rolls 2007, Pritchard et al. 2008, Machado et al. 2010). The OFC is thought to provide, in part, top–down control of risky behaviors and reward evaluation (see Noonan et al. 2012, Pujara and Koenigs 2014). Importantly, neurotoxic lesions of the OFC result in unrestrained eating in monkeys (Machado and Bachevalier 2007), underscoring the importance of cortico-striatal-limbic circuits in the regulation of feeding behavior. Understanding factors that impact cortico-striatal-limbic circuitry will provide insights into the complex regulation of appetite. As data largely from rodent models suggest, chronic stressor exposure induces significant changes of prefrontal cortex (PFC)–limbic–striatal circuits (Arnsten 2009, McEwen and Morrison 2013). Consequently, it is possible that unrestrained eating is a consequence of stress-induced functional disruption of cortico–striatal–limbic circuitry.

4.3   ADVERSE SOCIAL EXPERIENCE AND FEEDING BEHAVIOR

Supported by a substantial body of literature from rodent models (e.g., Dallman et al. 2007, Tamashiro et al. 2011), emotional feeding or stress-induced consumption of palatable diets is recognized as a significant contributor to unrestrained eating (Hemmingsson 2014), with reports even available in the popular press (Kenny 2013). This emotional eating phenomena goes beyond the notion of the rewarding value of food (Zheng and Berthoud 2007, Berridge 2009) but is based on the premise that acute but more typically chronic exposure to stressors increases vulnerability to unrestrained consumption of palatable, calorically dense diets to somehow alleviate the adverse consequences of the stress experience. Because chronic stressor exposure is a known risk factor for psychostimulant abuse in people (Sinha and Jastreboff 2013) or self-administration in animals (Goeders 2002, Morgan et al. 2002, Koob and Kreek 2007), a history of stress resulting from adverse social experience may also explain the variance in consumption of palatable diets and susceptibility to DIO.

It is important to appreciate that the effects of stressor exposure on food intake may be bidirectional, with the specific effect dependent on a number of factors such as a stress history and whether the stressor exposure is acute or chronic (Maniam and Morris 2012, Harris 2015). Macronutrient content of the diet is likely important for the directionality, as an extensive literature from rodent models indicates that stressor exposure in animals fed a typical low-calorie diet is anorexic (Harris et al. 1998), an effect reversed by central administration of a corticotropin releasing factor (CRF) receptor antagonist (Smagin et al. 1999). Indeed, central administration of CRF to adult macaques has immediate and lasting suppressive effects on food intake (Glowa and Gold 1991). On the other hand, an extensive literature in rodent models indicates that chronic exposure to stressors is a mitigating factor in the preference for and consumption of excess calories from high caloric, "comfort foods" (Tamashiro, Hegeman, and Sakai 2006, Warne 2009). These data underscore the importance of considering the dietary environment when assessing the consequences of stressor exposure or stress hormones on appetite. Importantly, findings from rodent models clearly show that having a dietary choice between a palatable, high-caloric diet and lab chow diet sustains unrestrained eating and increases risk for obesity (la Fleur et al. 2007), whereas access to only a palatable diet does not sustain increased caloric intake and weight gain (Rolls, Van Duijvenvoorde, and Rowe 1983, la Fleur et al. 2014).

Studies in rodents of stress-induced unrestrained eating of palatable diets are consistent with the notion of comfort food ingestion in people (Epel et al. 2000, Adam and Epel 2007). With the exception of a few studies (Solomon et al. 2011), the majority of studies in rodent models have used male subjects (Tamashiro, Nguyen, and Sakai 2005, Warne 2009), despite epidemiological data highlighting significantly higher incidence of stress-eating and obesity in women (Grunberg and Straub 1992, Kitraki, Soulis, and Gerozissis 2004, Soulis, Kitraki, and Gerozissis 2005, Soulis et al. 2007). One translational, ethologically relevant animal model that has been leveraged to further define mechanisms for emotional feeding in women is that of social subordination in female macaques. Social subordination in well-established macaque groups produces a number of stress-related phenotypes (Michopoulos et al. 2012a), including a dysregulation of the limbic–hypothalamic–pituitary–adrenal axis (Shively, Laber-Laird, and Anton 1997, Kaplan et al. 2010, Michopoulos et al. 2012b). Neuroimaging studies reveal differences in binding potential across a number of monoamine receptor subtypes (Shively et al. 1997, 2006; Grant et al. 1998, Michopoulos et al. 2014), as well as developmental differences in white matter integrity (Howell et al. 2014), which mimic particular stress-induced outcomes in humans or other species. Furthermore, there is evidence of structural effects on gray matter density (e.g., reduced in PFC, superior temporal sulcus [STS]) and amygdala measured by magnetic resonance imaging (MRI) in subordinate adult male rhesus monkeys (Sallet et al. 2011). Recent studies using resting-state functional MRI in macaques reveal dominance status-dependent differences in brain circuits involving some of these same regions such as the PFC and STS as well as a circuit that includes the amygdala, brain stem, and portions of the striatum (Noonan et al. 2014). Together, these data suggest that the experience of being subordinate produces differences in brain structure and function that, in turn, result in behavioral or physiological differences that may function to facilitate attending to cues to successfully navigate the social environment and minimize the risk of aggression from more dominant animals (Silk 2002). These data are consistent with findings of increased white matter tracts in ventromedial PFC of squirrel monkeys exposed to early life stress, an observation that was interpreted as "adaptive," preparing the individual to cope with challenges in their environment (Lyons et al. 2009).

Regression analyses of available data from macaque colonies provisioned with standard laboratory chow (a low-fat, high-fiber fortified diet) suggests that dominance status and activity levels are important predictors of body weight, with increased rates of obesity and increased time spent feeding observed in more dominant animals (Bauer et al. 2012). Other studies of captive monkeys underscore the importance of social status and food distribution within the animals' enclosure, with more subordinate animals developing different strategies of feeding behavior when food is less accessible (see Bauer et al. 2011 for a review). In addition to studies done with large breeding groups of macaques in captive environments (Walker, Wilson, and Gordon 1984, Wilson, Gordon, and Collins 1986, McCowan et al. 2011, Rommeck et al. 2011), smaller groups are used to study the adverse effects of subordination on behavior and physiology. More specifically, small groups can be safely formed with unfamiliar animals (Kaplan et al. 1982, 1984, Mook et al. 2005) while balancing group composition by previous social history and specific gene polymorphisms (Jarrell et al. 2008). A similar pattern of subordination effects on feeding behavior emerges with these small experimentally created groups in a dietary environment where a typical low-fat, high-fiber monkey chow diet is available, as adult subordinate female rhesus monkeys consistently show lower body weights than more dominant age-matched, group mates (Michopoulos and Wilson 2011). Employing automated feeding stations provides a tool to measure food acquired by individuals in these social groups (Wilson et al. 2008, Research_Diets 2015). Importantly, data suggest that animals consume what they obtain, with dominant females stealing pellets from more subordinate females ~1% of the time (Wilson et al. 2008). Furthermore, because food is available continually, dominant animals do not restrict subordinate animals from accessing the feeders. Analyses of feeding behavior suggests that the lower body weight observed, on average, in subordinate females is associated with slightly lower (Michopoulos et al. 2009) or similar calorie intake compared with dominant females (Michopoulos, Toufexis, and Wilson 2012). Dominance-status-related differences in energy expenditure are not known. Nonetheless, these data from adult female rhesus monkeys are consistent with the notion that stressor exposure consistently reduces body weight by a reduction in food intake of a laboratory chow diet or an increase in energy expenditure (Harris 2015).

However, a very different pattern emerges when animals are maintained in a rich dietary environment and given the choice between the low-calorie chow diet and a palatable, calorically dense diet (Arce et al. 2010, Michopoulos, Toufexis, and Wilson 2012). Under these conditions, all animals prefer the high-calorie diet. Interestingly, dominant females do not consume significantly more overall calories in this rich dietary environment compared to the chow-only condition. In contrast, subordinates consume significantly more overall calories in this choice dietary environment than in the chow-only phase and compared with dominant females (Arce et al. 2010, Michopoulos, Toufexis, and Wilson 2012). While these studies were short-term in nature, focusing on changes in appetite and not the consequences of consuming these diets on body composition, other studies of female macaques indicate that subordinates more typically show increases in visceral fat stores when fed a high-fat, atherogenic diet (Shively, Register, and Clarkson 2009). Together, these data suggest that female rhesus monkeys provide a unique model to better understand how psychosocial stressor exposure may account for variance in DIO in females.

4.4   ESTRADIOL AND DIET INTERACT WITH STRESS
HISTORY TO SHAPE FEEDING BEHAVIOR

Because a large literature from rodent models indicates that estradiol has a suppressive effect on food intake in females, notably by reducing the size of meals (Wade and Gray 1979, Eckel 2004, 2011), understanding how stressor exposure interacts with estradiol in females to affect feeding is important. Available data indicate that estradiol attenuates feeding by acting through estrogen receptor-α (Santollo, Wiley, and Eckel 2007) to target hindbrain and hypothalamic regions to alter processing and feedback signals (Roepke 2009, Van Vugt 2010). Studies show that increasing levels of estradiol direct motivation toward mating and away from eating as females approach ovulation (Schneider et al. 2013). Unlike rodents, humans and other old world primates have menstrual cycles characterized by an ~12 day follicular phase and a prolonged luteal phase following ovulation (Knobil 1980). A periovulatory nadir in food intake of a variety of diets is described in women (Lissner et al. 1988, Gong, Garrel, and Calloway 1989, Fong and Kretsch 1993, Johnson et al. 1994, Eck et al. 1997, Hirschberg 2012). A similar decrease in food intake is also described in monkeys on a laboratory chow diet (Gilbert and Gillman 1956, Czaja and Goy 1975, Czaja 1978, Rosenblatt et al. 1980, Bielert and Busse 1983, Kemnitz et al. 1989).

However, one issue not often systematically considered in evaluating estradiol effects on food intake is the macronutrient content of the diet, as most studies in animal models have used a laboratory diet that is quite unlike the more calorically dense diets consumed by people. In addition, it is unclear how the effects of estradiol on feeding behavior would be influenced by stressor exposure. Those studies in rodents and humans that have examined estradiol's effect on dietary preference show no consistent effect of estradiol on the selection of particular diet (for review, see Dye and Blundell 1997). However, a recent report in socially housed adult female rhesus monkeys suggests that the effect of estradiol on caloric intake varies as a function of the availability of a palatable, calorically dense diet and this response may be modified by social status (Johnson et al. 2013). Ovariectomized females were studied in two dietary conditions: a no choice condition where only laboratory chow diet was available and a choice condition where the chow diet and a palatable diet with increased fat and sugar was available. Furthermore, females were studied in both dietary conditions during estradiol replacement, which produced serum concentrations comparable to the mid-follicular phase, and no estradiol replacement. As shown in Figure 4.1, during the chow-only condition, estradiol significantly reduces total calorie intake compared to the no treatment condition due primarily to smaller meals but not fewer meals or less snacking between defined meals. All females consume significantly more calories during the condition when both the chow and high-caloric diet are available compared to the chow-only condition. However, during this dietary choice condition, estradiol does not attenuate food intake compared with the no treatment condition. Indeed, estradiol appears to increase consumption of the calorically dense diet compared with the no treatment condition, particularly for subordinate females (Johnson et al. 2013). These data suggest that the palatability and macronutrient content of the diet may engage neural circuitry that desensitizes the suppressive effects of estradiol on food intake.

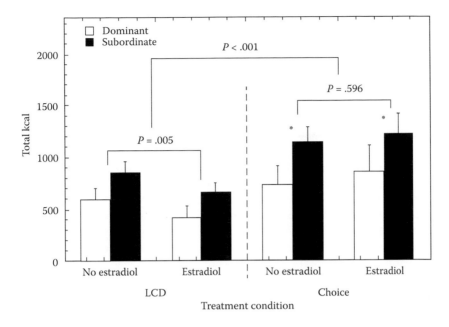

FIGURE 4.1 Mean ± SEM of total kcal intake of adult, ovariectomized dominant and subordinate adult female rhesus monkeys during both no estradiol replacement and estradiol treatment under two dietary conditions. Estradiol significantly reduces kcal intake when only a laboratory chow diet is available but not when animals have a choice between chow and a high-calorie diet. Subordinate females consume significantly more calories during the dietary choice condition compared with dominant females independent of estradiol replacement. (Redrawn from Johnson, ZP, Lowe, J, Michopoulos, V, Moore, CJ, Wilson, ME, Toufexis, D, *J Neuroendocrinol* 25, 729-741, 2013.)

Clearly more systematic research is needed to address these questions in female nonhuman primates.

4.5 SIGNALS SUSTAINING EMOTIONAL FEEDING

Recent studies employing rhesus monkeys have begun to investigate what initiates and sustains stress-induced feeding in a rich dietary environment. One possibility is that subordinate female monkeys may be more sensitive to orexigenic peptides. Although acute ghrelin administration increased the intake of the chow diet in subordinate but not dominant females (Michopoulos et al. 2010), it had no effect on consumption of a high-calorie diet. Alternatively, signals from the stress hormone axis may be critical in sustaining intake of these highly palatable diets. A number of studies in rats have confirmed that glucocorticoids dose dependently increase the intake of diets high in fat and sugar (Dallman, Pecoraro, and la Fleur 2005, Warne 2009), supporting the well-established notion that these steroids promote food intake (Sominsky and Spencer 2014). Although prospective studies assessing the direct effects of stress-like glucocorticoids concentrations on diet preference and caloric intake have not been performed in monkeys, the increase in cortisol following an acute stressor significantly predicts increased intake of a high-calorie diet and not a standard monkey diet immediately following the stressor exposure in female monkeys (Michopoulos, Toufexis, and Wilson 2012). Furthermore, serum cortisol levels following a dexamethasone suppression test also positively predict consumption of a high-caloric diet but not a monkey chow diet in female rhesus monkeys (Michopoulos, Toufexis, and Wilson 2012). These data suggest that female monkeys with reduced glucocorticoid negative feedback will consume more calories from a palatable, calorically denser diet.

Because reduced glucocorticoid negative feedback as a consequence of chronic exposure to stressors is characterized by an up-regulation of central CRF signaling (Dallman et al. 2004, Herman 2013), the use of CRF receptor antagonists could provide insights into the role of this neuropeptide in sustaining excessive palatable food consumption. Acute administration of a CRF type 1–2 receptor antagonist, which is unable to penetrate the blood–brain barrier, does not reduce this emotional feeding phenotype shown by subordinates in a choice dietary environment despite a significant reduction in serum cortisol (Michopoulos et al. 2010). However, different results are observed with the use of the CRF type 1 receptor antagonist, antalarmin, which does penetrate the brain when administered peripherally (Moore et al. 2014). During vehicle treatments, subordinate females consume significantly more calories in a dietary environment that includes a choice between a chow diet and a high-caloric diet than do dominant females. Two days of peripheral administration of antalarmin significantly reduces daily caloric intake in subordinate female monkeys to amounts comparable to those consumed by dominant group mates in the choice dietary environment (Moore et al. 2014). Moreover, examination of agonistic behaviors that define rank indicate that the animals that exhibited higher rates of submissive behaviors, most typically the more subordinate animals responding to aggression from group mates, and those animals that were the most aggressive were significantly more sensitive to the attenuation in emotional feeding by antalarmin (Moore et al. 2014). While one would expect dominant animals to be more aggressive to enforce their social status on lower ranking females (Bernstein 1976), the absolute frequency of aggression is unrelated to specific dominance ranks (Bernstein, Gordon, and Rose 1974) and may thus reflect a female's reaction to her social environment. This hypothesis is consistent with the notion that increased aggression, as a form of defensive behavior, may be a consequence of an animal's adaptation to its position is a social hierarchy (Honess and Marin 2006). While depression or behavioral inhibition may be an outcome of chronic stressor exposure (Nemeroff and Vale 2005), data from diverse species indicate that CRF increases social aggression (Tazi et al. 1987, Robison et al. 2004, Backstrom and Winberg 2013). Thus, it seems likely that increased rates of submission, typical of more subordinate animals, and aggression, most typical of more dominant monkeys, are behavioral manifestations of the socially induced stress in the context of a female macaque dominance hierarchy. This analysis highlights the role of a female's response to the social environment in the appetite suppressing effects of CRF_1 receptor antagonist in this rich dietary environment.

Because the dose and route of administration of antalarmin that effectively reduce caloric intake in these female monkeys do not affect peripheral cortisol secretion (Herod, Pohl, and Cameron 2011, Herod et al. 2011), the data suggest that activation of central CRF type 1 receptors may be important for sustaining this emotional feeding phenotype. These observations are consistent with data from rodents indicating that chronic activation of central CRF type 1 receptors are likely important for stress-induced overconsumption of palatable diets. In these rodent models, diet cycling or intermittent dietary availability to a palatable diet functions as a mild stressor, and immunohistochemistry reveals elevated CRF-positive cells in the central nucleus of the amygdala among diet cycled but not control rats (Cottone et al. 2009, Iemolo et al. 2013). Importantly, infusion of the CRF type 1 receptor antagonist, antalarmin, into the central nucleus of the amygdala of diet cycled male rats fully blocked hyperphagia of a palatable food with no effect on standard chow intake (Iemolo et al. 2013). Together, these data suggest that central CRF signaling is an important factor in perhaps initiating and sustaining excessive intake of palatable diets.

4.6 TARGETS OF STRESS SIGNALS MEDIATING EMOTIONAL FEEDING

The palatability value of food goes beyond its sensory properties given the emerging hypothesis that excess food consumption and resulting obesity in people are a form of addiction involving the same corticostriatal circuitry engaged by drugs of abuse (Tomasi and Volkow 2013). What is compelling are data from animal models showing that continual self-administration of psychostimulants (Nader et al. 2006, Thanos et al. 2007) or consumption of a palatable high-fat, high-sugar reduces mesolimbic dopamine 2 receptor (D2R) availability (Geiger et al. 2009, Lee et al. 2010, Johnson and Kenny 2010). Studies of people show attenuated D2R binding is associated with reduced activity of prefrontal regions involved in stimulus salience, inhibitory control, and emotional regulation (see Volkow et al. 2012). Decreased D2R levels are also associated with a disruption in the functional connectivity of prefrontal regions with limbic-ventral striatal targets, notably the amygdala and nucleus accumbens (Volkow and Baler 2015). Such neuroadaptions likely result in increased motivation to consume highly palatable diets and an inability to inhibit subsequent feeding behavior beyond satiety (Volkow et al. 2013). Furthermore, as observed in drug abuse (Koob and Le Moal 2005), intermittent consumption of these calorically dense diets produces adverse emotional states in rodent models (i.e., stress) that may be relieved, at least temporarily, by palatable food intake (Parylak, Koob, and Zorrilla 2011).

However, as noted earlier, not all people or animals with access to palatable diets show evidence of food addiction. Because chronic stressor exposure, possibly mediated through central CRF signaling, is a risk factor for psychostimulant abuse in people (Sinha and Jastreboff 2013) or self-administration in experimental animals (Goeders 2002, Koob and Kreek 2007), including monkeys (Morgan et al. 2002), it is possible that exposure to chronic stressors increases vulnerability to food addiction (Dallman, Pecoraro, and la Fleur 2005). Evidence from rodents and humans suggests that changes in dopamine (DA) activity are at least part of the mechanism linking stress exposure to comfort food ingestion (Martel and Fantino 1996a,b, Bassareo and Di Chiara 1999, Pelchat 2002, Rada, Avena, and Hoebel 2005). Based on studies in rodents, it is well established that signals from the stress axis, including glucocorticoids and CRF, target DA neurons in mesolimbic regions (Ambroggi et al. 2009, Burke and Miczek 2013, Koob et al. 2014), producing a dysregulation of DA neurotransmission (Izzo, Sanna, and Koob 2005) that increases the expression of anhedonia and the risk for developing an addictive phenotype (Koob and Le Moal 2001, Anisman and Matheson 2005, Koob and Kreek 2007). Indeed, the observation of a significant attenuation in palatable food consumption by more subordinate female monkeys following antalarmin administration is reminiscent of the effect of CRF_1 receptor antagonism on attenuating drug reinstatement in drug-dependent but not nondependent rats (see Koob and Le Moal 2001, Koob and Kreek 2007, Parylak, Koob, and Zorrilla 2011 for review).

Diet- and stress-induced DA dysfunction and resulting reduction in D2R binding or availability are referred to as a "reward deficiency syndrome" (Blum et al. 1996, 2014) that is both predictive of an addictive phenotype (Volkow, Fowler, and Wang 2003, Volkow and Wise 2005) and observed in human obesity (Wang et al. 2001). Whether the imposition of chronic stress by social subordination in macaque monkeys leads to this reward deficiency syndrome that predicts stress-induced consumption of calorically dense diets is not currently known. However, socially subordinate female macaques exhibit a widespread reduction in D2R binding potential throughout the reward network (Grant et al. 1998, Shively et al. 1997) that consists of DA-rich areas, including the striatum and PFC, and is critical for regulating reward-goal-directed behaviors and responses (Haber and Knutson 2010). Preliminary data suggest that social subordination in female macaques also reduces functional connectivity within the cingulo-opercular/limbic network, which includes the nucleus accumbens, amygdala, and PFC and has been linked to stimulus salience (Godfrey et al. 2013). Because stressor exposure affects structural and functional connectivity of the PFC and other regions regulating reward (Sanchez et al. 1998, Kaufman and Charney 2001, Teicher et al. 2002, Govindan et al. 2010), it is possible that exposure to chronic stress compromises DA modulation of prefrontal regulation of the striatum, thus increasing vulnerability for food addiction.

4.7 MISSING PIECES USING NONHUMAN PRIMATE MODELS

Available data suggest that the effects of gut and neuropeptides that generally regulate feeding do so similarly in nonprimate animals and nonhuman primates (see Wilson et al. 2014 for an overview). In addition, nonhuman primate models are of value for testing the efficacy of drugs that target gut and neuropeptide systems for the treatment of eating disorders in people and, in some cases, may be required for preclinical evaluation (Casper, Sullivan, and Tecott 2008, Foltin 2012, van Gestel et al. 2014, Lutter, Croghan, and Cui 2016). However, because feeding patterns are driven by factors other than just satiety and orexigenic signals, appreciating how the social context and dietary environment shape appetite in monkeys may be informative for understanding the complexity of feeding in people. Importantly, technology is now available that quantifies caloric intake in free-feeding, group housed monkeys (Wilson et al. 2008, Arce et al. 2010, Michopoulos, Toufexis, and Wilson 2012, Research_Diets 2015), thus facilitating our ability to determine the effects of dietary, social, or pharmacological interventions on meal structure (Moore et al. 2013) and changes in appetite (Johnson et al. 2013, Moore et al. 2014).

These novel methods in nonhuman primate models can also be used to examine how early exposure to particular dietary environments affects the neurobiological development of feeding behavior, as data are accumulating on how early exposure to a particular diet may program feeding behavior later in life (Grove et al. 2005, Vucetic et al. 2010, Zambrano and Nathanielsz 2013, Gali Ramamoorthy et al. 2015). In addition to a focus on maternal obesity and access to calorically rich diets, studies are showing how early social experience or maternal care influence appetite regulation through adulthood. For example, results from rodents clearly show that prenatal stress increases risk for obesity later in life (Tamashiro et al. 2009, Boersma et al. 2014). Although data from humans are limited, reports of stress are often comorbid with emotional eating in children (Mazur, Dzielska, and Malkowska-Szkutnik 2011). In addition, children from families reporting more distress have higher rates of obesity (Koch, Sepa, and Ludvigsson 2008, Moens et al. 2009, Gundersen et al. 2011, Anderson et al. 2012, Anderson and Whitaker 2011), particularly for girls (Noll et al. 2007, Schneiderman et al. 2012, Suglia et al. 2012). Consistent with these observations, juvenile bonnet macaques, whose mothers were required to forage for food in unpredictable conditions during the postnatal period, show elevated central concentrations of CRF (Coplan et al. 1996) and an obese phenotype (Kaufman et al. 2007). However, it is not known whether these metabolic differences are due to differences in food intake or feeding efficiency.

While peer versus mother rearing is also a well-validated approach to assess differences in early life experiences on a number of phenotypes during development and adulthood, including anxiety-like behavior and alcohol intake (Dettmer and Suomi 2014), its lasting effects on feeding and metabolism are unexplored. Because infant macaques assume the dominance rank of their mother (Chikazawa et al. 1979), the social subordination model provides an opportunity to examine how chronic stressor exposure during development impacts appetite, preference for calorically dense diets, and risk for obesity. However, limited data suggest that in female rhesus monkeys fed a monkey chow diet, subordinate females show slower growth through the juvenile period (Zehr, Van Meter, and Wallen 2005). It is not known whether this reflects differences in food intake or energy expenditure. Importantly, with the exception of a few studies (Sullivan, Koegler, and Cameron 2006, Sullivan and Cameron 2010), the consideration of activity and energy expenditure is largely missing from the analysis of appetite and resulting body composition in nonhuman primates. Thus, future studies must consider both sides of the energy balance equation to appreciate how changes in appetite affect body composition. Nonetheless, the use of nonhuman primate models of early adverse experience can illustrate how exposure to social stress during development may be an aggravating factor for DIO during childhood and other adverse health outcomes in adulthood (Evans, Fuller-Rowell, and Doan 2012).

Given that social group membership can be experimentally determined in macaques (Kaplan et al. 1982, 1984, Mook et al. 2005, Jarrell et al. 2008), the consequences of acute social instability (Manuck, Kaplan, and Clarkson 1983, Capitanio and Cole 2015) or the lasting effects of acquiring a new rank can be assessed (Shively, Laber-Laird, and Anton 1997). The latter strategy provides the opportunity to determine how a behavioral intervention aimed to alleviate stress in previously subordinate, but currently more dominant, group members affects appetite and diet preference and whether the residual effects of a previous rank reflect epigenetic differences. Previous studies show that several phenotypes track with an animal's current rank (Tung et al. 2012, Shively, Laber-Laird, and Anton 1997), but the effect of stress alleviation on appetite regulation has not yet been examined.

It is also important to note that studies assessing the impact of social factors on appetite in nonprimate models have predominantly used males, while the few studies conducted in nonhuman primates have used exclusively females. Given sex differences in stress hormone regulation in macaques and other species (Smith and Norman 1987a,b, Norman et al. 1992, Handa et al. 1994, Toufexis and Wilson 2012, Goel et al. 2014), it is possible that males may respond differently than females would to chronic stressor exposure, particularly with respect to appetite. For macaques in free-ranging conditions, males have a different life history than females, as males are frequently emigrating between groups and acquiring a new rank (Bernstein 1970). Females, on the other hand, typically remain in their natal group. While rates of obesity are higher in women than men (Haslam and James 2005), studies do not take into account evidence of preexisting stress. However, emotional feeding is more often reported in women compared to men (Laitinen, Ek, and Sovio 2002). Whether these sex differences reflect differences in coping strategies to social stressors or simply sex differences in metabolism is unknown.

Finally, what is incompletely understood is how reward-related signals and pathways that can be compromised by diet and/or stressor exposure interact with well-established canonical signals known to regulate appetite (Adam and Epel 2007). A series of studies in rodents are beginning to elucidate these interactions. For example, studies in male rats are illustrating how motivation to consume a palatable diet involves orexigenic neuropeptide signaling, including neuropeptide Y (NPY) and the melanocortins (van den Heuvel et al. 2015). Additional studies in rodents show stressor exposure alters melanocortin signaling in the hypothalamus that may augment food intake (Chagra et al. 2011). In contrast, other studies show that the glucocorticoid facilitation of food intake occurs in the absence of leptin-induced suppression of hypothalamic expression of NPY (Solano and Jacobson 1999). Thus, further studies are needed to determine how reward pathways interact with orexigenic and satiety-inducing neuropeptides to affect appetite and nonhuman primate models could help fill this gap in knowledge.

4.8 CONCLUSION

Animal models are critically important for defining the signals and neural circuitry that regulate appetite to help define effective treatment strategies for eating disorders in people (Harris 2015). Because social context and cognitive processes also have a significant impact on food intake and resulting body composition, the use of socially housed nonhuman primate models provides an unprecedented opportunity to define how these factors alter satiety and orexigenic signals to influence feeding behavior. Recent advances in technology to quantify caloric intake in free-feeding, socially housed monkeys (Wilson et al. 2008), coupled with wearable activity monitors (Sullivan, Koegler, and Cameron 2006), enable precise quantitation of energy intake and expenditure. Furthermore, neuroimaging (Fair et al. 2007, Miranda-Dominguez et al. 2014) and neuromodulation approaches such as optogenetics (Gerits et al. 2012, Ozden et al. 2013) can be applied to understand systems-level neural circuitry that influence appetite and that may affected by exposure to stress.

ACKNOWLEDGMENTS

Preparation of this chapter was supported in part by NIH grants R01DK096883, R01HD077623, R01MH094757, and ODP51001123. The authors report no conflicts of interest.

LITERATURE CITED

Adam, T. C., and E. S. Epel. 2007. Stress, eating and the reward system. *Physiol Behav* 91 (4):449–58.

Ambroggi, F., M. Turiault, A. Milet, V. Deroche-Gamonet, S. Parnaudeau, E. Balado, J. Barik, R. van der Veen, G. Maroteaux, T. Lemberger, G. Schutz, M. Lazar, M. Marinelli, P. V. Piazza, and F. Tronche. 2009. Stress and addiction: Glucocorticoid receptor in dopaminoceptive neurons facilitates cocaine seeking. *Nat Neurosci* 12 (3):247–9.

Anderson, S. E., and R. C. Whitaker. 2011. Attachment security and obesity in US preschool-aged children. *Arch Pediatr Adolesc Med* 165 (3):235–42.

Anderson, S. E., R. A. Gooze, S. Lemeshow, and R. C. Whitaker. 2012. Quality of early maternal–child relationship and risk of adolescent obesity. *Pediatrics* 129 (1):132–40.

Anisman, H., and K. Matheson. 2005. Stress, depression, and anhedonia: Caveats concerning animal models. *Neurosci Biobehav Rev* 29 (4–5):525–46.

Arce, M., V. Michopoulos, K. N. Shepard, Q. C. Ha, and M. E. Wilson. 2010. Diet choice, cortisol reactivity, and emotional feeding in socially housed rhesus monkeys. *Physiol Behav* 101:446–55.

Archer, Z. A., and J. G. Mercer. 2007. Brain responses to obesogenic diets and diet-induced obesity. *Proc Nutr Soc* 66 (1):124–30.

Arnsten, A. F. 2009. Stress signalling pathways that impair prefrontal cortex structure and function. *Nat Rev Neurosci* 10 (6):410–22.

Assaad, H., K. Yao, C. D. Tekwe, S. Feng, F. W. Bazer, L. Zhou, R. J. Carroll, C. J. Meininger, and G. Wu. 2014. Analysis of energy expenditure in diet-induced obese rats. *Front Biosci (Landmark Ed)* 19:967–85.

Backstrom, T., and S. Winberg. 2013. Central corticotropin releasing factor and social stress. *Front Neurosci* 7:117.

Bassareo, V., and G. Di Chiara. 1999. Differential responsiveness of dopamine transmission to food-stimuli in nucleus accumbens shell/core compartments. *Neuroscience* 89 (3):637–41.

Bauer, S. A., T. P. Arndt, K. E. Leslie, D. L. Pearl, and P. V. Turner. 2011. Obesity in rhesus and cynomolgus macaques: A comparative review of the condition and its implications for research. *Comp Med* 61 (6):514–26.

Bauer, S. A., D. L. Pearl, K. E. Leslie, J. Fournier, and P. V. Turner. 2012. Causes of obesity in captive cynomolgus macaques: Influence of body condition, social and management factors on behaviour around feeding. *Lab Anim* 46 (3):193–9.

Bernstein, I. S. 1970. Primate status hierachies. In *Primate Behavior: Developments in Field and laboratory Research*, edited by L. A. Rosenblum, 71–109. New York: Academic Press.

Bernstein, I. S. 1976. Dominance, aggression and reproduction in primate societies. *J Theor Biol* 60 (2):459–72.

Bernstein, I. S., T. P. Gordon, and R. M. Rose. 1974. Aggression and social controls in rhesus monkey (*Macaca mulatta*) groups revealed in group formation studies. *Folia Primatol (Basel)* 21 (2):81–107.

Berridge, K. C. 2009. 'Liking' and 'wanting' food rewards: Brain substrates and roles in eating disorders. *Physiol Behav* 97 (5):537–50.

Berthoud, H. R. 2012. The neurobiology of food intake in an obesogenic environment. *Proc Nutr Soc* 71 (4):478–87.

Bielert, C., and C. Busse. 1983. Influences of ovarian hormones on the food intake and feeding of captive and wild female chacma baboons (*Papio ursinus*). *Physiol Behav* 30 (1):103–11.

Blum, K., M. Febo, T. McLaughlin, F. J. Cronje, D. Han, and S. M. Gold. 2014. Hatching the behavioral addiction egg: Reward Deficiency Solution System (RDSS) as a function of dopaminergic neurogenetics and brain functional connectivity linking all addictions under a common rubric. *J Behav Addict* 3 (3):149–56.

Blum, K., P. J. Sheridan, R. C. Wood, E. R. Braverman, T. J. Chen, J. G. Cull, and D. E. Comings. 1996. The D2 dopamine receptor gene as a determinant of reward deficiency syndrome. *J R Soc Med* 89 (7):396–400.

Blundell, J. E., and J. Cooling. 2000. Routes to obesity: Phenotypes, food choices and activity. *Br J Nutr* 83 Suppl 1:S33–8.

Boersma, G. J., T. L. Bale, P. Casanello, H. E. Lara, A. B. Lucion, D. Suchecki, and K. L. Tamashiro. 2014. Long-term impact of early life events on physiology and behaviour. *J Neuroendocrinol* 26 (9):587–602.

Booth, D. A., and P. Booth. 2011. Targeting cultural changes supportive of the healthiest lifestyle patterns. A biosocial evidence-base for prevention of obesity. *Appetite* 56 (1):210–21.

Bremer, A. A., K. L. Stanhope, J. L. Graham, B. P. Cummings, W. Wang, B. R. Saville, and P. J. Havel. 2011. Fructose-fed rhesus monkeys: A nonhuman primate model of insulin resistance, metabolic syndrome, and type 2 diabetes. *Clin Transl Sci* 4 (4):243–52.

Bruce, L. J., and L. A. Ricciardelli. 2015. A systematic review of the psychosocial correlates of intuitive eating among adult women. *Appetite* 96:454–72.

Burdge, G. C., and K. A. Lillycrop. 2014. Environment-physiology, diet quality and energy balance: The influence of early life nutrition on future energy balance. *Physiol Behav* 134:119–22.

Burke, A. R., and K. A. Miczek. 2013. Stress in adolescence and drugs of abuse in rodent models: Role of dopamine, CRF, and HPA axis. *Psychopharmacology (Berl)*.

Capitanio, J. P., and S. W. Cole. 2015. Social instability and immunity in rhesus monkeys: The role of the sympathetic nervous system. *Philos Trans R Soc Lond B Biol Sci* May 26; 370 (1669). pii: 20140104.

Casper, R. C., E. L. Sullivan, and L. Tecott. 2008. Relevance of animal models to human eating disorders and obesity. *Psychopharmacology (Berl)* 199 (3):313–29.

Chagra, S. L., J. K. Zavala, M. V. Hall, and K. L. Gosselink. 2011. Acute and repeated restraint differentially activate orexigenic pathways in the rat hypothalamus. *Regul Pept* 167 (1):70–8.

Chikazawa, D., T. P. Gordon, C. A. Bean, and I. S. Bernstein. 1979. Mother–daughter dominance reversals in rhesus monkeys (*Macaca mulatta*). *Primates* 20 (2):301–5.

Cohen, D. A. 2008. Obesity and the built environment: Changes in environmental cues cause energy imbalances. *Int J Obes (Lond)* 32 Suppl 7:S137–42.

Cohen, D. A., and S. H. Babey. 2012. Contextual influences on eating behaviours: Heuristic processing and dietary choices. *Obes Rev* 13 (9):766–79.

Coplan, J. D., M. W. Andrews, L. A. Rosenblum, M. J. Owens, S. Friedman, J. M. Gorman, and C. B. Nemeroff. 1996. Persistent elevations of cerebrospinal fluid concentrations of corticotropin-releasing factor in adult nonhuman primates exposed to early-life stressors: Implications for the pathophysiology of mood and anxiety disorders. *Proc Natl Acad Sci U S A* 93 (4):1619–23.

Cottone, P., V. Sabino, M. Roberto, M. Bajo, L. Pockros, J. B. Frihauf, E. M. Fekete, L. Steardo, K. C. Rice, D. E. Grigoriadis, B. Conti, G. F. Koob, and E. P. Zorrilla. 2009. CRF system recruitment mediates dark side of compulsive eating. *Proc Natl Acad Sci U S A* 106 (47):20016–20.

Czaja, J. A. 1978. Ovarian influences on primate food intake: Assessment of progesterone actions. *Physiol Behav* 21 (6):923–8.

Czaja, J. A., and R. W. Goy. 1975. Ovarian hormones and food-intake in female guinea-pigs and rhesus-monkeys. *Horm Behav* 6 (4):329–49.

Dallman, M. F., S. F. Akana, N. C. Pecoraro, J. P. Warne, S. E. la Fleur, and M. T. Foster. 2007. Glucocorticoids, the etiology of obesity and the metabolic syndrome. *Curr Alzheimer Res* 4 (2):199–204.

Dallman, M. F., S. F. Akana, A. M. Strack, K. S. Scribner, N. Pecoraro, S. E. La Fleur, H. Houshyar, and F. Gomez. 2004. Chronic stress-induced effects of corticosterone on brain: Direct and indirect. *Ann N Y Acad Sci* 1018:141–50.

Dallman, M. F., N. C. Pecoraro, and S. E. la Fleur. 2005. Chronic stress and comfort foods: Self-medication and abdominal obesity. *Brain Behav Immun* 19 (4):275–80.

Dettmer, A. M., and S. J. Suomi. 2014. Nonhuman primate models of neuropsychiatric disorders: Influences of early rearing, genetics, and epigenetics. *ILAR J* 55 (2):361–70.

Dye, L., and J. E. Blundell. 1997. Menstrual cycle and appetite control: Implications for weight regulation. *Hum Reprod* 12 (6):1142–51.

Eck, L. H., A. G. Bennett, B. M. Egan, J. W. Ray, C. O. Mitchell, M. A. Smith, and R. C. Klesges. 1997. Differences in macronutrient selections in users and nonusers of an oral contraceptive. *Am J Clin Nutr* 65 (2):419–24.

Eckel, L. A. 2004. Estradiol: A rhythmic, inhibitory, indirect control of meal size. *Physiol Behav* 82 (1):35–41.

Eckel, L. A. 2011. The ovarian hormone estradiol plays a crucial role in the control of food intake in females. *Physiol Behav* 104 (4):517–24.

Epel, E. S., B. McEwen, T. Seeman, K. Matthews, G. Castellazzo, K. D. Brownell, J. Bell, and J. R. Ickovics. 2000. Stress and body shape: Stress-induced cortisol secretion is consistently greater among women with central fat. *Psychosom Med* 62 (5):623–32.

Evans, G. W., T. E. Fuller-Rowell, and S. N. Doan. 2012. Childhood cumulative risk and obesity: The mediating role of self-regulatory ability. *Pediatrics* 129 (1):e68–73.

Fair, D. A., B. L. Schlaggar, A. L. Cohen, F. M. Miezin, N. U. Dosenbach, K. K. Wenger, M. D. Fox, A. Z. Snyder, M. E. Raichle, and S. E. Petersen. 2007. A method for using blocked and event-related fMRI data to study "resting state" functional connectivity. *Neuroimage* 35 (1):396–405.

Feinle-Bisset, C. 2014. Modulation of hunger and satiety: Hormones and diet. *Curr Opin Clin Nutr Metab Care* 17 (5):458–64.

Foltin, R. W. 2012. The behavioral pharmacology of anorexigenic drugs in nonhuman primates: 30 years of progress. *Behav Pharmacol* 23 (5–6):461–77.

Fong, A. K., and M. J. Kretsch. 1993. Changes in dietary intake, urinary nitrogen, and urinary volume across the menstrual cycle. *Am J Clin Nutr* 57 (1):43–6.

Gali Ramamoorthy, T., G. Begum, E. Harno, and A. White. 2015. Developmental programming of hypothalamic neuronal circuits: Impact on energy balance control. *Front Neurosci* 9:126.

Gao, Q., and T. L. Horvath. 2007. Neurobiology of feeding and energy expenditure. *Annu Rev Neurosci* 30:367–98.

Geiger, B. M., M. Haburcak, N. M. Avena, M. C. Moyer, B. G. Hoebel, and E. N. Pothos. 2009. Deficits of mesolimbic dopamine neurotransmission in rat dietary obesity. *Neuroscience* 159 (4):1193–9.

Gerits, A., R. Farivar, B. R. Rosen, L. L. Wald, E. S. Boyden, and W. Vanduffel. 2012. Optogenetically induced behavioral and functional network changes in primates. *Curr Biol* 22 (18):1722–6.

Gilbert, C., and J. Gillman. 1956. The changing pattern of food intake and appetite during the menstrual cycle of the baboon (*Papio ursinus*) with a consideration of some of the controlling endocrine factors. *S Afr J Med Sci* 21 (3–4):75–88.

Glowa, J. R., and P. W. Gold. 1991. Corticotropin releasing hormone produces profound anorexigenic effects in the rhesus monkey. *Neuropeptides* 18 (1):55–61.

Godfrey, J., C. Kelly, X. Zhang, X. Castellanos, M. Wilson, and M. M. Sanchez. 2013. Cingulo-Opercular and Limbic Intrinsic Functional Connectivity is Affected by Delayed Puberty and Social Status in Female Rhesus Macaques. *Annual Meeting of the Society of Biological Psychiatry (SOBP). San Francisco, CA.* May, 2013.

Goeders, N. E. 2002. Stress and cocaine addiction. *J Pharmacol Exp Ther* 301 (3):785–9.

Goel, N., J. L. Workman, T. T. Lee, L. Innala, and V. Viau. 2014. Sex differences in the HPA axis. *Compr Physiol* 4 (3):1121–55.

Gong, E. J., D. Garrel, and D. H. Calloway. 1989. Menstrual cycle and voluntary food intake. *Am J Clin Nutr* 49 (2):252–8.

Govindan, R. M., M. E. Behen, E. Helder, M. I. Makki, and H. T. Chugani. 2010. Altered water diffusivity in cortical association tracts in children with early deprivation identified with tract-based spatial statistics (TBSS). *Cereb Cortex* 20 (3):561–9.

Grant, K. A., C. A. Shively, M. A. Nader, R. L. Ehrenkaufer, S. W. Line, T. E. Morton, H. D. Gage, and R. H. Mach. 1998. Effect of social status on striatal dopamine D2 receptor binding characteristics in cynomolgus monkeys assessed with positron emission tomography. *Synapse* 29 (1):80–3.

Grove, K. L., B. E. Grayson, M. M. Glavas, X. Q. Xiao, and M. S. Smith. 2005. Development of metabolic systems. *Physiol Behav* 86 (5):646–60.

Grunberg, N. E., and R. O. Straub. 1992. The role of gender and taste class in the effects of stress on eating. *Health Psychol* 11 (2):97–100.

Gundersen, C., D. Mahatmya, S. Garasky, and B. Lohman. 2011. Linking psychosocial stressors and childhood obesity. *Obes Rev* 12 (5):e54–63.

Haber, S. N., and B. Knutson. 2010. The reward circuit: Linking primate anatomy and human imaging. *Neuropsychopharmacology* 35 (1):4–26.

Handa, R. J., L. H. Burgess, J. E. Kerr, and J. A. O'Keefe. 1994. Gonadal steroid hormone receptors and sex differences in the hypothalamo–pituitary–adrenal axis. *Horm Behav* 28 (4):464–76.

Hansen, B. C., J. D. Newcomb, R. Chen, and E. H. Linden. 2013. Longitudinal dynamics of body weight change in the development of type 2 diabetes. *Obesity (Silver Spring)* 21 (8):1643–9.

Hariri, N., and L. Thibault. 2010. High-fat diet-induced obesity in animal models. *Nutr Res Rev* 23 (2):270–99.

Harris, R. B. 2015. Chronic and acute effects of stress on energy balance: Are there appropriate animal models? *Am J Physiol Regul Integr Comp Physiol* 308 (4):R250–65.

Harris, R. B., J. Zhou, B. D. Youngblood, Rybkin, II, G. N. Smagin, and D. H. Ryan. 1998. Effect of repeated stress on body weight and body composition of rats fed low- and high-fat diets. *Am J Physiol* 275 (6 Pt 2):R1928–38.

Haslam, D. W., and W. P. James. 2005. Obesity. *Lancet* 366 (9492):1197–209.

Heidbreder, C. A., and H. J. Groenewegen. 2003. The medial prefrontal cortex in the rat: Evidence for a dorso-ventral distinction based upon functional and anatomical characteristics. *Neurosci Biobehav Rev* 27 (6):555–79.

Hemmingsson, E. 2014. A new model of the role of psychological and emotional distress in promoting obesity: Conceptual review with implications for treatment and prevention. *Obes Rev* 15 (9):769–79.

Herman, J. P. 2013. Neural control of chronic stress adaptation. *Front Behav Neurosci* 7:61.

Herod, S. M., A. M. Dettmer, M. A. Novak, J. S. Meyer, and J. L. Cameron. 2011. Sensitivity to stress-induced reproductive dysfunction is associated with a selective but not a generalized increase in activity of the adrenal axis. *Am J Physiol Endocrinol Metab* 300 (1):E28–36.

Herod, S. M., C. R. Pohl, and J. L. Cameron. 2011. Treatment with a CRH-R1 antagonist prevents stress-induced suppression of the central neural drive to the reproductive axis in female macaques. *Am J Physiol Endocrinol Metab* 300 (1):E19–27.

Hirschberg, A. L. 2012. Sex hormones, appetite and eating behaviour in women *Maturitas* 71 (3):248–56.

Honess, P. E., and C. M. Marin. 2006. Behavioural and physiological aspects of stress and aggression in nonhuman primates. *Neurosci Biobehav Rev* 30 (3):390–412.

Howell, B. R., J. Godfrey, D. A. Gutman, V. Michopoulos, X. Zhang, G. Nair, X. Hu, M. E. Wilson, and M. M. Sanchez. 2014. Social subordination stress and serotonin transporter polymorphisms: Associations with brain white matter tract integrity and behavior in juvenile female macaques. *Cereb Cortex* 24 (12):3334–49.

Iemolo, A., A. Blasio, S. A. St Cyr, F. Jiang, K. C. Rice, V. Sabino, and P. Cottone. 2013. CRF-CRF receptor system in the central and basolateral nuclei of the amygdala differentially mediates excessive eating of palatable food. *Neuropsychopharmacology* 38:2456–66.

Izzo, E., P. P. Sanna, and G. F. Koob. 2005. Impairment of dopaminergic system function after chronic treatment with corticotropin-releasing factor. *Pharmacol Biochem Behav* 81 (4):701–8.

Jarrell, H., J. B. Hoffman, J. R. Kaplan, S. Berga, B. Kinkead, and M. E. Wilson. 2008. Polymorphisms in the serotonin reuptake transporter gene modify the consequences of social status on metabolic health in female rhesus monkeys. *Physiol Behav* 93 (4–5):807–19.

Johnson, P. M., and P. J. Kenny. 2010. Dopamine D2 receptors in addiction-like reward dysfunction and compulsive eating in obese rats. *Nat Neurosci* 13:635–41.

Johnson, W. G., S. A. Corrigan, C. R. Lemmon, K. B. Bergeron, and A. H. Crusco. 1994. Energy regulation over the menstrual cycle. *Physiol Behav* 56 (3):523–7.

Johnson, Z. P., J. Lowe, V. Michopoulos, C. J. Moore, M. E. Wilson, and D. Toufexis. 2013. Oestradiol differentially influences feeding behaviour depending on diet composition in female rhesus monkeys. *J Neuroendocrinol* 25 (8):729–41.

Kaplan, J. R., M. R. Adams, T. B. Clarkson, and D. R. Koritnik. 1984. Psychosocial influences on female 'protection' among cynomolgus macaques. *Atherosclerosis* 53 (3):283–95.

Kaplan, J. R., H. Chen, S. E. Appt, C. J. Lees, A. A. Franke, S. L. Berga, M. E. Wilson, S. B. Manuck, and T. B. Clarkson. 2010. Impairment of ovarian function and associated health-related abnormalities are attributable to low social status in premenopausal monkeys and not mitigated by a high-isoflavone soy diet. *Hum Repr* 25 (12):3083–94.

Kaplan, J. R., S. B. Manuck, T. B. Clarkson, F. M. Lusso, and D. M. Taub. 1982. Social status, environment, and atherosclerosis in cynomolgus monkeys. *Arteriosclerosis* 2 (5):359–68.

Kaufman, J., and D. Charney. 2001. Effects of early stress on brain structure and function: Implications for understanding the relationship between child maltreatment and depression. *Dev Psychopathol* 13 (3):451–71.

Kaufman, D., M. A. Banerji, I. Shorman, E. L. Smith, J. D. Coplan, L. A. Rosenblum, and J. G. Kral. 2007. Early-life stress and the development of obesity and insulin resistance in juvenile bonnet macaques. *Diabetes* 56 (5):1382–6.

Kemnitz, J. W., J. R. Gibber, K. A. Lindsay, and S. G. Eisele. 1989. Effects of ovarian hormones on eating behaviors, body weight, and glucoregulation in rhesus monkeys. *Horm Behav* 23 (2):235–50.

Kenny, P. J. 2013. The food addiction. *Sci Am* 309:44–9.

Kitraki, E., G. Soulis, and K. Gerozissis. 2004. Impaired neuroendocrine response to stress following a short-term fat-enriched diet. *Neuroendocrinology* 79 (6):338–45.

Knobil, E. 1980. The neuroendocrine control of the menstrual cycle. *Recent Prog Horm Res* 36:53–88.

Koch, F. S., A. Sepa, and J. Ludvigsson. 2008. Psychological stress and obesity. *J Pediatr* 153 (6):839–44.

Kolb, B. 1984. Functions of the frontal cortex of the rat: A comparative review. *Brain Res* 320 (1):65–98.

Koob, G. F., and M. Le Moal. 2001. Drug addiction, dysregulation of reward, and allostasis. *Neuropsychopharmacology* 24 (2):97–129.

Koob, G. F., and M. Le Moal. 2005. Plasticity of reward neurocircuitry and the 'dark side' of drug addiction. *Nat Neurosci* 8 (11):1442–4.

Koob, G., and M. J. Kreek. 2007. Stress, dysregulation of drug reward pathways, and the transition to drug dependence. *Am J Psychiatry* 164 (8):1149–59.

Koob, G. F., C. L. Buck, A. Cohen, S. Edwards, P. E. Park, J. E. Schlosburg, B. Schmeichel, L. F. Vendruscolo, C. L. Wade, T. W. Whitfield, Jr., and O. George. 2014. Addiction as a stress surfeit disorder. *Neuropharmacology* 76 Pt B:370–82.

la Fleur, S. E., M. C. Luijendijk, E. M. van der Zwaal, M. A. Brans, and R. A. Adan. 2014. The snacking rat as model of human obesity: Effects of a free-choice high-fat high-sugar diet on meal patterns. *Int J Obes (Lond)* 38 (5):643–9.

la Fleur, S. E., L. J. Vanderschuren, M. C. Luijendijk, B. M. Kloeze, B. Tiesjema, and R. A. Adan. 2007. A reciprocal interaction between food-motivated behavior and diet-induced obesity. *Int J Obes (Lond)* 31 (8):1286–94.

Laitinen, J., E. Ek, and U. Sovio. 2002. Stress-related eating and drinking behavior and body mass index and predictors of this behavior. *Prev Med* 34 (1):29–39.

Lee, A. K., M. Mojtahed-Jaberi, T. Kyriakou, E. Aldecoa-Otalora Astarloa, M. Arno, N. J. Marshall, S. D. Brain, and S. D. O'Dell. 2010. Effect of high-fat feeding on expression of genes controlling availability of dopamine in mouse hypothalamus. *Nutrition* 26:411–22.

Levin, B. E. 2000. Metabolic imprinting on genetically predisposed neural circuits perpetuates obesity. *Nutrition* 16 (10):909–15.

Levin, B. E. 2008. Epigenetic influences on food intake and physical activity level: Review of animal studies. *Obesity (Silver Spring)* 16 Suppl 3:S51–4.

Levin, B. E., A. A. Dunn-Meynell, B. Balkan, and R. E. Keesey. 1997. Selective breeding for diet-induced obesity and resistance in Sprague-Dawley rats. *Am J Physiol* 273 (2 Pt 2):R725–30.

Lissner, L., J. Stevens, D. A. Levitsky, K. M. Rasmussen, and B. J. Strupp. 1988. Variation in energy intake during the menstrual cycle: Implications for food-intake research. *Am J Clin Nutr* 48 (4):956–62.

Lutter, M., A. E. Croghan, and H. Cui. 2016. Escaping the golden cage: Animal models of eating disorders in the post-diagnostic and statistical manual era. *Biol Psychiatry* 79:17–24.

Lyons, D. M., K. J. Parker, M. Katz, and A. F. Schatzberg. 2009. Developmental cascades linking stress inoculation, arousal regulation, and resilience. *Front Behav Neurosci* Sep 18; 3:32.

Machado, C. J., and J. Bachevalier. 2007. Measuring reward assessment in a semi-naturalistic context: The effects of selective amygdala, orbital frontal or hippocampal lesions. *Neuroscience* 148 (3):599–611.

Machado, C. J., N. J. Emery, W. A. Mason, and D. G. Amaral. 2010. Selective changes in foraging behavior following bilateral neurotoxic amygdala lesions in rhesus monkeys. *Behav Neurosci* 124 (6):761–72.

Maniam, J., and M. J. Morris. 2012. The link between stress and feeding behaviour. *Neuropharmacology* 63 (1):97–110.

Manuck, S. B., J. R. Kaplan, and T. B. Clarkson. 1983. Social instability and coronary artery atherosclerosis in cynomolgus monkeys. *Neurosci Biobehav Rev* 7 (4):485–91.

Martel, P., and M. Fantino. 1996a. Influence of the amount of food ingested on mesolimbic dopaminergic system activity: A microdialysis study. *Pharmacol Biochem Behav* 55 (2):297–302.

Martel, P., and M. Fantino. 1996b. Mesolimbic dopaminergic system activity as a function of food reward: A microdialysis study. *Pharmacol Biochem Behav* 53 (1):221–6.

Mazur, J., A. Dzielska, and A. Malkowska-Szkutnik. 2011. Psychological determinants of selected eating behaviours in adolescents. *Med Wieku Rozwoj* 15 (3):240–9.

McCowan, B., B. A. Beisner, J. P. Capitanio, M. E. Jackson, A. N. Cameron, S. Seil, E. R. Atwill, and H. Fushing. 2011. Network stability is a balancing act of personality, power, and conflict dynamics in rhesus macaque societies. *PLoS One* 6 (8):e22350.

McEwen, B. S., and J. H. Morrison. 2013. The brain on stress: Vulnerability and plasticity of the prefrontal cortex over the life course. *Neuron* 79 (1):16–29.

Michopoulos, V., and M. E. Wilson. 2011. Body weight decreases induced by estradiol in female rhesus monkeys are dependent upon social status. *Physiol Behav* 102 (3–4):382–8.

Michopoulos, V., M. Higgins, D. Toufexis, and M. E. Wilson. 2012a. Social subordination produces distinct stress-related phenotypes in female rhesus monkeys. *Psychoneuroendocrinology* 37 (7):1071–85.

Michopoulos, V., T. Loucks, S. L. Berga, J. Rivier, and M. E. Wilson. 2010. Increased ghrelin sensitivity and calorie consumption in subordinate monkeys is affected by short-term astressin B administration. *Endocrine* 38 (2):227–34.

Michopoulos, V., M. Perez Diaz, M. Embree, K. Reding, J. R. Votaw, J. Mun, R. J. Voll, M. M. Goodman, M. Wilson, M. Sanchez, and D. Toufexis. 2014. Oestradiol alters central 5-HT1A receptor binding potential differences related to psychosocial stress but not differences related to 5-HTTLPR genotype in female rhesus monkeys. *J Neuroendocrinol* 26 (2):80–8.

Michopoulos, V., K. M. Reding, M. E. Wilson, and D. Toufexis. 2012b. Social subordination impairs hypothalamic–pituitary–adrenal function in female rhesus monkeys. *Horm Behav* 62 (4):389–99.

Michopoulos, V., K. N. Shepard, M. Arce, J. Whitley, and M. E. Wilson. 2009. Food history and diet choice affect food intake in monkeys. *Appetite* 52 (3):848.

Michopoulos, V., D. Toufexis, and M. E. Wilson. 2012. Social stress interacts with diet history to promote emotional feeding in females. *Psychoneuroendocrinology* 37 (9):1479–90.

Miranda-Dominguez, O., B. D. Mills, D. Grayson, A. Woodall, K. A. Grant, C. D. Kroenke, and D. A. Fair. 2014. Bridging the gap between the human and macaque connectome: A quantitative comparison of global interspecies structure-function relationships and network topology. *J Neurosci* 34 (16):5552–63.

Moens, E., C. Braet, G. Bosmans, and Y. Rosseel. 2009. Unfavourable family characteristics and their associations with childhood obesity: A cross-sectional study. *Eur Eat Disord Rev* 17 (4):315–23.

Mook, D., J. Felger, F. C. Graves, K. Wallen, and M. E. Wilson. 2005. Tamoxifen fails to affect central serotonergic tone but increases indices of anxiety in female rhesus monkeys. *Psychoneuroendocrinology* 30:273–83.

Moore, C. J., J. Lowe, V. Michopoulos, P. Ulam, D. Toufexis, M. E. Wilson, and Z. Johnson. 2013. Small changes in meal patterns lead to significant changes in total caloric intake. Effects of diet and social status on food intake in female rhesus monkeys. *Appetite* 62:60–9.

Moore, C. J., Z. P. Johnson, D. Toufexis, and M. E. Wilson. 2014. Antagonism of CRF type 1 receptors attenuates caloric intake of free feeding subordinate female rhesus monkeys in a rich dietary environment. *J Neuroendocrinol* 27:33–43

Morgan, D., K. A. Grant, H. D. Gage, R. H. Mach, J. R. Kaplan, O. Prioleau, S. H. Nader, N. Buchheimer, R. L. Ehrenkaufer, and M. A. Nader. 2002. Social dominance in monkeys: Dopamine D2 receptors and cocaine self-administration. *Nat Neurosci* 5 (2):169–74.

Nader, M. A., D. Morgan, H. D. Gage, S. H. Nader, T. L. Calhoun, N. Buchheimer, R. Ehrenkaufer, and R. H. Mach. 2006. PET imaging of dopamine D2 receptors during chronic cocaine self-administration in monkeys. *Nat Neurosci* 9 (8):1050–6.

Nemeroff, C. B., and W. W. Vale. 2005. The neurobiology of depression: Inroads to treatment and new drug discovery. *J Clin Psychiatry* 66 Suppl 7:5–13.

Nguyen-Rodriguez, S. T., J. B. Unger, and D. Spruijt-Metz. 2009. Psychological determinants of emotional eating in adolescence. *Eat Disord* 17 (3):211–24.

Noll, J. G., M. H. Zeller, P. K. Trickett, and F. W. Putnam. 2007. Obesity risk for female victims of childhood sexual abuse: A prospective study. *Pediatrics* 120 (1):e61–7.

Noonan, M. P., N. Kolling, M. E. Walton, and M. F. Rushworth. 2012. Re-evaluating the role of the orbitofrontal cortex in reward and reinforcement. *Eur J Neurosci* 35 (7):997–1010.

Noonan, M. P., J. Sallet, R. B. Mars, F. X. Neubert, J. X. O'Reilly, J. L. Andersson, A. S. Mitchell, A. H. Bell, K. L. Miller, and M. F. Rushworth. 2014. A neural circuit covarying with social hierarchy in macaques. *PLoS Biol* 12 (9):e1001940.

Norman, R. L., C. J. Smith, J. D. Pappas, and J. Hall. 1992. Exposure to ovarian steroids elicits a female pattern of plasma cortisol levels in castrated male macaques. *Steroids* 57 (1):37–43.

Ozden, I., J. Wang, Y. Lu, T. May, J. Lee, W. Goo, D. J. O'Shea, P. Kalanithi, I. Diester, M. Diagne, K. Deisseroth, K. V. Shenoy, and A. V. Nurmikko. 2013. A coaxial optrode as multifunction write–read probe for optogenetic studies in non-human primates. *J Neurosci Methods* 219 (1):142–54.

Panchal, S. K., and L. Brown. 2011. Rodent models for metabolic syndrome research. *J Biomed Biotechnol* 2011:351982.

Parylak, S. L., G. F. Koob, and E. P. Zorrilla. 2011. The dark side of food addiction. *Physiol Behav* 104 (1):149–56.

Pelchat, M. L. 2002. Of human bondage: Food craving, obsession, compulsion, and addiction. *Physiol Behav* 76 (3):347–52.

Petrides, M., F. Tomaiuolo, E. H. Yeterian, and D. N. Pandya. 2012. The prefrontal cortex: Comparative architectonic organization in the human and the macaque monkey brains. *Cortex* 48 (1):46–57.

Pound, L. D., P. Kievit, and K. L. Grove. 2014. The nonhuman primate as a model for type 2 diabetes. *Curr Opin Endocrinol Diabetes Obes* 21 (2):89–94.

Preuss, T. M. 1995. Do rats have prefrontal cortex? The Rose-Woolsey-Akert program reconsidered. *J Cogn Neurosci* 7 (1):1–24.

Pritchard, T. C., E. N. Nedderman, E. M. Edwards, A. C. Petticoffer, G. J. Schwartz, and T. R. Scott. 2008. Satiety-responsive neurons in the medial orbitofrontal cortex of the macaque. *Behav Neurosci* 122 (1):174–82.

Pujara, M., and M. Koenigs. 2014. Mechanisms of reward circuit dysfunction in psychiatric illness: Prefrontal–striatal interactions. *Neuroscientist* 20 (1):82–95.

Rada, P., N. M. Avena, and B. G. Hoebel. 2005. Daily bingeing on sugar repeatedly releases dopamine in the accumbens shell. *Neuroscience* 134 (3):737–44.

Reep, R. 1984. Relationship between prefrontal and limbic cortex: A comparative anatomical review. *Brain Behav Evol* 25 (1):5–80.

Research_Diets. 2015. BioDAQ NHP. http://www.researchdiets.com/biodaq/biodaq-nhp.

Robison, C. L., J. L. Meyerhoff, G. A. Saviolakis, W. K. Chen, K. C. Rice, and L. A. Lumley. 2004. A CRH1 antagonist into the amygdala of mice prevents defeat-induced defensive behavior. *Ann N Y Acad Sci* 1032:324–7.

Roepke, T. A. 2009. Oestrogen modulates hypothalamic control of energy homeostasis through multiple mechanisms. *J Neuroendocrinol* 21 (2):141–50.

Rolls, E. T. 2007. Sensory processing in the brain related to the control of food intake. *Proc Nutr Soc* 66 (1):96–112.

Rolls, B. J., P. M. Van Duijvenvoorde, and E. A. Rowe. 1983. Variety in the diet enhances intake in a meal and contributes to the development of obesity in the rat. *Physiol Behav* 31 (1):21–7.

Rommeck, I., J. P. Capitanio, S. C. Strand, and B. McCowan. 2011. Early social experience affects behavioral and physiological responsiveness to stressful conditions in infant rhesus macaques (*Macaca mulatta*). *Am J Primatol* 73 (7):692–701.

Rosenblatt, H., I. Dyrenfurth, M. Ferin, and R. L. vande Wiele. 1980. Food intake and the menstrual cycle in rhesus monkeys. *Physiol Behav* 24 (3):447–9.

Rosini, T. C., A. S. Silva, and Cd Moraes. 2012. Diet-induced obesity: Rodent model for the study of obesity-related disorders. *Rev Assoc Med Bras* 58 (3):383–7.

Sallet, J., R. B. Mars, M. P. Noonan, J. L. Andersson, J. X. O'Reilly, S. Jbabdi, P. L. Croxson, M. Jenkinson, K. L. Miller, and M. F. Rushworth. 2011. Social network size affects neural circuits in macaques. *Science* 334:697–700.

Sanchez, M. M., E. F. Hearn, D. Do, J. K. Rilling, and J. G. Herndon. 1998. Differential rearing affects corpus callosum size and cognitive function of rhesus monkeys. *Brain Res* 812 (1–2):38–49.

Santollo, J., M. D. Wiley, and L. A. Eckel. 2007. Acute activation of ER alpha decreases food intake, meal size, and body weight in ovariectomized rats. *Am J Physiol Regul Integr Comp Physiol* 293 (6):R2194–201.

Schneider, J. E., J. D. Wise, N. A. Benton, J. M. Brozek, and E. Keen-Rhinehart. 2013. When do we eat? Ingestive behavior, survival, and reproductive success. *Horm Behav* 64:702–28.

Schneiderman, J. U., F. E. Mennen, S. Negriff, and P. K. Trickett. 2012. Overweight and obesity among maltreated young adolescents. *Child Abuse Negl* 36 (4):370–8.

Shively, C. A., D. P. Friedman, H. D. Gage, M. C. Bounds, C. Brown-Proctor, J. B. Blair, J. A. Henderson, M. A. Smith, and N. Buchheimer. 2006. Behavioral depression and positron emission tomography-determined serotonin 1A receptor binding potential in cynomolgus monkeys. *Arch Gen Psychiatry* 63 (4):396–403.

Shively, C. A., K. A. Grant, R. L. Ehrenkaufer, R. H. Mach, and M. A. Nader. 1997. Social stress, depression, and brain dopamine in female cynomolgus monkeys. *Ann N Y Acad Sci* 807:574–7.

Shively, C. A., K. Laber-Laird, and R. F. Anton. 1997. Behavior and physiology of social stress and depression in female cynomolgus monkeys. *Biol Psych* 41 (8):871–82.

Shively, C. A., T. C. Register, and T. B. Clarkson. 2009. Social stress, visceral obesity, and coronary artery atherosclerosis in female primates. *Obesity (Silver Spring)* 17:1513–20.

Silk, J. B. 2002. Practice random acts of aggression and senseless acts of intimidation: The logic of status contests in social groups. *Evol Anthropol* 11: 221–5.

Sinha, R., and A. M. Jastreboff. 2013. Stress as a common risk factor for obesity and addiction. *Biol Psychiatry* 73 (9):827–35.

Smagin, G. N., L. A. Howell, S. Redmann, Jr., D. H. Ryan, and R. B. Harris. 1999. Prevention of stress-induced weight loss by third ventricle CRF receptor antagonist. *Am J Physiol* 276 (5 Pt 2):R1461–8.

Smith, C. J., and R. L. Norman. 1987a. Circadian periodicity in circulating cortisol is absent after orchidectomy in rhesus macaques. *Endocrinology* 121 (6):2186–91.

Smith, C. J., and R. L. Norman. 1987b. Influence of the gonads on cortisol secretion in female rhesus macaques. *Endocrinology* 121 (6):2192–8.

Solano, J. M., and L. Jacobson. 1999. Glucocorticoids reverse leptin effects on food intake and body fat in mice without increasing NPY mRNA. *Am J Physiol* 277 (4 Pt 1):E708–16.

Solomon, M. B., R. Jankord, J. N. Flak, and J. P. Herman. 2011. Chronic stress, energy balance and adiposity in female rats. *Physiol Behav* 102 (1):84–90.

Sominsky, L., and S. J. Spencer. 2014. Eating behavior and stress: A pathway to obesity. *Front Psychol* 5:434.

Soulis, G., E. Kitraki, and K. Gerozissis. 2005. Early neuroendocrine alterations in female rats following a diet moderately enriched in fat. *Cell Mol Neurobiol* 25 (5):869–80.

Soulis, G., E. Papalexi, C. Kittas, and E. Kitraki. 2007. Early impact of a fat-enriched diet on behavioral responses of male and female rats. *Behav Neurosci* 121 (3):483–90.

Suglia, S. F., C. S. Duarte, E. C. Chambers, and R. Boynton-Jarrett. 2012. Cumulative social risk and obesity in early childhood. *Pediatrics* 129 (5):e1173–9.

Sullivan, E. L., and J. L. Cameron. 2010. A rapidly occurring compensatory decrease in physical activity counteracts diet-induced weight loss in female monkeys. *Am J Physiol Regul Integr Comp Physiol* 298 (4):R1068–74.

Sullivan, E. L., F. H. Koegler, and J. L. Cameron. 2006. Individual differences in physical activity are closely associated with changes in body weight in adult female rhesus monkeys (*Macaca mulatta*). *Am J Physiol Regul Integr Comp Physiol* 291 (3):R633–42.

Tamashiro, K. L., M. A. Hegeman, and R. R. Sakai. 2006. Chronic social stress in a changing dietary environment. *Physiol Behav* 89 (4):536–42.

Tamashiro, K. L., M. M. Nguyen, and R. R. Sakai. 2005. Social stress: From rodents to primates. *Front Neuroendocrinol* 26 (1):27–40.

Tamashiro, K. L., R. R. Sakai, C. A. Shively, I. N. Karatsoreos, and L. P. Reagan. 2011. Chronic stress, metabolism, and metabolic syndrome. *Stress* 14 (5):468–74.

Tamashiro, K. L., C. E. Terrillion, J. Hyun, J. I. Koenig, and T. H. Moran. 2009. Prenatal stress or high-fat diet increases susceptibility to diet-induced obesity in rat offspring. *Diabetes* 58 (5):1116–25.

Tazi, A., R. Dantzer, M. Le Moal, J. Rivier, W. Vale, and G. F. Koob. 1987. Corticotropin-releasing factor antagonist blocks stress-induced fighting in rats. *Regul Pept* 18 (1): 37–42.

Teicher, M. H., S. L. Andersen, A. Polcari, C. M. Anderson, and C. P. Navalta. 2002. Developmental neurobiology of childhood stress and trauma. *Psychiatr Clin North Am* 25 (2):397–426, vii–viii.

Thanos, P. K., M. Michaelides, H. Benveniste, G. J. Wang, and N. D. Volkow. 2007. Effects of chronic oral methylphenidate on cocaine self-administration and striatal dopamine D2 receptors in rodents. *Pharmacol Biochem Behav* 87 (4):426–33.

Thivel, D., J. Aucouturier, E. Doucet, T. J. Saunders, and J. P. Chaput. 2013. Daily energy balance in children and adolescents. Does energy expenditure predict subsequent energy intake? *Appetite* 60 (1):58–64.

Thivel, D., L. Metz, A. Julien, B. Morio, and P. Duche. 2014. Obese but not lean adolescents spontaneously decrease energy intake after intensive exercise. *Physiol Behav* 123:41–6.

Tomasi, D., and N. D. Volkow. 2013. Striatocortical pathway dysfunction in addiction and obesity: Differences and similarities. *Crit Rev Biochem Mol Biol* 48 (1):1–19.

Toufexis, D. J., and M. E. Wilson. 2012. Dihydrotestosterone differentially modulates the cortisol response of the hypothalamic–pituitary–adrenal axis in male and female rhesus macaques, and restores circadian secretion of cortisol in females. *Brain Res* 1429:43–51.

Tsenkova, V., J. M. Boylan, and C. Ryff. 2013. Stress eating and health. Findings from MIDUS, a national study of US adults. *Appetite* 69:151–5.

Tung, J., L. B. Barreiro, Z. P. Johnson, K. D. Hansen, V. Michopoulos, D. Toufexis, K. Michelini, M. E. Wilson, and Y. Gilad. 2012. Social environment is associated with gene regulatory variation in the rhesus macaque immune system. *Proc Natl Acad Sci U S A* 109 (17):6490–5.

van den Heuvel, J. K., K. Furman, M. C. Gumbs, L. Eggels, D. M. Opland, B. B. Land, S. M. Kolk, S. Narayanan N, E. Fliers, A. Kalsbeek, R. J. DiLeone, and S. E. la Fleur. 2015. Neuropeptide Y activity in the nucleus accumbens modulates feeding behavior and neuronal activity. *Biol Psychiatry* 77 (7):633–41.

Van Eden, C. G., and R. M. Buijs. 2000. Functional neuroanatomy of the prefrontal cortex: Autonomic interactions. *Prog Brain Res* 126:49–62.

van Gestel, M. A., E. Kostrzewa, R. A. Adan, and S. K. Janhunen. 2014. Pharmacological manipulations in animal models of anorexia and binge eating in relation to humans. *Br J Pharmacol* 171 (20):4767–84.

Van Vugt, D. A. 2010. Brain imaging studies of appetite in the context of obesity and the menstrual cycle. *Hum Reprod Update* 16 (3):276–92.

Volkow, N. D., and R. D. Baler. 2015. NOW vs LATER brain circuits: Implications for obesity and addiction. *Trends Neurosci* 38 (6):345–52.

Volkow, N. D., and R. A. Wise. 2005. How can drug addiction help us understand obesity? *Nat Neurosci* 8 (5):555–60.

Volkow, N. D., J. S. Fowler, and G. J. Wang. 2003. The addicted human brain: Insights from imaging studies. *J Clin Invest* 111 (10):1444–51.

Volkow, N. D., G. J. Wang, J. S. Fowler, D. Tomasi, and R. Baler. 2012. Food and drug reward: Overlapping circuits in human obesity and addiction. *Curr Top Behav Neurosci* 11:1–24.

Volkow, N. D., G. J. Wang, D. Tomasi, and R. D. Baler. 2013. The addictive dimensionality of obesity. *Biol Psychiatry* 73 (9):811–8.

Vucetic, Z., J. Kimmel, K. Totoki, E. Hollenbeck, and T. M. Reyes. 2010. Maternal high-fat diet alters methylation and gene expression of dopamine and opioid-related genes. *Endocrinology* 151 (10):4756–64.

Wade, G. N., and J. M. Gray. 1979. Gonadal effects on food-intake and adiposity—metabolic hypothesis. *Physiol Behav* 22 (3):583–93.

Walker, M. L., M. E. Wilson, and T. P. Gordon. 1984. Endocrine control of the seasonal occurrence of ovulation in rhesus monkeys housed outdoors. *Endocrinology* 114 (4):1074–81.

Wang, G. J., N. D. Volkow, J. Logan, N. R. Pappas, C. T. Wong, W. Zhu, N. Netusil, and J. S. Fowler. 2001. Brain dopamine and obesity. *Lancet* 357 (9253):354–7.

Warne, J. P. 2009. Shaping the stress response: Interplay of palatable food choices, glucocorticoids, insulin and abdominal obesity *Mol Cell Endocrinol* 300 (1–2):137–46.

Williams, K. W., and J. K. Elmquist. 2012. From neuroanatomy to behavior: Central integration of peripheral signals regulating feeding behavior. *Nat Neurosci* 15 (10):1350–5.

Wilson, M. E., J. Fisher, A. Fischer, V. Lee, R. B. Harris, and T. J. Bartness. 2008. Quantifying food intake in socially housed monkeys: Social status effects on caloric consumption. *Physiol Behav* 94 (4):586–94.

Wilson, M. E., T. P. Gordon, and D. C. Collins. 1986. Ontogeny of luteinizing hormone secretion and first ovulation in seasonal breeding rhesus monkeys. *Endocrinology* 118 (1):293–301.

Wilson, M. E., C. J. Moore, K. F. Ethun, and Z. P. Johnson. 2014. Understanding the control of ingestive behavior in primates. *Horm Behav* 66 (1):86–94.

Woods, S. C., D. A. D'Alessio, P. Tso, P. A. Rushing, D. J. Clegg, S. C. Benoit, K. Gotoh, M. Liu, and R. J. Seeley. 2004. Consumption of a high-fat diet alters the homeostatic regulation of energy balance. *Physiol Behav* 83 (4):573–8.

Yazbek, S. N., S. H. Spiezio, J. H. Nadeau, and D. A. Buchner. 2010. Ancestral paternal genotype controls body weight and food intake for multiple generations. *Hum Mol Genet* 19 (21):4134–44.

Yeterian, E. H., D. N. Pandya, F. Tomaiuolo, and M. Petrides. 2012. The cortical connectivity of the prefrontal cortex in the monkey brain. *Cortex* 48 (1):58–81.

Zambrano, E., and P. W. Nathanielsz. 2013. Mechanisms by which maternal obesity programs offspring for obesity: Evidence from animal studies. *Nutr Rev* 71 Suppl 1:S42–54.

Zehr, J. L., P. E. Van Meter, and K. Wallen. 2005. Factors regulating the timing of puberty onset in female rhesus monkeys (*Macaca mulatta*): Role of prenatal androgens, social rank, and adolescent body weight. *Biol Reprod* 72 (5):1087–94.

Zheng, H., and H. R. Berthoud. 2007. Eating for pleasure or calories. *Curr Opin Pharmacol* 7 (6):607–12.

5 Untangling Appetite Circuits with Optogenetics and Chemogenetics

Michael J. Krashes

CONTENTS

5.1 BACKGROUND

5.1.1 Hunger Evolution

The word "hunger" encapsulates many concepts. At its core, the interoceptive detection of hunger, foraging to locate a potential food source, and ensuing consumption of calories and nutrients are the most primitive and conserved behavior across Kingdom Animalia. In mammals, the homeostatic maintenance of energetic state is highlighted by a sensorimotor feedback system that strives to maintain stability through the concerted regulation of both energy intake (via caloric consumption) and energy expenditure (via basal metabolism, adaptive thermogenesis, and physical exertion). This simple formula, whose unbalanced equilibrium results in alterations in body weight and subsequent maladaptive physiology, has influenced our genes, lifestyles, and landscapes throughout human history.

However, hunger is not merely a homeostatic process; it is a dynamic transaction that commands profound power across cognitive, emotional, and physiological processes (Rolls 2000). It is positioned at the heart of numerous public health concerns that span multiple disciplines of modern medicine. These include ailments on opposite ends of the caloric consumption spectrum, from malnutrition to obesity, and the negative consequences of these states to our cognitive, emotional, and physiological well-being. The omnipresence of food-related complications in the world we live in underscores the importance for experimental research. A fundamental comprehension of the biological manifestation of hunger in the brain could provide potentially unifying information about these disease states and lead to groundbreaking new frameworks in which to approach these problems.

5.1.2 Experimentally Assessing Feeding Behavior

Undoubtedly, the central authority of appetite regulation has garnered our attention and has been the subject of countless studies throughout human history. Yet, only in the past two centuries have investigators turned to the utilization of animal models rather than simply evaluating the relative intensity of hunger levels in man to probe complicated questions within this discipline. Such studies in genetically tractable organisms allow for unprecedented access and control of precise neural circuits in order to address inquiries such as how a combination of internal and external signals govern the selection and intake of foods and how feeding behavior is integrated into the overall process of nutritional homeostasis.

Major goals in the experimental exploration of feeding behavior are initially to break down and subsequently attempt to identify the underlying mechanisms by which an animal (a) is stimulated to eat; (b) eats a fixed amount of a certain food during a meal, or bout of eating, until satiety occurs; and (c) ceases feeding behavior due to various satiety signals. This is accomplished using a variety of feeding paradigms in animal models, such as free-feeding (ad libitum), scheduled feeding, instrumental motivational feeding, and food deprivation states while recording the ensuing eating patterns. Furthermore, food palatability, external sensory cues, and learned responses all play major roles in both the attainment and ingestion of calories. The overarching complexity and multiple layers of eating behavior, in addition to increased interest from the general public at large, make understanding the molecular, cellular, and neural machinery controlling feeding imperative to both our health and curiosity. To this end, the last century has made significant progress toward this goal using a variety of approaches. For the purposes of this chapter, emphasis will be placed on real-time methods, namely, optogenetics and chemogenetics, to rapidly and reversibly tune cellular activity with unparalleled jurisdiction.

5.1.3   Benchmark Food Intake Studies

Classic work revealed a vital role of the hypothalamus in appetite control via lesions (Anand, Dua, and Shoenberg 1955, Aravich and Sclafani 1983, Bergen et al. 1998, Gold, Jones, and Sawchenko 1977, Gold, Quackenbush, and Kapatos 1972, Holzwarth-McBride, Hurst, and Knigge 1976, Holzwarth-McBride, Sladek, and Knigge 1976, Leibowitz, Hammer, and Chang 1981, Teitelbaum and Epstein 1962), intracranial drug delivery (Boghossian, Park, and York 2010, Booth 1968, de Backer et al. 2011, Grill et al. 1998, Grossman 1960, Leibowitz 1970, Williams, Kaplan, and Grill 2000) and electric brain stimulation in animal models (Hoebel and Teitelbaum 1962, Tenen and Miller 1964). This work culminated into a theory that attributed the balance between hunger and satiety to distinct nuclei of the hypothalamus, including the lateral hypothalamus (LH), paraventricular hypothalamus (PVH), ventral medial hypothalamus (VMH), dorsal medial hypothalamus (DMH), and arcuate nucleus (ARC).

For example, electrical brain stimulation of the LH produced increases in feeding, while lesions of this structure led to decreases in feeding (Hoebel and Teitelbaum 1962, Teitelbaum and Epstein 1962, Tenen and Miller 1964). Although these results seem straightforward and conclusive, other classic nonfeeding research revealed that this was an oversimplification of the findings. Animals engaged in other motivated behaviors such as copulation and aggression under LH brain stimulation in the absence of food (Panksepp 1971, Valenstein, Cox, and Kakolewski 1970, Vaughan and Fisher 1962). Additionally, this classic electric brain stimulation work revealed an intriguing paradox: stimulation of the LH seemed to make animals hungry, but animals would readily work to self-stimulate this brain region, suggesting that it was a rewarding sensation. These findings pose the question: Why would animals actively work to become hungry? The diversity of rewarding behaviors associated with LH stimulation along with this hunger/reward paradox led to a variety of theories regarding hunger and reward in the brain, ranging from activation of reward related fixed action patterns to incentive motivation to incentive salience (Berridge and Valenstein 1991, Trowill, Panksepp, and Gandelman 1969, Valenstein, Cox, and Kakolewski 1970). Interestingly, similar observations of alternative behaviors, beyond simple fluctuations of food intake, have been made for other hypothalamic structures after these types of manipulations.

Another insightful lesion experiment found that destruction of the ARC promptly initiated massive weight gain (Holzwarth-McBride, Hurst, and Knigge 1976, Holzwarth-McBride, Sladek, and Knigge 1976). Yet given the heterogeneity of cell types compartmentalized in this area, its proximity to the third ventricle, and ensuing communication with bloodborne signals and circulating factors from the periphery, one might expect the manifestation of disparate neural populations that respond to caloric surfeit and deficit and subsequently transmit satiety and hunger signals to downstream regions of the brain. Therefore, such a resolute phenotype as a consequence of a structural lesion may miss critical components of appetite control.

Although this work clearly demonstrated a role for the LH, PVH, VMH, DMH, and ARC in appetite and reward, the techniques used in these studies carry significant limitations. While electrical stimulation and lesion strategies elicited robust responses, they lacked specificity. For example, electric brain stimulation activates all neurons within the radius of the electrode as well as all axons passing through the region, which has grave implications for downstream targets. Conversely, lesions destroy all cell types in the affected area, including both afferent and efferent processes outside the targeted lesion zone. Moreover, the past approaches often lacked anatomical precision, resulting in off-target effects, because discrete nuclei of the hypothalamus border one another and are roughly defined. Additionally, many of the methods lacked reversibility, making it difficult to interpret direct versus indirect outcomes of the initial manipulation as well as the inability to reproduce results in the same animals over a number of trials or observe bidirectional control over a defined behavior. The paucity of specificity in these techniques has likely led to the diversity of effects found among different behavioral paradigms, which has given us a broad and disjointed understanding of the role of the hypothalamus in regulating appetite.

5.1.4 UTILIZING GENETICS TO EXPLORE FOOD INTAKE

Genetic strategies to globally knock out, selectively delete, or overexpress genes encoding critical peptides and receptors using transgenic mice driving the expression of Cre-recombinase under endogenous regulatory elements (Figure 5.1A) further aided in our overall understanding of energy balance, placing importance on the adipocyte-derived hormone leptin and its cognate leptin receptor (LEPR) (Cohen et al. 2001, Halaas et al. 1995, Zhang et al. 1994) as well as the melanocortin system (Butler et al. 2000, Fan et al. 1997, Huszar et al. 1997, Ollmann et al. 1997, Yaswen et al. 1999). While these approaches and studies have significantly increased our understanding of the precise cell types and signaling schemes underlying feeding behavior, they are associated with their own set of limitations. Namely, these manipulations occur throughout development, and thus, compensation for genetic perturbations is difficult to detect.

To both bring attention to these compensatory mechanisms and bypass this drawback, several studies aimed to inactivate neurons acutely in adulthood. Diphtheria toxin-mediated ablation approaches have been used to test the functional role of a number of neuronal subpopulations within the hypothalamus (Figure 5.1B) (Gropp et al. 2005, Luquet et al. 2005, Wu et al. 2012, Xi et al. 2012, Zhan et al. 2013). Although these approaches help address temporal concerns, the kinetics of the manipulation is not immediate. Moreover, neural ablation is permanent, and thus, the resulting phenotypes cannot be reversed. Finally, the methodology can only be used to answer questions of cell-type necessity, and not sufficiency, in mediating behaviors. Given these caveats, alternative techniques need to be employed for

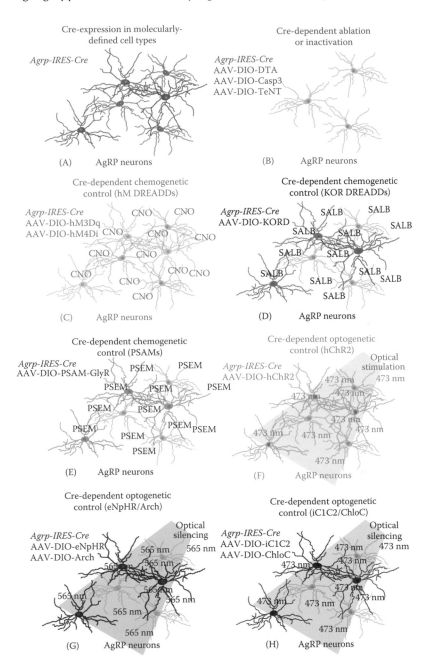

FIGURE 5.1 Selective manipulation of neural subtypes employing Cre-expressing mice with Cre-dependent viral tools. (A) Marking ARC^AgRP neurons with *Agrp-IRES-Cre* mouse line expressing Cre-recombinase under endogenous regulatory elements. (B) Methods of permanent ARC^AgRP neural inactivation. (C–E) Chemogenetic methods to reversibly activate or silence neural activity using chemical ligand actuators. (F–H) Optogenetic methods to reversibly activate or silence neural activity using distinct wavelengths of light.

molecular-defined neural circuit analysis. Fortunately, recent breakthroughs in neuroscience allow for more targeted approaches to tackle these empirical questions.

Studying the mechanisms of homeostatic food intake is challenging due to slow temporal kinetics of the parameters mediating the switch between hunger and satiety. Hormones need to be released from peripheral tissues, travel to the brain, and signal nutrient-sensing neurons to direct food-seeking and consumption behavior. These prolonged changes in energy deficit considerably hamper the examination of the contributing relationships between deprivation-sensitive sensory systems and the downstream brain circuits they engage. To side step this difficulty, manipulations of molecularly circumscribed nutrient-sensing neurons can be used to prove the central control of feeding. Once identified, the afferent and efferent pathways modulating both hunger and satiety can be further analyzed in detail (Sternson 2013).

5.2 INTRODUCTION TO CHEMOGENETIC AND OPTOGENETIC STRATEGIES

5.2.1 Overcoming Hypothalamic Heterogeneity

This need to obtain discrete access to defined neurons is essential given the diversity and complexity of the neural circuits that underlie feeding behaviors. For example, two of the most heavily studied cell types involved in appetite regulation, the agouti-related peptide (AgRP) and proopiomelanocortin (POMC) populations in the ARC, marked by the expression of *Agrp* and *Pomc*, are not only adjacent to one another but also anatomically intermingled. Given that these separate neural subtypes are thought to evoke opposing functions on appetite, gaining command over each unique population is essential to unraveling their respective behavioral contributions.

A common way to achieve such explicit specificity is through a two-pronged approach using genetically-engineered mice that express Cre-recombinase in defined neurons, often driven off the endogenous gene promoter, in combination with Cre-dependent viral vectors expressing activity modulators to stimulate or silence neuronal activity using particular wavelengths of light or pharmacologically inert, chemical ligands (Figure 5.1) (Luo, Callaway, and Svoboda 2008). These adeno-associated viruses are designed in such a way that the open reading frame of the coding sequence is inverted, in the antisense orientation, flanked by two pairs of heterotypic, antiparallel loxP-type recombination sites. In the presence of Cre-recombinase, the recombination sites first undergo an inversion of the coding sequence, followed by excision of two sites, leading to one of each orthogonal recombination site oppositely oriented and incapable of further recombination (Atasoy et al. 2008, Schnutgen et al. 2003). This Cre-dependent viral approach is commonly referred to as a FLEX switch or double-floxed inverse open reading frame (DIO) (Atasoy et al. 2008, Witten et al. 2010) and is used to target specific cell types with spatial precision via intracranial surgeries in distinct Cre driver mouse lines.

Two methods, optogenetics and chemogenetics, devised for manipulating neural activity in vivo have benefited tremendously from this viral approach. Optogenetics involves the use of microbial and chimeric-vertebrate opsin genes that have been developed to control highly defined electrical activity with cell-type selectivity, high temporal precision, and rapid reversibility. As most neurons in the brain are not naturally light-sensitive, selective expression of opsin genes in targeted neural populations makes it possible to specifically control the activity in these populations through optical light delivery, and the resulting fast on–off kinetics make it possible to evoke or inhibit neural activity within milliseconds, on a timescale relevant to physiological brain function (Tye and Deisseroth 2012, Yizhar et al. 2011).

The most widely used opsin to stimulate neural activity is channelrhodopsin2 (ChR2), a nonselective cation channel isolated from algae, which leads to action potential firing upon blue light photostimulation (Figure 5.1F) (Boyden et al. 2005). For cell silencing, common opsins are the chloride pump halorhodopsin (eNpHR) (Gradinaru, Thompson, and Deisseroth 2008, Zhang et al. 2007) and the hydrogen pump archaerhodopsin-3 (Arch) (Chow et al. 2010) that enables hyperpolarization of membranes to eliminate the production of action potentials upon yellow light photoinhibition (Figure 5.1G). Recently, structure guided protein engineering was utilized to convert ChR2 (originally cation-conducting) into chloride-conducting anion channels, resulting in more physiological, efficient, and sensitive optogenetic inhibition (Figure 5.1H) (Berndt et al. 2014, Wietek et al. 2014).

These channels and pumps are membranous and are expressed on the soma as well as neural processes from dendritic arborizations to long-range axonal projections. Optical fibers are then implanted into the animal and an external light source, such as a laser or light-emitting diode, is used to supply the appropriate wavelength of light to the targeted tissue. Depending on the location of the optical fiber implant, experimenters have meticulous control over cell body stimulation or specific trajectory-defined projections and can then evaluate the effect of such manipulation on behavioral output (Tye et al. 2011).

Chemogenetics is a system to control neuronal activity noninvasively in the mammalian brain by regulating signaling through a G-protein-coupled receptor (GPCR) (Armbruster et al. 2007, Luo, Callaway, and Svoboda 2008) or recently using ligand-activated ion channels (Atasoy et al. 2012, Magnus et al. 2011, Stachniak, Ghosh, and Sternson 2014). These pharmacological approaches to manipulate neuronal activity through GPCR signaling pathways in neurons both in vitro and in vivo include ectopic expression of either GPCRs with engineered binding sites such as receptors activated solely by synthetic ligands (RASSLs) (Redfern et al. 1999, Zhao et al. 2003) or nonnative GPCRs such as the *Drosophila* allatostatin receptor (AlstR) (Lechner, Lein, and Callaway 2002, Tan et al. 2006).

Despite the vast contributions utilizing these methods, continued improvements are needed to facilitate regulation of activity of discrete populations of CNS neurons selectively and noninvasively in vivo. RASSLs, for example, are activated by nonselective, pharmacologically active small molecules and in some tissues exhibit high levels of signaling in the absence of exogenous small-molecule agonists, which can result in pathologic phenotypes (Hsiao et al. 2008, Peng et al. 2008, Redfern et al. 2000, Sweger et al. 2007). Although AlstR displays no evidence of basal signaling, it does not allow for remote manipulations of neuronal activity, as its ligand is unlikely to cross the blood–brain barrier and must be directly infused into brain tissue (Tan et al. 2006). Furthermore, AlstR is coupled only to neuronal silencing so it cannot be used for neuronal activation.

Advancing on these methods, designer receptors exclusively activated by designer drug (DREADDs) were developed to provided researchers with a system for neuronal regulation in which (1) the exogenous ligand would be pharmacologically inert, (2) the exogenous ligand could be administered in the periphery and cross the blood–brain barrier to access receptors in deep brain structures and/or widely distributed neuronal populations, (3) receptor expression alone would not induce pathology, (4) neuronal activity could be both increased and decreased, and (5) both spatial and temporal resolution would be sufficient to facilitate study of brain function in health and disease (Alexander et al. 2009).

The most commonly employed DREADDs are molecularly evolved GPCRs derived from human muscarinic receptors that have lost the ability to bind the endogenous ligand, acetylcholine, and instead have been mutated so they are only activated by the pharmacologically inert compound, clozapine-N-oxide (CNO) (Figure 5.1C) (Armbruster et al. 2007, Conklin et al. 2008). Importantly, distinct DREADD receptors have been generated to stimulate neural activity, through the canonical G_q (Alexander et al. 2009, Armbruster et al. 2007) or G_s (Farrell et al. 2013) signaling pathways, or inhibit neural activity, via $G_{i/o}$ molecular signaling (Armbruster et al. 2007, Ferguson et al. 2013). Recently, a structure-based approach was applied to develop a new $G_{i/o}$-coupled DREADD using the kappa-opiod receptor (KORD) as a template that is activated by the otherwise inert ligand salvinorin B (Figure 5.1D) (Vardy et al. 2015). These tools can be used synergistically to facilitate the sequential and bidirectional remote control of behavior. Additionally, ligand-gated ion channels with orthogonal pharmacologic selectivity and divergent functional properties have been developed which grant more refined temporal precision (Figure 5.1E) (Magnus et al. 2011).

5.2.2 BENEFITS AND DRAWBACKS

The ideal platform for manipulating neuronal activity would require no specialized equipment and would provide noninvasive, multiplexed spatiotemporal control of neuronal activity in domains ranging from single synapses to ensembles of neurons. Although both optogenetic and chemogenetic technologies are now extensively utilized, leading to thousands of publications, both technologies in their current incarnations suffer from inherent limitations hindering their ability to fulfill this particular ideal.

Each method possesses its own unique advantages and disadvantages. For instance, many optogenetic approaches, as opposed to chemogenetic strategies, are integrally invasive, requiring the implantation of an optical fiber into the brain, and involve specialized equipment such as multichannel programmable light sources, cleanly cleaved optical fiber implants, and expensive patchcords used to transmit the light from the source to the implant. Additionally, intervention can lead to brain tissue damage through overheating from the photon source, which is problematic for long-term manipulations. Furthermore, the scalability of the size or number of neurons in the brain is limited due to the absorption, scattering, and distance-dependent decay of light through brain tissue and subsequent attenuation of light delivered to a target site. Finally, much of the photoactivation and photoinhibition is nonphysiologic because artificially synchronized patterns of excitation/inhibition are commonly induced with varying degrees of effect on behavior (Kravitz and Bonci 2013), as compared to the canonical GPCR signaling of DREADDs.

Despite these apparent caveats, optogenetics, unlike chemogenetic approaches, provides precise spatiotemporal millisecond-scale control, does not undergo desensitization, is capable of multiplexing with remarkable spectral diversity (although KORD now allows for chemogenetic multiplexing; that is, employing distinct tools to simultaneously or sequentially manipulate different neural subpopulations) (Vardy et al. 2015), and importantly allows for neuronal subdomain-specific modulation via excitation of opsins in axonal fibers (although backpropagating action potentials have been reported). Thus, both schemes of acute neuronal manipulation comprise of benefits and shortcomings depending on the particular application. However, these methodologies are constantly being modified and expanded upon to continually provide researchers with the latest and greatest tools to control molecularly circumscribed cell types and to direct behavior.

Merging viral-assisted, Cre-dependent strategies to deliver optogenetic and chemogenetic tools with various Cre-recombinase expressing mouse lines grants researchers with unprecedented, demarcated control of neuronal subtypes allowing for the probing of causal relationships of defined, cellular manipulation with a myriad of behaviors, a task unheard of before the advent of these methodologies. Since the introduction of these novel techniques, the feeding field has made significant progress in the understanding of neural circuits underlying the homeostatic and hedonic processes of appetite regulation. Given the immense heterogeneity that exists in the brain, particularly in elaborate structures such as the hypothalamus, it is absolutely essential to have tools that ensure specific manipulation of delineated cell types. The key to dissecting a complex anatomical neural circuit is to find a key node in which to start. Once identified, additional strategies can be used to deconstruct these multifaceted networks and unravel functional connectivity, ultimately helping us comprehend just how these circuits guide behavior. The natural question is where do we begin?

5.3 AN ENTRY POINT INTO FEEDING CIRCUITRY—ARC^{AgRP} NEURONS

5.3.1 Appetite-State Dependent Activity Changes

ARC^{AgRP} neurons are unique in that they are state dependent, meaning that their neural activity differs depending on the caloric condition of the animal. As assessed in ex vivo brain slices, these neurons are relatively quiescent when mice are sated and fire at a much higher frequency when the animals are physiologically hungry or fasted (Krashes et al. 2013, Takahashi and Cone 2005), which is related to increased excitatory transmission onto ARC^{AgRP} neurons (Liu et al. 2012, Yang et al. 2011). However, it should be noted that a major limitation to acute, brain slice electrophysiology experiments is the inevitable severing of neural processes, and thus, disconnection in the intact brain network should be considered when interpreting results. Recently, in vivo photometry- and endoscopy-based imaging of these cells using genetically encoded calcium indicators (GCaMP) as well as in vivo electrode recordings demonstrated high activity levels in hungry animals and an immediate cessation of firing due to the detection of a food source, a response that was potentiated with calorically rich food, and one that could be conditioned through expectation of caloric reward (Betley et al. 2015, Chen et al. 2015, Mandelblat-Cerf et al. 2015). Importantly, this permanent shut down of ARC^{AgRP} neural activity was dependent on the subsequent consumption of caloric sustenance after detection (Betley et al. 2015, Chen et al. 2015, Mandelblat-Cerf et al. 2015).

Additionally, pharmacological administration of the peptides released by these neurons (AgRP and neuropeptide Y [NPY]) (Clark et al. 1984, Rossi et al. 1998, Semjonous et al. 2009) or GABA receptor agonists (Stratford and Kelley 1997) systemically or into downstream ARC^{AgRP} target regions induces a robust hyperphagic response. Finally, given the severe reduction in body weight and food intake observed following acute ARC^{AgRP} cell ablation in adults (Gropp et al. 2005, Luquet et al. 2005), ARC^{AgRP} neurons were the ideal testing ground for these innovative, remote, and reversible tools.

5.3.2　RAPID, REMOTE, AND REVERSIBLE NEURAL ACTIVATION

Optogenetic and chemogenetic ARC^{AgRP} neuronal stimulation evoked rapid feeding in naïve animals (Figure 5.2) (Aponte, Atasoy, and Sternson 2011, Krashes et al.

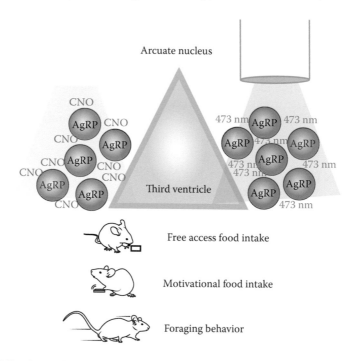

FIGURE 5.2　Acute chemogenetic or optogenetic activation of ARC^{AgRP} neurons lining the third ventricle is sufficient to elicit both ad libitum and motivated food intake and foraging behavior in the absence of food.

2011). Importantly, this induction of feeding occurred in calorically replete mice with no homeostatic motive to consume food. Remarkably, activation of as little as 800 out of 10,000 ARC^{AgRP} neurons, with a 1-second burst of light pulses at a frequency of 20 Hz, was sufficient to drive a "ceiling" feeding effect with sated mice eating up to 1 gram of food in an hour (Aponte, Atasoy, and Sternson 2011, Betley et al. 2013). Both the amount of food consumed and the latency to first meal were dependent on the number of ARC^{AgRP} neurons activated (Aponte, Atasoy, and Sternson 2011). Furthermore, the initial hour of feeding during optogenetic ARC^{AgRP} photoactivation was independent of the melanocortin pathway (Aponte, Atasoy, and Sternson 2011).

Chemogenetic DREADD-mediated ARC^{AgRP} stimulation resulted in escalated feeding over several hours as a single injection of CNO (0.3 mg/kg) continued to activate the targeted receptor (predicted half-life ~8 hours) (Alexander et al. 2009, Krashes et al. 2011). Interestingly, after the acute activation of ARC^{AgRP} neurons with DREADD technology, both GABA and NPY were found to be required for the rapid stimulation of feeding, and the neuropeptide AgRP, through action on melanocortin-4 receptors (MC4Rs), was sufficient to induce feeding over a delayed yet prolonged period. It should be noted that these experiments were done in genetic knockout (KO) models and significant compensation may impact the interpretation of the findings (Krashes et al. 2013). Chronic activation of ARC^{AgRP} neurons over 5 days caused marked weight gain, accompanied by increased fat stores, due to hyperphagia and most likely decreased energy expenditure, and acute ARC^{AgRP} activation drastically reduced energy expenditure (Krashes et al. 2011). Remarkably, following drug withdrawal, the CNO-induced obesity and increased fat mass were normalized, and this reversal was associated with compensatory hypophagia (Krashes et al. 2011). A similar magnitude of food consumption was observed using an alternative chemogenetic approach relying on the Trpv1 cation channel and the exogenous agonist capsaicin (Caterina et al. 1997, Dietrich et al. 2015).

It has been suggested that the hypothalamic neurocircuitry responsible for integrating metabolic signals is embedded within a complex network that permits both the adaptation and synchronization of nutrient needs to conditions in the animal's local environment (Shin, Zheng, and Berthoud 2009). It is likely that these same neurons invoke neural mechanisms of reward, motivation, and decision making, all of which are integrated to serve the ultimate goal of obtaining and ingesting food.

Of note, ARC^{AgRP} neurons not only drive homeostatic feeding when food is freely available but also engage a behavioral program to work for and seek out food. Chemogenetic or optogenetic ARC^{AgRP} activation significantly increased a sated animal's willingness to work for food as determined through an instrumental nosepoke or leverpress assay, in a similar magnitude to that induced by the calorically deficient, fasted state (Atasoy et al. 2012, Krashes et al. 2011). To further investigate goal-directed behavior aimed at food acquisition, physical activity was measured during the light cycle, when mice normally are relatively inactive. Chemogenetic stimulation of ARC^{AgRP} neurons in the absence of food led to intense, unrelenting activity, a behavioral state that continued unabated for hours (Krashes et al. 2011). This was interpreted as food-seeking behavior for two major reasons. First, the mice were often seen visiting areas of the cage where food was normally located or accumulated and they engaged in vigorous digging-type behaviors. Second, when the same mice were again given CNO on a different day in the presence of food, this sharp increase in activity was completely absent, indicating that the activity was directed toward the acquisition and consumption of food (Krashes et al. 2011). This finding was validated when the increased exploratory behavior was replicated using the Trpv1/capsaicin system (Dietrich et al. 2015).

5.3.3 IDENTIFYING DOWNSTREAM NODES

In addition to probing behavioral outcomes in vivo during acute optogenetic manipulation, channelrhodpsin2-assisted circuit mapping (CRACM) can be used to establish monosynaptic connectivity between two sets of neurons through ex vivo acute brain slice electrophysiology (Petreanu et al. 2007). To determine if neurons are functionally connected, "upstream" neurons expressing ChR2 are photostimulated and candidate "downstream" neurons are assessed for coincident postsynaptic currents: excitatory postsynaptic currents (EPSCs) in the case of glutamatergic inputs or inhibitory postsynaptic currents in the case of GABAergic inputs. The advantage of ChR2 is that it is trafficked to the terminals so that when these experiments are done in brain slices, the soma of the transduced cell is not required. Therefore, long-range connections can be properly analyzed.

A number of studies have employed a multitude of optogenetic and chemogenetic approaches to investigate downstream ARC[AgRP] connections and circuits, respective functional contributions on feeding behavior, and anatomical architecture (Atasoy et al. 2012, Betley et al. 2013, Garfield et al. 2015). Photoactivation of ARC[AgRP] terminal fields in the PVH, LH, anterior bed nucleus of the stria terminalus (aBNST), and to a lesser extent the paraventricular thalamus (PVT) was sufficient to elicit feeding behavior in calorically replete mice, while ARC[AgRP] terminal field photostimulation of the periaqueductal grey (PAG), central nucleus of the amygdala (CeA) or parabrachial nucleus (PBN) failed to induce food intake (Figure 5.3) (Atasoy et al. 2012, Betley et al. 2013, Garfield et al. 2015). Interestingly, pharmacological blockade of the NPY receptor Y_1 or of $GABA_A$ receptors abrogated the ARC[AgRP] → PVH neuron-evoked elevation of food intake, suggesting that selective antagonism of either of the inhibitory signals, NPY or GABA, was required for acute food intake (Atasoy et al. 2012). This finding suggests that NPY and GABA are not redundant and supports the idea of compensatory mechanisms in genetic deletion models. In fact, circuit characterization experiments in NPY KO mice displayed marked strengthening of GABA signaling in ARC[AgRP] → PVH circuitry (Atasoy et al. 2012). This could explain the rapid (GABA and NPY) versus delayed (AgRP) stimulation of feeding by ARC[AgRP] neuromediators following chemogenetic activation in KO backgrounds (Krashes et al. 2013).

Circuit mapping was used to investigate monosynaptic connectivity between ARC[AgRP] neurons and potential downstream anatomical brain sites, revealing inhibitory, monosynaptic connections to the ARC, PVH, LH, aBNST, PVT, and PBN, which were blocked by the $GABA_A$-R antagonist, PTX (Atasoy et al. 2008, 2012, Garfield et al. 2015). More specifically, ARC[AgRP] neurons synapse directly onto nearby ARC[POMC] neurons, without forming autaptic (self-sensing) connections (Atasoy et al.

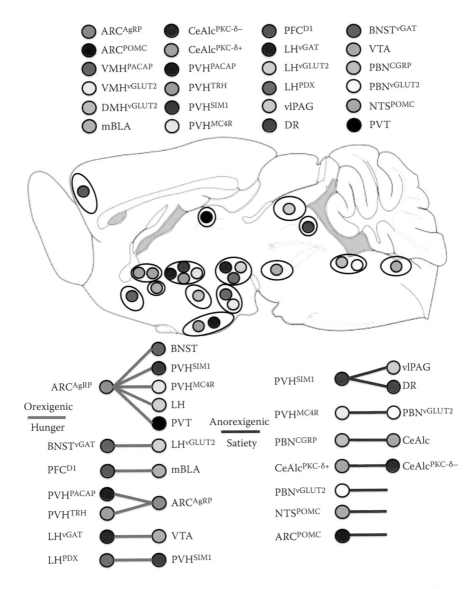

FIGURE 5.3 Multiple brain nodes implicated in feeding behavior via chemogenetic and optogenetic techniques.

2012). Although acute ARC[POMC] activation induced satiety and subsequent diminished feeding over days (Figure 5.3) (Aponte, Atasoy, and Sternson 2011, Atasoy et al. 2012, Zhan et al. 2013), simultaneous optogenetic activation of ARC[AgRP] and ARC[POMC] neurons still remained sufficient to promote acute food intake, strongly suggesting alternative downstream targets of ARC[AgRP] neurons and the slower temporal kinetics of satiety signals released by ARC[POMC] neurons (Aponte, Atasoy, and Sternson 2011, Atasoy et al. 2012, Zhan et al. 2013). It should be noted that chemogenetic silencing of ARC[POMC] neurons evoked increases in feeding, but this also occurred over 24 hours, further supporting the slower temporal kinetics of *Pomc*-derived peptides (Atasoy et al. 2012).

5.3.3.1 Putting the PVH on the Map

To pinpoint the relevant downstream ARC[AgRP] circuits mediating feeding behavior, a variety of optogenetic and chemogenetic strategies were employed. The majority of studies focused on the PVH, based on (a) pharmacology, (b) lesion, (c) microscopy, and (d) mapping data, strongly implicating this structure as a putative downstream target of ARC[AgRP] neurons (Aravich and Sclafani 1983, Atasoy et al. 2014, Broberger et al. 1998, Gold, Jones, and Sawchenko 1977). The majority of PVH neurons are marked by the transcription factor *Single-minded 1* (SIM1), which is required for proper development (Michaud et al. 1998). Both knock out of *Sim1* or ablation of PVH[SIM1] neurons trigger obesity (Tolson et al. 2010, Xi et al. 2012). To demonstrate sufficiency of these PVH[SIM1] neurons as well as their direct influence on the ARC[AgRP] neural circuit, ChR2 was used to costimulate the ARC[AgRP] → PVH projections and PVH[SIM1] neurons, which completely suppressed the ARC[AgRP] neuron-induced eating (Atasoy et al. 2012). Concordantly, deletion of the GABA-A receptor γ2 subunit in PVH[SIM1] neurons impaired GABAergic input and reduced feeding (Wu et al. 2015).

In attempts to determine which specific subset of PVH[SIM1] neurons were responsible for this occlusion, it was reported that simultaneous photostimulation of ARC[AgRP] → PVH projections and neurons marked by a mouse *oxytocin* (OXT) promoter fragment completely suppressed the ARC[AgRP] → PVH-evoked increase in food intake (Atasoy et al. 2012). However, a similar experiment using a knock-in mouse driving Cre expression under endogenous *Oxt* regulatory elements failed to find an attenuation of the ARC[AgRP] → PVH-driven feeding, which was consistent with the lack of detectable direct connectivity between ARC[AgRP] → PVH[OXT] neurons (Garfield et al. 2015). These inconsistencies could be explained by the different reagents used to label PVH[OXT] neurons. Interestingly, bilateral photoactivation of PVH[OXT] neurons alone in calorically deficient animals was not sufficient to inhibit feeding following reintroduction to food after deprivation, which is consistent with the lack of feeding effect described after acute ablation or bidirectional chemogenetic manipulation of OXT[PVH] neurons (Atasoy et al. 2012, Garfield et al. 2015, Sutton et al. 2014, Wu et al. 2012).

Although a recent report failed to detect direct ARC[AgRP] → PVH[OXT] or ARC[AgRP] → PVH[CRH] (corticotropin-releasing hormone) connectivity, neurons expressing MC4R represent a highly enriched population of PVH cells that received monosynaptic input from ARC[AgRP] neurons (Garfield et al. 2015). Functional occlusion studies demonstrated that these PVH[MC4R] neurons, but not aBNST[MC4R] or LH[MC4R] neurons, are a key second-order node in the ARC[AgRP] circuitry. Furthermore, bidirectional chemogenetic activation or inhibition of PVH[SIM1] or PVH[MC4R] neurons (a small subset of the former) rapidly evoked decreases and increases in food consumption (Atasoy et al. 2012, Garfield et al. 2015, Sutton et al. 2014). Of note, silencing of these neurons elevated motivational food consumption using instrumental operant tasks, indicating behavioral programs beyond free feeding (Atasoy et al. 2012, Garfield et al. 2015). These two PVH populations were utilized to further examine the downstream circuits required to disentangle the complex neural networks coordinating feeding behavior (Garfield et al. 2015, Stachniak, Ghosh, and Sternson 2014).

5.3.3.2 Pinpointing Third-Order Nodes

A recent study engineered an inhibitory DREADD targeted to neural processes to silence synapses (Stachniak, Ghosh, and Sternson 2014). Through the use of cannula implantations, CNO was infused to specific downstream PVH^{SIM1} projection sites and food intake was measured. Synaptic silencing of PVH^{SIM1} axons to the midbrain, near the ventral-lateral portion of the PAG and dorsal raphe, promptly and robustly stimulated feeding in sated animals, while suppressing signaling to the PBN and nucleus of the solitary tract (NTS) had no significant effect on food intake (Figure 5.3) (Stachniak, Ghosh, and Sternson 2014). Another study employed gain-of-function experiments to rapidly activate PVH^{MC4R} neural projections to these downstream brain sites and found that the PVH^{MC4R} → lateral parabrachial nucleus (LPBN) circuit primarily mediated the satiety effects of these neurons (Figure 5.3) (Garfield et al. 2015). Further synaptic loss-of-function studies will be vital to establish the necessity of the PVH^{MC4R} → LPBN axis in feeding behavior. Of note, no feeding effect was observed from stimulation of PVH^{MC4R} terminals within the NTS/DMV, suggesting that these projections may influence other aspects of PVH^{MC4R}-regulated physiology, potentially concerning facets of autonomic nervous system function such as gastric motility or insulin release. Furthermore, this explicit pathway encoded positive valence in hungry animals, consistent with the negative teaching signal transmitted from upstream ARC^{AgRP} neurons (Betley et al. 2015, Garfield et al. 2015).

5.3.4 SILENCING LEADS TO APPETITE SUPPRESSION

These studies convincingly demonstrated the sufficiency of ARC^{AgRP} neurons in promoting feeding behavior. To further address whether these same neurons were acutely required for feeding behavior, a chemogenetic approach was used to inhibit ARC^{AgRP} activity, which attenuated firing rate in brain slices and resulted in reduced food intake in calorically deficient mice in vivo (Betley et al. 2015, Krashes et al. 2011, Vardy et al. 2015). This finding was consistent with the observation that adult animals with acute ARC^{AgRP} ablation displayed cessation of feeding to the point of starvation (Gropp et al. 2005, Luquet et al. 2005). However, since acute chemogenetic inhibition was restricted to the cell soma, the necessity of discrete axonal projection targets has yet to be elucidated.

5.4 NOVEL PBN CIRCUITS UNDERLYING FEEDING

5.4.1 DOWNSTREAM OF ARC^{AgRP} NEURONS

Interestingly, the termination of feeding behavior as a result of diphtheria-toxin directed deletion of ARC^{AgRP} neurons can be rescued by the delivery of the GABA$_A$ receptor partial agonist bretazenil, specifically to the PBN, suggesting that hyperactivity within the PBN following loss of GABAergic input from ARC^{AgRP} neurons promotes anorexia (Wu, Boyle, and Palmiter 2009). Of note, although ARC[AgRP] neurons are monosynaptically connected to PBN cells, optogenetic photostimulation of this discrete terminal field was insufficient to orchestrate food intake (Atasoy et al. 2012). However, these ARC[AgRP] ablation studies unveiled the PBN as a critical structural relay in signaling satiety. It is hypothesized that the loss of GABA signaling from ARC[AgRP] within the PBN results in unopposed excitation of the PBN, which in turn inhibits feeding. A pivotal study uncovered the source of excitatory inputs to the PBN coming from glutamatergic neurons, marked by vesicular glutamate transporter 2 (vGLUT2) in the NTS. These NTS[vGLUT2] neurons, via a caudal serotonergic signaling pathway, project to and control the excitability of PBN neurons and inhibit feeding. Further strengthening these results, genetic inactivation of glutamatergic signaling by the NTS onto N-methyl-D-aspartate-type glutamate receptors (NMDARs) in the PBN prevents starvation (Wu, Clark, and Palmiter 2012).

5.4.2 PBN[CGRP]-MEDIATED APPETITE SUPPRESSION

The importance of the PBN in modulating satiety led to the discovery of a neural population marked by calcitonin gene-related peptide (CGRP) that suppresses appetite (Carter et al. 2013). Fos expression in the PBN following the ablation of ARC[AgRP] neurons, intraperitoneal injection of lithium chloride (LiCl), injection of lipopolysaccharide (LPS), or the administration of the satiety hormones amylin or cholecystokinin (CCK) highly colocalized with immunohistochemical detection of CGRP, suggesting a key node for dampening appetite following a meal or during illness or exposure to toxins. Employing a toolbox of genetically encoded actuators, it was demonstrated that the activation of PBN[CGRP] neurons severely reduced food intake, while inhibition increased food intake during adverse conditions that normally subdue appetite (Figure 5.3) (Carter et al. 2013). Furthermore, these neurons mediated conditioned taste aversion, implying the encoding of a negative valence state (Carter, Han, and Palmiter 2015). Optogenetic photoactivation of PBN[CGRP] neurons projecting to the CeA (CeAlc), but not to the bed nucleus of the stria terminalus (BNST), recapitulated the loss of feeding observed after stimulation of PBN[CGRP] soma, while an innovative "collision" strategy combining the retrograde properties of a canine adenovirus (CAV2) carrying Cre recombinase with Cre-dependent inhibitory DREADD receptors, established the necessity of this projection to elevate feeding in circumstances that curb appetite (Carter et al. 2013).

Although the direct target of the anorectic PBN[CGRP] → CeAlc pathway has yet to be elucidated, another study characterized a subpopulation of GABAergic neurons marked by protein kinase C-δ (PKC-δ) that were activated in vivo by diverse anorexigenic signals (Cai et al. 2014). PBN[CGRP] neurons were identified monosynaptic inputs to this amygdala subpopulation using a retrograde modified rabies mapping technique (Wall et al. 2010, Wickersham et al. 2007). Furthermore, CeAlc[PKC-s] neural activity was required for the appetite-suppressing influences of CCK (which mimics satiety), LiCl (which induces nausea and visceral malaise), and LPS (which triggers a wide range of inflammatory and sickness responses). Finally, bidirectional control of food intake was achieved through optogenetic stimulation or inhibition of

CeAlc[PKC-δ] neurons, leading to respective decreases and increases in intake independent of anxiety (Figure 5.3) (Cai et al. 2014).

5.5 ARC[AgRP] NEURAL PLASTICITY

5.5.1 Evaluating Glutamatergic Action on ARC[AgRP] Neurons

Fasting-induced activation of ARC[AgRP] neurons is associated with increased frequency of EPSCs (Liu et al. 2012, Yang et al. 2011). To investigate the physiologic significance of glutamatergic neurotransmission to ARC[AgRP] neurons, and more specifically its plasticity as regulated by NMDARs, mice lacking NMDARs specifically in ARC[AgRP] neurons were generated. Body weight and fat stores were markedly reduced in these mice, and this was due, at least in part, to reduced 24-hour ad libitum food intake (Liu et al. 2012). Additionally, rates of refeeding following a 24-hour fast were also significantly decreased. Interestingly, this same NMDAR deletion approach in ARC[POMC] neurons had no effect on energy homeostasis. Consistent with this, ARC[AgRP] neurons, but not ARC[POMC] neurons, were found to have abundant dendritic spines, the postsynaptic specializations where most excitatory synapses reside and within which NMDARs operate to control plasticity (Bito 2010, Higley and Sabatini 2008, Yuste 2011). Removal of NMDARs from ARC[AgRP] neurons reduced the number of spines by ~50% and modestly decreased the spine head size and spine neck length, suggesting that NMDARs positively affect the number and size of spines (Liu et al. 2012). Furthermore, fasting-induced increases in Fos protein as well as *Agrp* and *Npy* neuropeptide mRNAs were greatly attenuated in mice lacking functional NMDARs, specifically in ARC[AgRP] neurons (Liu et al. 2012). Fasting markedly increased spine number on ARC[AgRP] neuron dendrites, and this stimulatory effect on spine number was significantly reduced in mice lacking NMDARs on ARC[AgRP] neurons (Liu et al. 2012). Finally, fasting doubled the frequency of α-amino-3-hydroxy-5-methyl-4-isoxazolepropionic acid receptor (AMPAR)-isolated spontaneous and miniature EPSCs, and this effect was absent in brain slices from mice lacking postsynaptic NMDARs on ARC[AgRP] neurons (Liu et al. 2012, Yang et al. 2011).

5.5.2 Identifying Sources of Excitatory Input to ARC[AgRP] Neurons

These studies provided evidence that glutamatergic transmission onto ARC[AgRP] neurons was important for regulating this appetite-stimulating cell population, but the anatomical and molecular sources of this excitatory input were unclear. Modified rabies tracing in combination with ex vivo circuit mapping (CRACM) was employed to mark and verify functional monosynaptic connections to ARC[AgRP] neurons, revealing that intrahypothalmic, glutamatergic projections, marked by vGLUT2, emanating from the DMH and PVH directly synapse onto ARC[AgRP] neurons (Krashes et al. 2014). Interestingly, the synaptic strength of these two inputs differs dramatically, with PVH[vGLUT2] inputs displaying 3-fold higher amplitudes than DMH[vGLUT2] inputs, a 0% failure rate of light-evoked EPSCs (compared to ~35% for DMH inputs) and the ability to evoke action potentials in ARC^AgRP neurons ~75% of the time (versus 0% for DMH inputs).

Using a battery of knock-in Cre-expressing lines, it was demonstrated that specific subsets of PVH neurons marked by thyrotropin-releasing hormone (PVH^TRH) and pituitary adenylate cyclase-activating polypeptide (PVH^PACAP) were monosynaptically connected to ARC^AgRP neurons (Krashes et al. 2014). Laser-evoked EPSCs were detected in every ARC^AgRP neuron recorded following blue-light photostimulation of PVH^TRH or PVH^PACAP terminal fields in the ARC. Furthermore, chemogenetic stimulation of these afferent neurons in sated mice markedly activated ARC^AgRP neurons, detected by Fos induction, and generated significant feeding in sated animals (Figure 5.3) (Krashes et al. 2014). Conversely, acute inhibition of PVH^TRH neurons decreased food intake in physiologically hungry mice. Discovery of these afferent and efferent neurons capable of triggering hunger helps advance our understanding of how this intense motivational state is regulated.

5.6 INTRAHYPOTHALAMIC AND EXTRAHYPOTHALAMIC NEURAL MODULATION OF APPETITE

5.6.1 POMC-Mediated Satiety

Although the studies discussed earlier specifically focus on the contributions of hypothalamic nuclei in guiding feeding behavior, new findings have implicated a role for limbic and cortical regions as well as the hindbrain in governing food consumption. To further explore the respective contributions of ARC^POMC and NTS^POMC neurons in regulating feeding behavior and metabolism, chemogenetic strategies were applied to either acutely or chronically activate these distinct neural populations, which led to the identification that both subsets of POMC cells suppressed feeding behavior on different time scales. Acute activation of NTS^POMC neurons produced an immediate inhibition of food intake, while chronic stimulation was required for ARC^POMC neurons to suppress feeding, demonstrating discrete temporal kinetics and possibly neuromodulator-mediated responses of these two disparate POMC populations (Figure 5.3) (Zhan et al. 2013). Further divergence of these POMC subgroups was exhibited when diphtheria toxin-induced ablation of ARC^POMC, but not NTS^POMC, neurons increased food intake, reduced energy expenditure, and ultimately resulted in obesity and metabolic and endocrine disorders (Zhan et al. 2013).

5.6.2 Molecular Identification of a BNST → LH Feeding Circuit

As reviewed previously, the LH was known to be a crucial substrate for motivated behavior, including feeding, but the exact circuitry presiding over such control remained elusive. A recent study found that inhibitory, GABAergic-mediated synaptic inputs from the BNST, demarked by the expression of vesicular GABA transporter (vGAT), to the LH, particularly to neurons expressing vGLUT2, form a functional circuit underlying feeding (Figure 5.3) (Jennings et al. 2013). Bidirectional optogenetic manipulations of BNST^vGAT → LH terminal fields directed food intake, whereby photoactivation induced feeding in well-fed mice, but photoinhibition diminished feeding in food-deprived mice. Moreover, the motivational valence of this pathway revealed that animals found the stimulation of this inhibitory circuit appetitive and the suppression of the BNST^{vGAT}→LH pathway aversive, consistent with previous electrical stimulation experiments. Finally, after identifying that the downstream LH neurons targeted by this BNST^{vGAT} inhibitory circuit preferentially synapse onto glutamatergic cell types, ChR2-assisted circuit mapping, combined with single-cell gene expression profiling, showed that acute activation or inactivation of LH^{vGLUT2} neurons resulted in decreased or increased food consumption, respectively (Jennings et al. 2013).

5.6.3 Genetic Discovery of a LH → Ventral Tegmental Area Feeding Circuit

To further unravel the basal ganglia circuitry behind the control of food intake, two studies focused on real-time monitoring and manipulation of LH neurons. Activation of LH^{vGAT} neurons, molecularly distinct from cells expressing hypocretin (orexin) and melanin-concentrating hormone, produced appetitive and consummatory behaviors, while selective ablation attenuated weight gain, consumption, and motivation (Jennings et al. 2015). In vivo calcium imaging in freely behaving mice was used to record activity dynamics from hundreds of cells and identified LH^{vGAT} neurons that preferentially encoded aspects of either appetitive or consummatory behaviors, but rarely both (Jennings et al. 2015). Further supporting this, in vivo electrical recordings revealed a reciprocal pathway between the LH and the ventral tegmental area (VTA), which is involved in reward processing, whereby LH→VTA neurons encode the learned action of seeking a reward, independent of reward availability, and VTA→LH neurons encode reward-predictive cues and unexpected reward omission (Nieh et al. 2015). Moreover, excitation of LH-VTA projections promoted, whereas inhibition attenuated, compulsive sucrose seeking (Nieh et al. 2015). Finally, photoactivation of LH^{vGAT} → VTA neurons, but not LH^{vGLUT2} → VTA neurons, increased feeding behaviors, directed toward calorie consumption as well as nonspecific gnawing on nonedible objects (Figure 5.3) (Nieh et al. 2015). Corroborating these findings, postnatal deletion of *Vgat* from the LH significantly reduced feeding and body weight (Wu et al. 2015). Furthermore, photoactivation of PVH-projecting LH neurons expressing pancreas duodenum homeobox 1 promoter (Pdx) rapidly evoked robust food intake, an effect dependent on functional GABAergic signaling (Figure 5.3) (Wu et al. 2015).

5.6.4 Uncovering a Cortex → Amygdala Feeding Circuit

In mammals, the prefrontal cortex (PFC) plays a crucial role in decision making and regulation of behavior, and although it has been implicated in controlling food intake, a direct circuit underlying this mechanism was only recently described (Miller and Cohen 2001, Rangel, Camerer, and Montague 2008). After it was found out that D1 dopamine receptor (D1R) neural activity in the PFC was increased during feeding events, stimulatory or inhibitory opsins were selectively targeted to D1R^{PFC} neurons and found to drive and restrain food intake, respectively (Land et al. 2014).

Moreover, based on axonal projection mapping techniques, an important network was established between D1R^{PFC} neurons and caudal-medial basolateral nuclei of the amygdala (mBLA). The augmented feeding following cell body stimulation of D1R^{PFC} neurons was recapitulated when terminals to the mBLA were explicitly photostimulated (Figure 5.3). To experimentally verify the role of the mBLA in mediating this response, an occlusion study was carried out whereby D1R^{PFC} → mBLA terminals were photoactivated (a manipulation that normally drives food intake alone) with simultaneous photoinhibition of mBLA neurons, which resulted in food intake returning to baseline levels (Land et al. 2014).

5.7 CONCLUSIONS

The previously mentioned studies highlight the recent advances in understanding the neural circuits controlling food intake and food-seeking behavior that have been made possible by the development of novel genetic tools and techniques that acutely, remotely, and reversibly manipulate neural function. Employing these circuit-specific methodologies has and will continue to lead to a better understanding of how discrete subsets of neurons communicate with one another, link up to form complex networks and ultimately guide feeding behavior. Advances in comprehending these intricate circuits underlying appetite will steer potential therapeutic targets to successfully combat the multitude of food-related afflictions affecting people all over the globe.

LITERATURE CITED

Alexander, G. M., S. C. Rogan, A. I. Abbas, B. N. Armbruster, Y. Pei, J. A. Allen, R. J. Nonneman, J. Hartmann, S. S. Moy, M. A. Nicolelis, J. O. McNamara, and B. L. Roth. 2009. Remote control of neuronal activity in transgenic mice expressing evolved G protein-coupled receptors. *Neuron* 63:27–39.

Anand, B. K., S. Dua, and K. Shoenberg. 1955. Hypothalamic control of food intake in cats and monkeys. *J Physiol* 127:143–52.

Aponte, Y., D. Atasoy, and S. M. Sternson. 2011. AGRP neurons are sufficient to orchestrate feeding behavior rapidly and without training. *Nat Neurosci* 14:351–5.

Aravich, P. F., and A. Sclafani. 1983. Paraventricular hypothalamic lesions and medial hypothalamic knife cuts produce similar hyperphagia syndromes. *Behav Neurosci* 97:970–83.

Armbruster, B. N., X. Li, M. H. Pausch, S. Herlitze, and B. L. Roth. 2007. Evolving the lock to fit the key to create a family of G protein-coupled receptors potently activated by an inert ligand. *Proc Natl Acad Sci USA* 104:5163–8.

Atasoy, D., Y. Aponte, H. H. Su, and S. M. Sternson. 2008. A FLEX switch targets Channelrhodopsin-2 to multiple cell types for imaging and long-range circuit mapping. *J Neurosci* 28:7025–30.

Atasoy, D., J. N. Betley, W. P. Li, H. H. Su, S. M. Sertel, L. K. Scheffer, J. H. Simpson, R. D. Fetter, and S. M. Sternson. 2014. A genetically specified connectomics approach applied to long-range feeding regulatory circuits. *Nat Neurosci* 17:1830–9.

Atasoy, D., J. N. Betley, H. H. Su, and S. M. Sternson. 2012. Deconstruction of a neural circuit for hunger. *Nature* 488:172–7.

Bergen, H. T., T. M. Mizuno, J. Taylor, and C. V. Mobbs. 1998. Hyperphagia and weight gain after gold-thioglucose: Relation to hypothalamic neuropeptide Y and proopiomelanocortin. *Endocrinology* 139:4483–8.

Berndt, A., S. Y. Lee, C. Ramakrishnan, and K. Deisseroth. 2014. Structure-guided transformation of channelrhodopsin into a light-activated chloride channel. *Science* 344:420–4.

Berridge, K. C., and E. S. Valenstein. 1991. What psychological process mediates feeding evoked by electrical stimulation of the lateral hypothalamus? *Behav Neurosci* 105:3–14.

Betley, J. N., Z. F. Cao, K. D. Ritola, and S. M. Sternson. 2013. Parallel, redundant circuit organization for homeostatic control of feeding behavior. *Cell* 155:1337–50.

Betley, J. N., S. Xu, Z. F. Cao, R. Gong, C. J. Magnus, Y. Yu, and S. M. Sternson. 2015. Neurons for hunger and thirst transmit a negative-valence teaching signal. *Nature* 521:180–5.

Bito, H. 2010. The chemical biology of synapses and neuronal circuits. *Nat Chem Biol* 6:560–3.

Boghossian, S., M. Park, and D. A. York. 2010. Melanocortin activity in the amygdala controls appetite for dietary fat. *Am J Physiol Regul Integr Comp Physiol* 298:R385–93.

Booth, D. A. 1968. Mechanism of action of norepinephrine in eliciting an eating response on injection into the rat hypothalamus. *J Pharmacol Exp Ther* 160:336–48.

Boyden, E. S., F. Zhang, E. Bamberg, G. Nagel, and K. Deisseroth. 2005. Millisecond-timescale, genetically targeted optical control of neural activity. *Nat Neurosci* 8:1263–8.

Broberger, C., J. Johansen, C. Johansson, M. Schalling, and T. Hokfelt. 1998. The neuropeptide Y/agouti gene-related protein (AGRP) brain circuitry in normal, anorectic, and monosodium glutamate-treated mice. *Proc Natl Acad Sci USA* 95:15043–8.

Butler, A. A., R. A. Kesterson, K. Khong, M. J. Cullen, M. A. Pelleymounter, J. Dekoning, M. Baetscher, and R. D. Cone. 2000. A unique metabolic syndrome causes obesity in the melanocortin-3 receptor-deficient mouse. *Endocrinology* 141:3518–21.

Cai, H., W. Haubensak, T. E. Anthony, and D. J. Anderson. 2014. Central amygdala PKC-delta(+) neurons mediate the influence of multiple anorexigenic signals. *Nat Neurosci* 17:1240–8.

Carter, M. E., S. Han, and R. D. Palmiter. 2015. Parabrachial calcitonin gene-related peptide neurons mediate conditioned taste aversion. *J Neurosci* 35:4582–6.

Carter, M. E., M. E. Soden, L. S. Zweifel, and R. D. Palmiter. 2013. Genetic identification of a neural circuit that suppresses appetite. *Nature* 503:111–4.

Caterina, M. J., M. A. Schumacher, M. Tominaga, T. A. Rosen, J. D. Levine, and D. Julius. 1997. The capsaicin receptor: A heat-activated ion channel in the pain pathway. *Nature* 389:816–24.

Chen, Y., Y. C. Lin, T. W. Kuo, and Z. A. Knight. 2015. Sensory detection of food rapidly modulates arcuate feeding circuits. *Cell* 160:829–41.

Chow, B. Y., X. Han, A. S. Dobry, X. Qian, A. S. Chuong, M. Li, M. A. Henninger, G. M. Belfort, Y. Lin, P. E. Monahan, and E. S. Boyden. 2010. High-performance genetically targetable optical neural silencing by light-driven proton pumps. *Nature* 463:98–102.

Clark, J. T., P. S. Kalra, W. R. Crowley, and S. P. Kalra. 1984. Neuropeptide Y and human pancreatic polypeptide stimulate feeding behavior in rats. *Endocrinology* 115:427–9.

Cohen, P., C. Zhao, X. Cai, J. M. Montez, S. C. Rohani, P. Feinstein, P. Mombaerts, and J. M. Friedman. 2001. Selective deletion of leptin receptor in neurons leads to obesity. *J Clin Invest* 108:1113–21.

Conklin, B. R., E. C. Hsiao, S. Claeysen, A. Dumuis, S. Srinivasan, J. R. Forsayeth, J. M. Guettier, W. C. Chang, Y. Pei, K. D. McCarthy, R. A. Nissenson, J. Wess, J. Bockaert, and B. L. Roth. 2008. Engineering GPCR signaling pathways with RASSLs. *Nat Meth* 5:673–8.

de Backer, M. W., S. E. la Fleur, M. A. Brans, A. J. van Rozen, M. C. Luijendijk, M. Merkestein, K. M. Garner, E. M. van der Zwaal, and R. A. Adan. 2011. Melanocortin receptor-mediated effects on obesity are distributed over specific hypothalamic regions. *Int J Obes (Lond)* 35:629–41.

Dietrich, M. O., M. R. Zimmer, J. Bober, and T. L. Horvath. 2015. Hypothalamic Agrp neurons drive stereotypic behaviors beyond feeding. *Cell* 160:1222–32.

Fan, W., B. A. Boston, R. A. Kesterson, V. J. Hruby, and R. D. Cone. 1997. Role of melanocortinergic neurons in feeding and the agouti obesity syndrome. *Nature* 385:165–8.

Farrell, M. S., Y. Pei, Y. Wan, P. N. Yadav, T. L. Daigle, D. J. Urban, H. M. Lee, N. Sciaky, A. Simmons, R. J. Nonneman, X. P. Huang, S. J. Hufeisen, J. M. Guettier, S. S. Moy, J. Wess, M. G. Caron, N. Calakos, and B. L. Roth. 2013. A Galphas DREADD mouse for selective modulation of cAMP production in striatopallidal neurons. *Neuropsychopharmacology* 38:854–62.

Ferguson, S. M., P. E. Phillips, B. L. Roth, J. Wess, and J. F. Neumaier. 2013. Direct-pathway striatal neurons regulate the retention of decision-making strategies. *J Neurosci* 33:11668–76.

Garfield, A. S., C. Li, J. C. Madara, B. P. Shah, E. Webber, J. S. Steger, J. N. Campbell, O. Gavrilova, C. E. Lee, D. P. Olson, J. K. Elmquist, B. A. Tannous, M. J. Krashes, and B. B. Lowell. 2015. A neural basis for melanocortin-4 receptor-regulated appetite. *Nat Neurosci* 18:863–71.

Gold, R. M., A. P. Jones, and P. E. Sawchenko. 1977. Paraventricular area: Critical focus of a longitudinal neurocircuitry mediating food intake. *Physiol Behav* 18:1111–9.

Gold, R. M., P. M. Quackenbush, and G. Kapatos. 1972. Obesity following combination of rostrolateral to VMH cut and contralateral mammillary area lesion. *J Comp Physiol Psychol* 79:210–8.

Gradinaru, V., K. R. Thompson, and K. Deisseroth. 2008. eNpHR: A Natronomonas halorhodopsin enhanced for optogenetic applications. *Brain Cell Biol* 36:129–39.

Grill, H. J., A. B. Ginsberg, R. J. Seeley, and J. M. Kaplan. 1998. Brainstem application of melanocortin receptor ligands produces long-lasting effects on feeding and body weight. *J Neurosci* 18:10128–35.

Gropp, E., M. Shanabrough, E. Borok, A. W. Xu, R. Janoschek, T. Buch, L. Plum, N. Balthasar, B. Hampel, A. Waisman, G. S. Barsh, T. L. Horvath, and J. C. Bruning. 2005. Agouti-related peptide-expressing neurons are mandatory for feeding. *Nat Neurosci* 8:1289–91.

Grossman, S. P. 1960. Eating or drinking elicited by direct adrenergic or cholinergic stimulation of hypothalamus. *Science* 132:301–2.

Halaas, J. L., K. S. Gajiwala, M. Maffei, S. L. Cohen, B. T. Chait, D. Rabinowitz, R. L. Lallone, S. K. Burley, and J. M. Friedman. 1995. Weight-reducing effects of the plasma protein encoded by the obese gene. *Science* 269:543–6.

Higley, M. J., and B. L. Sabatini. 2008. Calcium signaling in dendrites and spines: Practical and functional considerations. *Neuron* 59:902–13.

Hoebel, B. G., and P. Teitelbaum. 1962. Hypothalamic control of feeding and self-stimulation. *Science* 135:375–7.

Holzwarth-McBride, M. A., E. M. Hurst, and K. M. Knigge. 1976. Monosodium glutamate induced lesions of the arcuate nucleus. I. Endocrine deficiency and ultrastructure of the median eminence. *Anat Rec* 186:185–205.

Holzwarth-McBride, M. A., J. R. Sladek, Jr., and K. M. Knigge. 1976. Monosodium glutamate induced lesions of the arcurate nucleus. II. Fluorescence histochemistry of catecholamines. *Anat Rec* 186:197–205.

Hsiao, E. C., B. M. Boudignon, W. C. Chang, M. Bencsik, J. Peng, T. D. Nguyen, C. Manalac, B. P. Halloran, B. R. Conklin, and R. A. Nissenson. 2008. Osteoblast expression of an engineered Gs-coupled receptor dramatically increases bone mass. *Proc Natl Acad Sci USA* 105:1209–14.

Huszar, D., C. A. Lynch, V. Fairchild-Huntress, J. H. Dunmore, Q. Fang, L. R. Berkemeier, W. Gu, R. A. Kesterson, B. A. Boston, R. D. Cone, F. J. Smith, L. A. Campfield, P. Burn, and F. Lee. 1997. Targeted disruption of the melanocortin-4 receptor results in obesity in mice. *Cell* 88:131–41.

Jennings, J. H., G. Rizzi, A. M. Stamatakis, R. L. Ung, and G. D. Stuber. 2013. The inhibitory circuit architecture of the lateral hypothalamus orchestrates feeding. *Science* 341:1517–21.

Jennings, J. H., R. L. Ung, S. L. Resendez, A. M. Stamatakis, J. G. Taylor, J. Huang, K. Veleta, P. A. Kantak, M. Aita, K. Shilling-Scrivo, C. Ramakrishnan, K. Deisseroth, S. Otte, and G. D. Stuber. 2015. Visualizing hypothalamic network dynamics for appetitive and consummatory behaviors. *Cell* 160:516–27.

Krashes, M. J., S. Koda, C. Ye, S. C. Rogan, A. C. Adams, D. S. Cusher, E. Maratos-Flier, B. L. Roth, and B. B. Lowell. 2011. Rapid, reversible activation of AgRP neurons drives feeding behavior in mice. *J Clin Invest* 121:1424–8.

Krashes, M. J., B. P. Shah, S. Koda, and B. B. Lowell. 2013. Rapid versus delayed stimulation of feeding by the endogenously released AgRP neuron mediators GABA, NPY, and AgRP. *Cell Metab* 18:588–95.

Krashes, M. J., B. P. Shah, J. C. Madara, D. P. Olson, D. E. Strochlic, A. S. Garfield, L. Vong, H. Pei, M. Watabe-Uchida, N. Uchida, S. D. Liberles, and B. B. Lowell. 2014. An excitatory paraventricular nucleus to AgRP neuron circuit that drives hunger. *Nature* 507:238–42.

Kravitz, A. V., and A. Bonci. 2013. Optogenetics, physiology, and emotions. *Front Behav Neurosci* 7:169.

Land, B. B., N. S. Narayanan, R. J. Liu, C. A. Gianessi, C. E. Brayton, D. M. Grimaldi, M. Sarhan, D. J. Guarnieri, K. Deisseroth, G. K. Aghajanian, and R. J. DiLeone. 2014. Medial prefrontal D1 dopamine neurons control food intake. *Nat Neurosci* 17:248–53.

Lechner, H. A., E. S. Lein, and E. M. Callaway. 2002. A genetic method for selective and quickly reversible silencing of Mammalian neurons. *J Neurosci* 22:5287–90.

Leibowitz, S. F. 1970. Reciprocal hunger-regulating circuits involving alpha- and beta-adrenergic receptors located, respectively, in the ventromedial and lateral hypothalamus. *Proc Natl Acad Sci USA* 67:1063–70.

Leibowitz, S. F., N. J. Hammer, and K. Chang. 1981. Hypothalamic paraventricular nucleus lesions produce overeating and obesity in the rat. *Physiol Behav* 27:1031–40.

Liu, T., D. Kong, B. P. Shah, C. Ye, S. Koda, A. Saunders, J. B. Ding, Z. Yang, B. L. Sabatini, and B. B. Lowell. 2012. Fasting activation of AgRP neurons requires NMDA receptors and involves spinogenesis and increased excitatory tone. *Neuron* 73:511–22.

Luo, L., E. M. Callaway, and K. Svoboda. 2008. Genetic dissection of neural circuits. *Neuron* 57:634–60.

Luquet, S., F. A. Perez, T. S. Hnasko, and R. D. Palmiter. 2005. NPY/AgRP neurons are essential for feeding in adult mice but can be ablated in neonates. *Science* 310:683–5.

Magnus, C. J., P. H. Lee, D. Atasoy, H. H. Su, L. L. Looger, and S. M. Sternson. 2011. Chemical and genetic engineering of selective ion channel-ligand interactions. *Science* 333:1292–6.

Mandelblat-Cerf, Y., R. N. Ramesh, C. R. Burgess, P. Patella, Z. Yang, B. B. Lowell, and M. L. Andermann. 2015. Arcuate hypothalamic AgRP and putative POMC neurons show opposite changes in spiking across multiple timescales. *Elife* 10;4 doi:10.7554/elife .07122.

Michaud, J. L., T. Rosenquist, N. R. May, and C. M. Fan. 1998. Development of neuroendocrine lineages requires the bHLH-PAS transcription factor SIM1. *Genes Dev* 12:3264–75.

Miller, E. K., and J. D. Cohen. 2001. An integrative theory of prefrontal cortex function. *Annu Rev Neurosci* 24:167–202.

Nieh, E. H., G. A. Matthews, S. A. Allsop, K. N. Presbrey, C. A. Leppla, R. Wichmann, R. Neve, C. P. Wildes, and K. M. Tye. 2015. decoding neural circuits that control compulsive sucrose seeking. *Cell* 160:528–41.

Ollmann, M. M., B. D. Wilson, Y. K. Yang, J. A. Kerns, Y. Chen, I. Gantz, and G. S. Barsh. 1997. Antagonism of central melanocortin receptors in vitro and in vivo by agouti-related protein. *Science* 278:135–8.

Panksepp, J. 1971. Aggression elicited by electrical stimulation of the hypothalamus in albino rats. *Physiol Behav* 6:321–9.

Peng, J., M. Bencsik, A. Louie, W. Lu, S. Millard, P. Nguyen, A. Burghardt, S. Majumdar, T. J. Wronski, B. Halloran, B. R. Conklin, and R. A. Nissenson. 2008. Conditional expression of a Gi-coupled receptor in osteoblasts results in trabecular osteopenia. *Endocrinology* 149:1329–37.

Petreanu, L., D. Huber, A. Sobczyk, and K. Svoboda. 2007. Channelrhodopsin-2-assisted circuit mapping of long-range callosal projections. *Nat Neurosci* 10:663–8.

Rangel, A., C. Camerer, and P. R. Montague. 2008. A framework for studying the neurobiology of value-based decision making. *Nat Rev Neurosci* 9:545–56.

Redfern, C. H., P. Coward, M. Y. Degtyarev, E. K. Lee, A. T. Kwa, L. Hennighausen, H. Bujard, G. I. Fishman, and B. R. Conklin. 1999. Conditional expression and signaling of a specifically designed Gi-coupled receptor in transgenic mice. *Nat Biotech* 17:165–9.

Redfern, C. H., M. Y. Degtyarev, A. T. Kwa, N. Salomonis, N. Cotte, T. Nanevicz, N. Fidelman, K. Desai, K. Vranizan, E. K. Lee, P. Coward, N. Shah, J. A. Warrington, G. I. Fishman, D. Bernstein, A. J. Baker, and B. R. Conklin. 2000. Conditional expression of a Gi-coupled receptor causes ventricular conduction delay and a lethal cardiomyopathy. *Proc Natl Acad Sci USA* 97:4826–31.

Rolls, E. T. 2000. Precis of The brain and emotion. *Behav Brain Sci* 23:177–91; discussion 192–233.

Rossi, M., M. S. Kim, D. G. Morgan, C. J. Small, C. M. Edwards, D. Sunter, S. Abusnana, A. P. Goldstone, S. H. Russell, S. A. Stanley, D. M. Smith, K. Yagaloff, M. A. Ghatei, and S. R. Bloom. 1998. A C-terminal fragment of agouti-related protein increases feeding and antagonizes the effect of alpha-melanocyte stimulating hormone in vivo. *Endocrinology* 139:4428–31.

Schnutgen, F., N. Doerflinger, C. Calleja, O. Wendling, P. Chambon, and N. B. Ghyselinck. 2003. A directional strategy for monitoring Cre-mediated recombination at the cellular level in the mouse. *Nat Biotech* 21:562–5.

Semjonous, N. M., K. L. Smith, J. R. Parkinson, D. J. Gunner, Y. L. Liu, K. G. Murphy, M. A. Ghatei, S. R. Bloom, and C. J. Small. 2009. Coordinated changes in energy intake and expenditure following hypothalamic administration of neuropeptides involved in energy balance. *Int J Obesity* 33:775–85.

Shin, A. C., H. Zheng, and H. R. Berthoud. 2009. An expanded view of energy homeostasis: Neural integration of metabolic, cognitive, and emotional drives to eat. *Physiol Behav* 97:572–80.

Stachniak, T. J., A. Ghosh, and S. M. Sternson. 2014. Chemogenetic synaptic silencing of neural circuits localizes a hypothalamus→midbrain pathway for feeding behavior. *Neuron* 82:797–808.

Sternson, S. M. 2013. Hypothalamic survival circuits: Blueprints for purposive behaviors. *Neuron* 77:810–24.

Stratford, T. R., and A. E. Kelley. 1997. GABA in the nucleus accumbens shell participates in the central regulation of feeding behavior. *J Neurosci* 17:4434–40.

Sutton, A. K., H. Pei, K. H. Burnett, M. G. Myers, Jr., C. J. Rhodes, and D. P. Olson. 2014. Control of food intake and energy expenditure by nos1 neurons of the paraventricular hypothalamus. *J Neurosci* 34:15306–18.

Sweger, E. J., K. B. Casper, K. Scearce-Levie, B. R. Conklin, and K. D. McCarthy. 2007. Development of hydrocephalus in mice expressing the G(i)-coupled GPCR Ro1 RASSL receptor in astrocytes. *J Neurosci* 27:2309–17.

Takahashi, K. A., and R. D. Cone. 2005. Fasting induces a large, leptin-dependent increase in the intrinsic action potential frequency of orexigenic arcuate nucleus neuropeptide Y/ agouti-related protein neurons. *Endocrinology* 146:1043–7.

Tan, E. M., Y. Yamaguchi, G. D. Horwitz, S. Gosgnach, E. S. Lein, M. Goulding, T. D. Albright, and E. M. Callaway. 2006. Selective and quickly reversible inactivation of mammalian neurons in vivo using the Drosophila allatostatin receptor. *Neuron* 51:157–70.

Teitelbaum, P., and A. N. Epstein. 1962. The lateral hypothalamic syndrome: Recovery of feeding and drinking after lateral hypothalamic lesions. *Psychol Rev* 69:74–90.

Tenen, S. S., and N. E. Miller. 1964. Strength of electrical stimulation of lateral hypothalamus, food deprivation, and tolerance for quinine in food. *J Comp Physiol Psychol* 58:55–62.

Tolson, K. P., T. Gemelli, L. Gautron, J. K. Elmquist, A. R. Zinn, and B. M. Kublaoui. 2010. Postnatal Sim1 deficiency causes hyperphagic obesity and reduced Mc4r and oxytocin expression. *J Neurosci* 30:3803–12.

Trowill, J. A., J. Panksepp, and R. Gandelman. 1969. An incentive model of rewarding brain stimulation. *Psychol Rev* 76:264–81.

Tye, K. M., and K. Deisseroth. 2012. Optogenetic investigation of neural circuits underlying brain disease in animal models. *Nat Rev Neurosci* 13:251–66.

Tye, K. M., R. Prakash, S. Y. Kim, L. E. Fenno, L. Grosenick, H. Zarabi, K. R. Thompson, V. Gradinaru, C. Ramakrishnan, and K. Deisseroth. 2011. Amygdala circuitry mediating reversible and bidirectional control of anxiety. *Nature* 471:358–62.

Valenstein, E. S., V. C. Cox, and J. W. Kakolewski. 1970. Reexamination of the role of the hypothalamus in motivation. *Psychol Rev* 77:16–31.

Vardy, E., J. E. Robinson, C. Li, R. H. Olsen, J. F. DiBerto, P. M. Giguere, F. M. Sassano, X. P. Huang, H. Zhu, D. J. Urban, K. L. White, J. E. Rittiner, N. A. Crowley, K. E. Pleil, C. M. Mazzone, P. D. Mosier, J. Song, T. L. Kash, C. J. Malanga, M. J. Krashes, and B. L. Roth. 2015. A New DREADD facilitates the multiplexed chemogenetic interrogation of behavior. *Neuron* 86:936–46.

Vaughan, E., and A. E. Fisher. 1962. Male sexual behavior induced by intracranial electrical stimulation. *Science* 137:758–60.

Wall, N. R., I. R. Wickersham, A. Cetin, M. De La Parra, and E. M. Callaway. 2010. Monosynaptic circuit tracing in vivo through Cre-dependent targeting and complementation of modified rabies virus. *Proc Natl Acad Sci USA* 107:21848–53.

Wickersham, I. R., S. Finke, K. K. Conzelmann, and E. M. Callaway. 2007. Retrograde neuronal tracing with a deletion-mutant rabies virus. *Nature Methods* 4:47–9.

Wietek, J., J. S. Wiegert, N. Adeishvili, F. Schneider, H. Watanabe, S. P. Tsunoda, A. Vogt, M. Elstner, T. G. Oertner, and P. Hegemann. 2014. Conversion of channelrhodopsin into a light-gated chloride channel. *Science* 344:409–12.

Williams, D. L., J. M. Kaplan, and H. J. Grill. 2000. The role of the dorsal vagal complex and the vagus nerve in feeding effects of melanocortin-3/4 receptor stimulation. *Endocrinology* 141:1332–7.

Witten, I. B., S. C. Lin, M. Brodsky, R. Prakash, I. Diester, P. Anikeeva, V. Gradinaru, C. Ramakrishnan, and K. Deisseroth. 2010. Cholinergic interneurons control local circuit activity and cocaine conditioning. *Science* 330:1677–81.

Wu, Q., M. P. Boyle, and R. D. Palmiter. 2009. Loss of GABAergic signaling by AgRP neurons to the parabrachial nucleus leads to starvation. *Cell* 137:1225–34.

Wu, Q., M. S. Clark, and R. D. Palmiter. 2012. Deciphering a neuronal circuit that mediates appetite. *Nature* 483:594–7.

Wu, Z., E. R. Kim, H. Sun, Y. Xu, L. R. Mangieri, D. P. Li, H. L. Pan, Y. Xu, B. R. Arenkiel, and Q. Tong. 2015. GABAergic projections from lateral hypothalamus to paraventricular hypothalamic nucleus promote feeding. *J Neurosci* 35:3312–8.

Wu, Z., Y. Xu, Y. Zhu, A. K. Sutton, R. Zhao, B. B. Lowell, D. P. Olson, and Q. Tong. 2012. An obligate role of oxytocin neurons in diet induced energy expenditure. *PloS One* 7:e45167.

Xi, D., N. Gandhi, M. Lai, and B. M. Kublaoui. 2012. Ablation of Sim1 neurons causes obesity through hyperphagia and reduced energy expenditure. *PloS One* 7:e36453.

Yang, Y., D. Atasoy, H. H. Su, and S. M. Sternson. 2011. Hunger states switch a flip-flop memory circuit via a synaptic AMPK-dependent positive feedback loop. *Cell* 146:992–1003.

Yaswen, L., N. Diehl, M. B. Brennan, and U. Hochgeschwender. 1999. Obesity in the mouse model of pro-opiomelanocortin deficiency responds to peripheral melanocortin. *Nat Med* 5:1066–70.

Yizhar, O., L. E. Fenno, T. J. Davidson, M. Mogri, and K. Deisseroth. 2011. Optogenetics in neural systems. *Neuron* 71:9–34.

Yuste, R. 2011. Dendritic spines and distributed circuits. *Neuron* 71:772–81.

Zhan, C., J. Zhou, Q. Feng, J. E. Zhang, S. Lin, J. Bao, P. Wu, and M. Luo. 2013. Acute and long-term suppression of feeding behavior by POMC neurons in the brainstem and hypothalamus, respectively. *J Neurosci* 33:3624–32.

Zhang, Y., R. Proenca, M. Maffei, M. Barone, L. Leopold, and J. M. Friedman. 1994. Positional cloning of the mouse obese gene and its human homologue. *Nature* 372:425–32.

Zhang, F., L. P. Wang, M. Brauner, J. F. Liewald, K. Kay, N. Watzke, P. G. Wood, E. Bamberg, G. Nagel, A. Gottschalk, and K. Deisseroth. 2007. Multimodal fast optical interrogation of neural circuitry. *Nature* 446:633–9.

Zhao, G. Q., Y. Zhang, M. A. Hoon, J. Chandrashekar, I. Erlenbach, N. J. Ryba, and C. S. Zuker. 2003. The receptors for mammalian sweet and umami taste. *Cell* 115:255–66.

6 The Use of Functional Magnetic Resonance Imaging in the Study of Appetite and Obesity

Selin Neseliler, Jung-Eun Han, and Alain Dagher

CONTENTS

6.1 INTRODUCTION

The brain regulates food intake in order to maintain energy homeostasis, which is required for survival (Woods, 2009). Information about the immediate and long-term state of energy balance in the body comes from three main sources: peptide hormones from the gut and adipose tissue, circulating nutrients such as glucose and lipids, and vagal afferents. These signals are integrated in the nucleus of the solitary tract (NTS) in the medulla, which is the major afferent target of the vagus nerve, and in the hypothalamus (Morton et al., 2014). They modulate eating behavior by communicating with the brain centers involved in learning, motivation, and decision making (Begg and Woods, 2013). However, food choices not *only* are under the influence of current energy balance but are also guided by the presence of food cues such as the sight, the smell, or the taste of food, which signal availability; by habits and social factors (e.g., eating at specific times); and by cognitive factors, such as a desire for health or the cost of food (Zheng et al., 2009).

    Here, we will review how the function of these systems can be studied in humans by functional magnetic resonance imaging (fMRI). fMRI relies on a measure called blood oxygenation level dependent (BOLD) contrast, which signals the activity-dependent change in the ratio of deoxyhemoglobin to oxyhemoglobin concentration due to increased neural activity (Kwong et al., 1992). It essentially measures energy usage by active neurons. The most common approach to study appetite with fMRI has been using food cues that have gained predictive value through previous experiences (Dagher, 2012). BOLD subtraction analyses are generally employed to investigate food-specific brain activations in different states (i.e., fasted vs. fed; lean vs. obese) and their modulation by peripheral signals of energy, personality traits (e.g., eating style, impulsivity), and outside influences such as stress or health information. In addition, the functional connectivity between brain areas can be assessed both during food tasks and rest. Connectivity analyses give information on how interactions between brain areas may underlie abnormalities in eating behavior (Carnell et al., 2012).

6.2 APPETITIVE BRAIN SYSTEMS PROMOTE FOOD INTAKE

The decision to eat results from the interaction between homeostatic signals and environmental signals of food availability (Rangel, 2013). Three interrelated brain systems regulate eating behavior (Figure 6.1): (1) the hypothalamus, implicated in

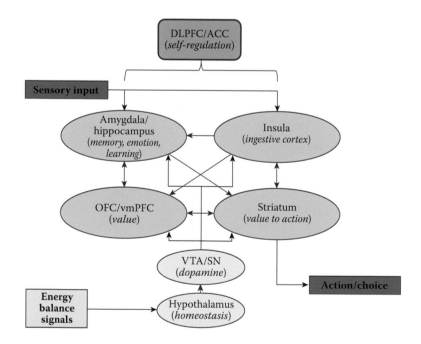

FIGURE 6.1 Appetitive and self-control brain networks. Four core regions (insula, medial temporal lobe, OFC/vmPFC, and striatum) encode the current incentive salience of sensed and available food rewards. Prefrontal regions may modulate appetitive network activity, enacting higher-level cognitive control of eating. Homeostatic signals influence this network in part via the hypothalamus and ascending dopaminergic projections.

energy homeostasis (Morton et al., 2006); (2) an "appetitive network" consisting of limbic and cortical systems that encode the incentive salience of foods (Dagher, 2012); and (3) the ventromedial, dorsomedial, and dorsolateral prefrontal cortices, which control goal-oriented and self-regulated behavior (Rangel, 2013).

Energy balance information from the body conveyed by the vagus nerve and blood-borne peptide hormones and nutrients enters the central nervous system (CNS) via the NTS and hypothalamus (Begg and Woods, 2013; Morton et al., 2006; Woods, 2009). The hypothalamus integrates the input from both long-term signals of peripheral energy stores (e.g., leptin, insulin, ghrelin) and short-term meal-related signals (e.g., macronutrients and gut-derived satiety signals, including, once again, insulin and ghrelin) to modulate the activity of higher-order brain networks that encode the incentive salience of available foods, a measure of both their intrinsic reward value and the current motivational state they produce. Our understanding of the role of the hypothalamus in food intake is mostly derived from animal research, as imaging this structure with fMRI has been a difficult technical challenge. Its proximity to air/tissue boundaries leads to distortion in the signal, and its location is especially prone to physiological artifact from pulse and respiration (Ojemann et al., 1997). Nonetheless, a few fMRI studies have utilized specialized scanning methods to show that the peripheral metabolic state is communicated to the hypothalamus. For example, glucose administration results in decreases in the hypothalamus BOLD signal in a dose-dependent matter (Little et al., 2014; Smeets et al., 2005, 2007, but see Purnell et al., 2011) and is reduced in patients with anorexia nervosa compared to controls (Van Opstal et al., 2015). Consistent with the role of the hypothalamus in communicating the metabolic state to the rest of the brain, resting state functional connectivity studies with fMRI show that it is connected with the appetitive and goal-directed systems described in Section 6.2 (Kullmann et al., 2014).

The NTS in the medulla is even more difficult to image with fMRI due to small size and physiological artifacts (Henderson and Macefield, 2013). However, a few studies have demonstrated changes in BOLD in the medulla in response to manipulations of intragastric nutrients such as glucose (Little et al., 2014) or lipids (Lassman et al., 2010) or responses to the gut peptides cholecystokinin (Lassman et al., 2010; Little et al., 2014) or ghrelin (Jones et al., 2012). These effects may represent gut to hindbrain signaling of energy balance information via the vagus nerve.

The appetitive network in the brain (Figure 6.1) is a set of interconnected regions whose activity as measured by fMRI consistently encodes the incentive salience of food cues (Figure 6.2). It consists of the hippocampus and the amygdala in the medial temporal lobe; the insula; the striatum; and the orbitofrontal cortex (OFC) and ventromedial prefrontal cortex (vmPFC) (Dagher, 2012). All these structures receive dopaminergic input from the midbrain and are implicated in emotion and reward processing. The shared dopamine signaling further supports their role in motivation, as this neurotransmitter has been consistently shown to encode incentive salience (Berridge, 2006; Berridge et al., 2010). When subjects are shown food pictures, the fMRI signal in this appetitive network correlates with the preference for highly palatable foods and predicts subsequent caloric intake (Mehta et al., 2012; Tryon et al., 2013) and weight gain (Demos et al., 2012; Lawrence et al., 2012).

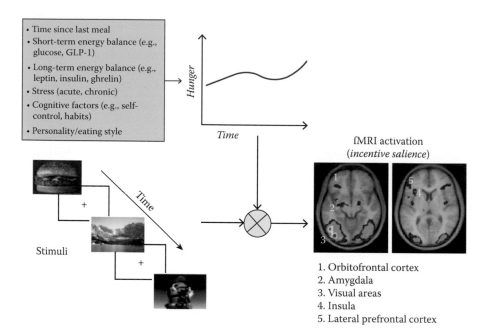

- Time since last meal
- Short-term energy balance (e.g., glucose, GLP-1)
- Long-term energy balance (e.g., leptin, insulin, ghrelin)
- Stress (acute, chronic)
- Cognitive factors (e.g., self-control, habits)
- Personality/eating style

Hunger

Time

Stimuli

Time

fMRI activation
(*incentive salience*)

1. Orbitofrontal cortex
2. Amygdala
3. Visual areas
4. Insula
5. Lateral prefrontal cortex

FIGURE 6.2 Functional MRI paradigms. Here, fMRI measures the brain response to food pictures. This reflects both a trait aspect of the individual and a state aspect, which reflects rapidly changing appetite in response to different factors. The factors that influence the neural response to food cues have vastly different time course: they may change hourly or be relatively stable over the lifespan.

6.2.1 HIPPOCAMPUS AND AMYGDALA

The hippocampus is traditionally linked to learning and memory; however, it also appears to play a role in motivation and in linking energy balance information to incentive behavior. There is greater BOLD signal in the hippocampus while viewing food pictures compared to nonfood pictures; moreover, the signal is modulated by hunger, craving and energy balance signals (Davidson et al., 2007; Malik et al., 2008; Pelchat et al., 2004). This signal is also greater in obese compared to lean individuals (Bragulat et al., 2010; Stoeckel et al., 2008).

The amygdala receives input from the sensory cortex (notably visual, gustatory, and olfactory) and hypothalamus and thus acts as a center for homeostatic-hedonic interactions. It also plays an important role in emotional learning and assigning incentive value to sensory stimuli such as food cues (Baxter and Murray, 2002; Mahler and Berridge, 2011; Yasoshima et al., 2015; Zhang et al., 2011). In humans, fMRI meta-analyses reveal consistent amygdala responses to gustatory and visual food cues (Jastreboff et al., 2013; Tang et al., 2012). Without an intact amygdala, the taste cortex is no longer able to encode the palatability of food cues (Piette et al., 2012).

Neural activity in the amygdala reflects the incentive value of foods and their cues. The amygdala fMRI response to food cues is modulated by factors that affect incentive salience such as outcome devaluation, hunger, and stress (Gottfried et al., 2003; Li et al., 2012; Malik et al., 2008; Rudenga et al., 2012; Van der Laan et al., 2011). It is also affected by cognitive information such as health-related food labels (Grabenhorst et al., 2013). Relative insensitivity of the amygdala to satiation induced by caloric load is predictive of subsequent weight gain (Sun et al., 2015).

6.2.2 INSULA

In humans, the mid-insula forms the taste cortex that encodes the features of pure taste stimuli, such as quality and intensity (Bender et al., 2009; Small, 2010). The anterior insula and adjacent frontal-operculum (sometimes named "fronto-insula") also respond to taste information and appear to encode the incentive value of taste stimuli. In addition to gustatory stimuli, insula activity encodes the somatosensory (e.g., oral texture) and olfactory properties of food (De Araujo and Rolls, 2004). The signals related to diverse sensory properties of foods (gustatory, olfactory, visual, and somatosensory) converge in the mid and anterior insula to form a flavor percept (De Araujo et al., 2012). In a recent fMRI meta-analysis, the insula was the only region that responded to food cues in all sensory modalities (Huerta et al., 2014).

The insula also appears to be sensitive to a number of functions that reflect value, including perceived pleasantness (Small et al., 2003; Sun et al., 2015), internal state (Small et al., 2001; Smeets et al., 2006), ghrelin concentration (Malik et al., 2008), blood glucose concentration (Simmons et al., 2013), and expected taste quality (Nitschke et al., 2006). Moreover, BOLD activity in the insula at rest correlates with the changes in plasma concentrations of several gut hormones (Li et al., 2012). Finally, flavor-energy conditioning, by which flavors paired with calories gain hedonic value, is reflected in insula activation (De Araujo et al., 2013).

Craving for a favorite food activates the insula (Pelchat et al., 2004), and its activity is modulated by higher-order cognitive functions such as attention. In one fMRI study, subjects who were instructed to detect a taste in a tasteless solution showed increased insular activation compared to passive sampling of the solution (Veldhuizen et al., 2007). Rodent experiments further confirm the role of insula in incentive processing of food cues (Balleine and Dickinson, 2000). The anticipation of sucrose produces sucrose-like activation in the insular cortex in the absence of sucrose (Gardner and Fontanini, 2014) and silencing insular neurons with optogenetics inhibits food-approach behavior (Kusumoto-Yoshida et al., 2015). In conclusion, the insula is more than only a taste cortex: it encodes the reward value of foods and the expectation of nutrients associated with visual and flavor cues, information that drives feeding behavior.

6.2.3 ORBITOFRONTAL CORTEX AND VENTROMEDIAL PREFRONTAL CORTEX

The OFC and adjacent vmPFC respond consistently to food cues and are implicated in decision making based on value. While there is some confusion in the imaging literature regarding the anatomy and naming of these two structures (Wallis, 2012), here, we follow recent nomenclature and refer to the OFC as the orbital portion of the frontal lobe and the vmPFC as the region on the medial wall of the frontal lobe that includes Brodmann area 14 as well as the subgenual anterior cingulate cortex (areas 25 and 32) (Haber and Behrens, 2014). Functionally, the vmPFC is more interconnected with limbic and visceral regions such as the hypothalamus, hippocampus, amygdala, and ventral striatum, while the OFC, especially in its central and lateral aspects, connects more to sensory and associative cortex (Haber and Behrens, 2014).

The OFC, along with the insula, contributes to the neural origin of the flavor percept of a food (Small and Prescott, 2005). Like the insula, it receives polymodal input from sensory cortices. OFC activity tracks both pleasantness ratings of ingested foods (Kringelbach et al., 2003) and the anticipated reward value of food as signaled by cues (Gottfried et al., 2003). The OFC response to food cues measured by fMRI is sensitive to current energy balance information (Van der Laan et al., 2011). This suggests a key role for the OFC in driving food choice toward those that have gained incentive salience (Berridge et al., 2010), possibly due to their caloric content. Interestingly, obese individuals may have a relative inability to down-regulate the OFC response to high-calorie food cues following satiation (Dimitropoulos et al., 2012). While both OFC and vmPFC respond to food cues, the vmPFC appears to play a distinct role in encoding stimulus value. In fMRI meta-analysis studies, vmPFC is the area where BOLD most consistently correlates with the subjective value of different types of stimuli, including foods (Bartra et al., 2013; Clithero and Rangel, 2014).

The vmPFC has diverse connections with regions implicated in visceral and emotional processing as well as self-control. There is a limbic/cognitive caudal/rostral gradient in the vmPFC, with caudal regions being interconnected with limbic areas and rostral ones having connections to lateral prefrontal areas. The caudal parts of the vmPFC receive inputs from the hypothalamus, amygdala, hippocampus, and insula and project densely to ventral striatum, amygdala, and hypothalamus. The caudal vmPFC is tightly coupled with the rostal vmPFC, which is in turn connected to anterior cingulate cortex, dorsolateral prefrontal cortex (dlPFC), and inferior frontal gyrus (IFG) (Haber and Behrens, 2014). Thus, a value signal in the vmPFC may be computed based on the integration of sensory attributes and palatability of food stimuli, the current state of energy balance, previous memories, and cognitively determined plans or self-control. The fMRI signal in the vmPFC during exposure to food cues is modulated by the caloric density of the items (Tang et al., 2014) and by hunger level (Thomas et al., 2015), and the vmPFC exhibits functional connectivity with the appetitive network structures at the time of decision, notably the striatum (Tang et al., 2014; Thomas et al., 2015). Interestingly, obese individuals, compared to lean controls, demonstrate increased functional connectivity at rest between the striatum and the vmPFC (Coveleskie et al., 2015). vmPFC activation is higher for cues associated with high-calorie foods (Stoeckel et al., 2008; Tang et al., 2014) and predicts subsequent ad libitum choosing of high-fat foods (Mehta et al., 2012) and future weight gain (Yokum et al., 2011).

6.2.4 STRIATUM

The striatum is the entrance to the basal ganglia and consists of the caudate nucleus, putamen, and nucleus accumbens. There is a dorsal/ventral and medial/lateral topography in the striatum that reflects functionality and connectivity with limbic, associative, and motor subregions (Haber, 2011). It is interconnected with all the other brain regions implicated in the organization of appetitive behavior: the amygdala, hippocampus, insula, OFC, vmPFC, anterior cingulate cortex, and lateral prefrontal cortex (PFC). It is thus suited to integrating information about food stimuli, transforming it into an action or motivated behavior, and learning from the consequences of these actions to shape future behavior (Haber and Behrens, 2014). fMRI meta-analyses show that the striatum is consistently activated by food cues (Van der Laan et al., 2011; Tang et al., 2012). This activation correlates with subjective craving (Pelchat et al., 2004) and is higher for subjectively tasty foods (Hollmann et al., 2012) and in the fasted state (Goldstone et al., 2009). In sum, it depends on both the internal state and the extrinsic (learned) reward value of the foods. The degree of striatal activation to food cues predicts subsequent food intake (Frankort et al., 2015), weight gain (Demos et al., 2012; Stice et al., 2011), or less successful voluntary weight loss (Murdaugh et al., 2012). Obesity is consistently associated with increased striatal reactivity to food cues (Carnell et al., 2014; DelParigi et al., 2004; Rothemund et al., 2007; Stoeckel et al., 2008), especially highly palatable (calorically dense) foods.

Striatal activity reflects the incentive salience of visual objects or cues. This response may interact with poor self-control signaling from lateral PFC to ultimately lead to increased food consumption and weight gain, paralleling findings from personality literature where an interaction between high emotional reactivity to food reward and poor self-control predicts body weight (Vainik et al., 2013). Indeed, striatal cue fMRI reactivity (perhaps representing emotional cue reactivity) predicts increased snack consumption through an interaction with reduced self-control as measured by questionnaires (Lawrence et al., 2012). Cognitive self-control may manifest in fMRI studies as inhibition of striatal activation mediated by the lateral PFC (Siep et al., 2012).

6.2.5 DORSOLATERAL PREFRONTAL CORTEX

The decision to eat is influenced by appetitive drive (hunger), but it also depends on cultural and social factors, habits (e.g., time of day), and health concerns, among others. These higher-level rules and cognitive influences depend on information integration and processing within the PFC, notably the dlPFC and Brodmann areas 9 and 46. Recently, researchers in the field of neuroeconomics have conceived of food choice as deriving from a comparison of the basic attributes of foods (taste, palatability) and the individual's long-term goals (i.e., health, diet). This area of research mostly uses fMRI to map the neural computations that relate what, when, and how much we eat to our explicit goals and current physiological state (Hare et al., 2011; Rangel, 2013). A useful approach introduced into the fMRI literature by the Rangel group is the combination of an auction paradigm with fMRI (Plassmann et al., 2007). The auction paradigm can be used to calculate the willingness to pay for food items, which measures the current value of a food item to the individual and thereby to identify neural processes involved in value computations. As stated previously, several lines of research suggest that the current value of food cues is represented in the vmPFC. This region may not only track value, it also appears to be crucial to its computation by the brain.

As for the striatum, vmPFC activity can be modulated by the lateral PFC: the down-regulation of a vmPFC value signal by the lateral PFC has been postulated to represent the neural correlate of self-control (Hare et al., 2009). In fMRI studies, where a participant is asked to consider the healthiness of foods or to regulate their craving, the cognitive manipulation increases activity in the dlPFC, which modulates the activity of the vmPFC (Hare et al., 2011; Hollmann et al., 2012; Siep et al., 2012). Increased reactivity in dlPFC to highly palatable foods predicts reduced subsequent chocolate intake (Frankort et al., 2015) and better weight loss from dieting (Murdaugh et al., 2012) or bariatric surgery (Goldman et al., 2013).

6.3   fMRI STUDIES OF OBESITY SUPPORT THE SELF-CONTROL MODEL

Obesity and overeating persist in our society despite the enormous amount of information about food and health that is available to us (Malhotra et al., 2015). There is some evidence that individuals with higher body mass index (BMI) may make maladaptive decisions due to impaired executive function (Fitzpatrick et al., 2013). Moreover, a comprehensive review identifies a consistent correlation between BMI and personality and cognitive tests of executive function (Vainik et al., 2013). Numerous fMRI studies of executive function implicate the PFC (notably dlPFC) and its corticostriatal connections in the control of motivated behavior (e.g., Kouneiher et al., 2009).

Self-control capacity is especially taxed by the modern obesogenic environment, consisting of abundant, palatable, and cheap calorically dense foods and their cues (e.g., advertising). This environment is thought to be an important contributor to the increased incidence of obesity over the last three decades (Levitsky and Youn, 2004; Wansink and Payne, 2008; Wansink et al., 2006). One aspect of the obesogenic environment that can be tested in the fMRI context is the neural response to food cues, which are presumed to act as conditioned stimuli that trigger food craving and consumption (Dagher, 2009). Individuals with obesity or a tendency to overeat tend to show greater emotional and physiological reactivity to food cues: when confronted with food odors or images, they show greater salivation and insulin release (the so-called cephalic phase of feeding), greater appetite, and greater food consumption (Hays and Roberts, 2008; Jansen et al., 2003; Wardle, 1990; Woods, 1991).

We make many food-related decisions every day; they often require weighing the value of immediate, tempting foods against a desire for health (Wansink and Sobal, 2007). Dietary self-control protects against weight gain and obesity. Reduced or depleted self-control leads individuals to state a greater desire for food, to consume more unhealthy food, and to fail at dieting (Allan et al., 2010; Allom and Mullan, 2014; Guerrieri et al., 2007, 2008; Hofmann et al., 2007; Jasinska et al., 2012; Nederkoorn et al., 2010; Vohs and Heatherton, 2000). On the other hand, successful self-controllers are more likely to succeed in making dietary changes and lose more weight (Allan et al., 2011; Hall et al., 2008; Johnson et al., 2012).

The lateral PFC is most frequently implicated in self-control generally and dietary self-control more specifically. Damage to the frontal cortex has been shown to lead to binge eating and cravings for sweet foods (Mendez et al., 2008; Piguet, 2011). In fMRI studies, volitionally suppressing a desire for tasty foods induces increased activity in the lateral PFC, including the IFG and dlPFC (Giuliani et al., 2014; Hollmann et al., 2012). Also, inhibiting prepotent responses to appetizing foods is associated with increased activity in the dlPFC and IFG (Batterink et al., 2010; He et al., 2014). An ecological paradigm showed that IFG activity measured with fMRI during response inhibition predicted lower levels of food desire, greater ability to resist food temptations, and a tendency to consume less food in everyday life (Lopez et al., 2014). Furthermore, activation of the left dlPFC while viewing food pictures was greater in individuals who place higher value on diet (Smeets et al., 2013) or who succeeded in achieving weight loss (Goldman et al., 2013; Jensen and Kirwan, 2015). Left dlPFC activation while viewing pictures of chocolate predicted less chocolate intake immediately after the scan (Frankort et al., 2015). Obese individuals compared to the nonobese and the previously obese showed reduced brain activity in the left dlPFC after a satiating meal, and this effect correlated with percentage adiposity (Le et al., 2009). Passive viewing of food images is typically associated with increased fMRI activity in prefrontal brain regions (Van der Laan et al., 2011); however, abnormalities in lateral PFC have been reported in obese individuals (see Brooks et al., 2013; Pursey et al., 2014, for reviews).

Rangel et al. have provided evidence in several studies that individuals adept at dietary self-control avoid selecting unhealthy but tasty foods by recruiting the left dlPFC to down-modulate value-related activity in the vmPFC (Hare et al., 2009, 2011). In support of this model, stronger functional connectivity between the vmPFC and dlPFC predicted dieting success (Weygandt et al., 2013). Moreover, connectivity between these two regions, as well as the ability to down-regulate the OFC response to food cues, was found to be vulnerable to cognitive resource depletion by a demanding attentional task (Wagner et al., 2013). This may explain how cognitive demands or psychosocial stress can lead to failure of self-control and overeating.

6.4   NEUROIMAGING OF HOMEOSTATIC SIGNALS

Peptides from the gut and adipose tissue signal long- and short-term energy balance to the CNS to affect feeding behavior (Begg and Woods, 2013). They act on the appetitive network both directly and indirectly via the brainstem, hypothalamus, and dopaminergic system (Salem and Dhillo, 2015). Leptin is secreted by adipocytes and signals information about long-term energy stores. Insulin and ghrelin convey information about both long-term energy balance and acute meal-related information related to caloric intake and satiety. Glucagon-like peptide (GLP-1) and peptide YY (PYY) are short-term signals implicated in meal termination (Begg and Woods, 2013; Salem and Dhillo, 2015; Woods, 2009).

After calorie ingestion, insulin levels rise and act as a satiety signal to terminate the meal. fMRI studies suggest that insulin reduces the rewarding effects of food (Davis et al., 2010; Kroemer et al., 2013a; Kullmann et al., 2012). This may be partly mediated through inhibition of dopamine neurons (Labouebe et al., 2013).

Parenteral insulin administration reduces the BOLD signal in the visual cortex, hypothalamus, PFC (Kullmann et al., 2015), and hippocampus (Guthoff et al., 2010). The fMRI response of the appetitive network to food cues is affected by acute insulin levels in a way that is consistent with a role in reducing appetite (Kullmann et al., 2015): BOLD signals in the visual cortex, insula, striatum, and OFC all decrease as a function of insulin levels (Guthoff et al., 2010; Kroemer et al., 2013a; Li et al., 2012; Luo et al., 2015).

Leptin is an adiposity signal that reduces food intake. It can reduce the hedonic value of food and favor cognitive self-control (Baicy et al., 2007; Farooqi et al., 2007; Farr et al., 2014; Grosshans et al., 2012). fMRI studies in patients with congenital leptin deficiency found that leptin replacement reduced the ventral striatum response to food cues (Farooqi et al., 2007). Leptin administration in patients who were leptin deficient due to lipodystrophy also reduced the BOLD response to food pictures in the amygdala, hippocampus, and striatum (Aotani et al., 2012). In subjects with normal leptin signaling, leptin levels negatively correlate with ventral striatal BOLD response to food cues (Grosshans et al., 2012).

In contrast to insulin and leptin, ghrelin increases hunger and food intake (Müller et al., 2015). Ghrelin levels correlate with resting state BOLD in the OFC, amygdala, and insula (Li et al., 2012). Fasting ghrelin levels correlate with the BOLD response to food pictures in visual areas and in the amygdala, striatum, insula, midbrain, and hypothalamus (Kroemer et al., 2013b), suggesting that ghrelin increases the incentive salience of food cues. Intravenous ghrelin also increases BOLD responses to food cues in these same brain areas proportionally to self-reported hunger (Goldstone et al., 2014; Malik et al., 2008).

GLP-1 and PYY are gut peptides that signal short-term satiety, and fMRI studies suggest that they act on the entire appetitive system. Postprandial GLP-1 levels negatively correlated with resting state BOLD activity in the OFC and insula (Li et al., 2012), and GLP-1 and PYY coadministration reduced the BOLD response to food pictures in the entire appetitive network (De Silva et al., 2011).

6.5   CONCLUSIONS

fMRI identifies a consistent set of brain regions we refer to as an appetitive network, centered around the insula, medial temporal lobe, OFC, vmPFC, and striatum. The response of this network to visual or flavor food cues appears to reflect current hunger and energy balance. Self-control involves a reduction in appetitive network reactivity, mediated in part by the lateral PFC. fMRI consistently identifies increases in appetitive system reactivity and reductions in either lateral PFC activity, or connectivity with appetitive regions, in obesity.

LITERATURE CITED

Allan, J.L., M. Johnston, and N. Campbell, 2010. Unintentional eating. What determines goal-incongruent chocolate consumption? *Appetite* 54, 422–425.
Allan, J.L., M. Johnston, and N. Campbell, 2011. Missed by an inch or a mile? Predicting the size of intention-behaviour gap from measures of executive control. *Psychol Health* 26, 635–650.

Allom, V. and B. Mullan, 2014. Individual differences in executive function predict distinct eating behaviours. *Appetite* 80, 123–130.

Aotani, D., K. Ebihara, N. Sawamoto, T. Kusakabe, M. Aizawa-Abe, S. Kataoka, T. Sakai, H. Iogawa, C. Ebihara, J. Fujikura et al., 2012. Functional magnetic resonance imaging analysis of food-related brain activity in patients with lipodystrophy undergoing leptin replacement therapy. *J Clin Endocrinol Metab* 97, 3663–3671.

De Araujo, I.E. and E.T. Rolls, 2004. Representation in the human brain of food texture and oral fat. *J Neurosci* 24, 3086–3093.

De Araujo, I.E., P. Geha, and D.M. Small, 2012. Orosensory and Homeostatic Functions of the Insular Taste Cortex. *Chemosens Percept* 5, 64–79.

De Araujo, I.E., T. Lin, M.G. Veldhuizen, and D.M. Small, 2013. Metabolic regulation of brain response to food cues. *Curr Biol CB* 23, 878–883.

Baicy, K., E.D. London, J. Monterosso, M-L. Wong, T. Delibasi, A. Sharma, and J. Licinio, 2007. Leptin replacement alters brain response to food cues in genetically leptin-deficient adults. *Proc Natl Acad Sci U S A* 104, 18276–18279.

Balleine, B.W. and A. Dickinson, 2000. The effect of lesions of the insular cortex on instrumental conditioning: Evidence for a role in incentive memory. *J Neurosci* 20, 8954–8964.

Bartra, O., J.T. McGuire, and J.W. Kable, 2013. The valuation system: A coordinate-based meta-analysis of BOLD fMRI experiments examining neural correlates of subjective value. *NeuroImage* 76, 412–427.

Batterink, L., S. Yokum, and E. Stice, 2010. Body mass correlates inversely with inhibitory control in response to food among adolescent girls: An fMRI study. *NeuroImage* 52, 1696–1703.

Baxter, M.G. and E.A. Murray, 2002. The amygdala and reward. *Nat Rev Neurosci* 3, 563–573.

Begg, D.P. and S.C. Woods, 2013. The endocrinology of food intake. *Nat Rev Endocrinol* 9, 584–597.

Bender, G., M.G. Veldhuizen, J.A. Meltzer, D.R. Gitelman, and D.M. Small, 2009. Neural correlates of evaluative compared with passive tasting. *Eur J Neurosci* 30, 327–338.

Berridge, K.C., 2006. The debate over dopamine's role in reward: The case for incentive salience. *Psychopharmacology (Berl)* 191, 391–431.

Berridge, K.C., C.Y. Ho, J.M. Richard, and A.G. Difeliceantonio, 2010. The tempted brain eats: Pleasure and desire circuits in obesity and eating disorders. *Brain Res* 1350: 43–64.

Bragulat, V., M. Dzemidzic, C. Bruno, C.A. Cox, T. Talavage, R.V. Considine, and D.A. Kareken, 2010. Food-related odor probes of brain reward circuits during hunger: A pilot fMRI study. *Obesity* 18, 1566–1571.

Brooks, S.J., J. Cedernaes, and H.B. Schiöth, 2013. Increased prefrontal and parahippocampal activation with reduced dorsolateral prefrontal and insular cortex activation to food images in obesity: A meta-analysis of fMRI studies. *PloS One* 8, e60393.

Carnell, S., C. Gibson, L. Benson, C.N. Ochner, and A. Geliebter, 2012. Neuroimaging and obesity: Current knowledge and future directions. *Obes Rev* 13, 43–56.

Carnell, S., L. Benson, S.P. Pantazatos, J. Hirsch, and A. Geliebter, 2014. Amodal brain activation and functional connectivity in response to high-energy-density food cues in obesity. *Obesity* 22:2370–2378.

Clithero, J.A. and A. Rangel, 2014. Informatic parcellation of the network involved in the computation of subjective value. *Soc Cogn Affect Neurosci* 9, 1289–1302.

Coveleskie, K., A. Gupta, L.A. Kilpatrick, E.D. Mayer, C. Ashe-McNalley, J. Stains, J.S. Labus, and E.A. Mayer, 2015. Altered functional connectivity within the central reward network in overweight and obese women. *Nutr Diabetes* 5, e148.

Dagher, A., 2009. The neurobiology of appetite: Hunger as addiction. *Int J Obes* 33, S30–S33.

Dagher, A., 2012. Functional brain imaging of appetite. *Trends Endocrinol Metab* 23, 250–260.

Davidson, T.L., S.E. Kanoski, L.A. Schier, D.J. Clegg, and S.C. Benoit, 2007. A potential role for the hippocampus in energy intake and body weight regulation. *Curr Opin Pharmacol* 7, 613–616.

Davis, J.F., D.L. Choi, and S.C. Benoit, 2010. Insulin, leptin and reward. *Trends Endocrinol Metab* 21, 68–74.

De Silva, A., V. Salem, C.J. Long, A. Makwana, R.D. Newbould, E.A. Rabiner, M.A. Ghatei, S.R. Bloom, P.M. Matthews, J.D. Beaver et al., 2011. The gut hormones PYY 3–36 and GLP-1 7–36 amide reduce food intake and modulate brain activity in appetite centers in humans. *Cell Metab* 14, 700–706.

DelParigi, A., K. Chen, A.D. Salbe, J.O. Hill, R.R. Wing, E.M. Reiman, and P.A. Tataranni, 2004. Persistence of abnormal neural responses to a meal in postobese individuals. *Int J Obes Relat Metab Disord* 28, 370–377.

Demos, K.E., T.F. Heatherton, and W.M. Kelley, 2012. Individual differences in nucleus accumbens activity to food and sexual images predict weight gain and sexual behavior. *J Neurosci* 32, 5549–5552.

Dimitropoulos, A., J. Tkach, A. Ho, and J. Kennedy, 2012. Greater corticolimbic activation to high-calorie food cues after eating in obese vs. normal-weight adults. *Appetite* 58, 303–312.

Farooqi, I.S., E. Bullmore, J. Keogh, J. Gillard, S. O'Rahilly, and P.C. Fletcher, 2007. Leptin regulates striatal regions and human eating behavior. *Science* 317, 1355.

Farr, O.M., C. Fiorenza, P. Papageorgiou, M. Brinkoetter, F. Ziemke, B.-B. Koo, R. Rojas, and C.S. Mantzoros, 2014. Leptin therapy alters appetite and neural responses to food stimuli in brain areas of leptin sensitive subjects without altering brain structure. *J Clin Endocrinol Metab* 99:E2529–E2538.

Fitzpatrick, S., S. Gilbert, and L. Serpell, 2013. Systematic Review: are overweight and obese individuals impaired on behavioural tasks of executive functioning? *Neuropsychol Rev* 23, 138–156.

Frankort, A., A. Roefs, N. Siep, A. Roebroeck, R. Havermans, and A. Jansen, 2015. Neural predictors of chocolate intake following chocolate exposure. *Appetite* 87, 98–107.

Gardner, M.P.H. and A. Fontanini, 2014. Encoding and tracking of outcome-specific expectancy in the gustatory cortex of alert rats. *J Neurosci* 34, 13000–13017.

Giuliani, N.R., T. Mann, A.J. Tomiyama, and E.T. Berkman, 2014. Neural systems underlying the reappraisal of personally craved foods. *J Cogn Neurosci* 26, 1390–1402.

Goldman, R.L., M. Canterberry, J.J. Borckardt, A. Madan, T.K. Byrne, M.S. George, P.M. O'Neil, and C.A. Hanlon, 2013. Executive control circuitry differentiates degree of success in weight loss following gastric-bypass surgery. *Obesity* 21, 2189–2196.

Goldstone, A.P., C.G. Prechtl de Hernandez, J.D. Beaver, K. Muhammed, C. Croese, G. Bell, G. Durighel, E. Hughes, A.D. Waldman, G. Frost et al., 2009. Fasting biases brain reward systems towards high-calorie foods. *Eur J Neurosci* 30, 1625–1635.

Goldstone, A.P., C.G. Prechtl, S. Scholtz, A.D. Miras, N. Chhina, G. Durighel, S.S. Deliran, C. Beckmann, M.A. Ghatei, D.R. Ashby et al., 2014. Ghrelin mimics fasting to enhance human hedonic, orbitofrontal cortex, and hippocampal responses to food. *Am J Clin Nutr* 99, 1319–1330.

Gottfried, J.A., J. O'Doherty, and R.J. Dolan, 2003. Encoding predictive reward value in human amygdala and orbitofrontal cortex. *Science* 301, 1104–1107.

Grabenhorst, F., F.P. Schulte, S. Maderwald, and M. Brand, 2013. Food labels promote healthy choices by a decision bias in the amygdala. *NeuroImage* 74, 152–163.

Grosshans, M., C. Vollmert, S. Vollstädt-Klein, H. Tost, S. Leber, P. Bach, M. Bühler, C. von der Goltz, J. Mutschler, S. Loeber et al., 2012. Association of leptin with food cue-induced activation in human reward pathways. *Arch Gen Psychiatry* 69, 529–537.

Guerrieri, R., C. Nederkoorn, and A. Jansen, 2007. How impulsiveness and variety influence food intake in a sample of healthy women. *Appetite* 48, 119–122.

Guerrieri, R., C. Nederkoorn, and A. Jansen, 2008. The interaction between impulsivity and a varied food environment: Its influence on food intake and overweight. *Int J Obes* 32, 708–714.

Guthoff, M., Y. Grichisch, C. Canova, O. Tschritter, R. Veit, M. Hallschmid, H.-U. Häring, H. Preissl, A.M. Hennige, and A. Fritsche, 2010. Insulin modulates food-related activity in the central nervous system. *J Clin Endocrinol Metab* 95, 748–755.

Haber, S.N., 2011. *Neuroanatomy of Reward: A View from the Ventral Striatum*. Boca Raton, FL: CRC Press.

Haber, S.N. and T.E.J. Behrens, 2014. The neural network underlying incentive-based learning: Implications for interpreting circuit disruptions in psychiatric disorders. *Neuron* 83, 1019–1039.

Hall, P.A., G.T. Fong, L.J. Epp, and L.J. Elias, 2008. Executive function moderates the intention-behavior link for physical activity and dietary behavior. *Psychol Health* 23, 309–326.

Hare, T.A., C.F. Camerer, and A. Rangel, 2009. Self-control in decision-making involves modulation of the vmPFC valuation system. *Science* 324, 646–648.

Hare, T.A., J. Malmaud, and A. Rangel, 2011. Focusing attention on the health aspects of foods changes value signals in vmPFC and improves dietary choice. *J Neurosci* 31, 11077–11087.

Hays, N.P. and S.B. Roberts, 2008. Aspects of eating behaviors "disinhibition" and "restraint" are related to weight gain and BMI in women. *Obesity* 16, 52–58.

He, Q., L. Xiao, G. Xue, S. Wong, S.L. Ames, S.M. Schembre, and A. Bechara, 2014. Poor ability to resist tempting calorie rich food is linked to altered balance between neural systems involved in urge and self-control. *Nutr J* 13, 92.

Henderson, L.A. and V.G. Macefield, 2013. Functional imaging of the human brainstem during somatosensory input and autonomic output. *Front Hum Neurosci* 7, 569.

Hofmann, W., W. Rauch, and B. Gawronski, 2007. And deplete us not into temptation: Automatic attitudes, dietary restraint, and self-regulatory resources as determinants of eating behavior. *J Exp Soc Psychol* 43, 497–504.

Hollmann, M., L. Hellrung, B. Pleger, H. Schlögl, S. Kabisch, M. Stumvoll, A. Villringer, and A. Horstmann, 2012. Neural correlates of the volitional regulation of the desire for food. *Int J Obes* 36, 648–655.

Huerta, C.I., P.R. Sarkar, T.Q. Duong, A.R. Laird, and P.T. Fox, 2014. Neural bases of food perception: Coordinate-based meta-analyses of neuroimaging studies in multiple modalities. *Obesity* 22, 1439–1446.

Jansen, A., N. Theunissen, K. Slechten, C. Nederkoorn, B. Boon, S. Mulkens, and A. Roefs, 2003. Overweight children overeat after exposure to food cues. *Eat Behav* 4, 197–209.

Jasinska, A.J., M. Yasuda, C.F. Burant, N. Gregor, S. Khatri, M. Sweet, and E.B. Falk, 2012. Impulsivity and inhibitory control deficits are associated with unhealthy eating in young adults. *Appetite* 59, 738–747.

Jastreboff, A.M., R. Sinha, C. Lacadie, D.M. Small, R.S. Sherwin, and M.N. Potenza, 2013. Neural correlates of stress- and food cue-induced food craving in obesity: Association with insulin levels. *Diabetes Care* 36, 394–402.

Jensen, C.D. and C.B. Kirwan, 2015. Functional brain response to food images in successful adolescent weight losers compared with normal-weight and overweight controls. *Obesity* 23, 630–636.

Johnson, F., M. Pratt, and J. Wardle, 2012. Dietary restraint and self-regulation in eating behavior. *Int J Obes* 36, 665–674.

Jones, R.B., S. McKie, N. Astbury, T.J. Little, S. Tivey, D.J. Lassman, J. McLaughlin, S. Luckman, S.R. Williams, G.J. Dockray et al., 2012. Functional neuroimaging demonstrates that ghrelin inhibits the central nervous system response to ingested lipid. *Gut* 61, 1543–1551.

Kouneiher, F., S. Charron, and E. Koechlin, 2009. Motivation and cognitive control in the human prefrontal cortex. *Nat Neurosci* 12:939–945.

Kringelbach, M.L., J. O'Doherty, E.T. Rolls, and C. Andrews, 2003. Activation of the human orbitofrontal cortex to a liquid food stimulus is correlated with its subjective pleasantness. *Cereb Cortex* 13, 1064–1071.

Kroemer, N.B., L. Krebs, A. Kobiella, O. Grimm, M. Pilhatsch, M. Bidlingmaier, U.S. Zimmermann, and M.N. Smolka, 2013b. Fasting levels of ghrelin covary with the brain response to food pictures. *Addict Biol* 18, 855–862.

Kroemer, N.B., L. Krebs, A. Kobiella, O. Grimm, S. Vollstädt-Klein, U. Wolfensteller, R. Kling, M. Bidlingmaier, U.S. Zimmermann, and M.N. Smolka, 2013a. (Still) longing for food: Insulin reactivity modulates response to food pictures. *Hum Brain Mapp* 34, 2367–2380.

Kullmann, S., M. Heni, A. Fritsche, and H. Preissl, 2015. Insulin action in the human brain: Evidence from neuroimaging studies. *J Neuroendocrinol* 27, 419–423.

Kullmann, S., M. Heni, K. Linder, S. Zipfel, H.-U. Häring, R. Veit, A. Fritsche, and H. Preissl, 2014. Resting-state functional connectivity of the human hypothalamus. *Hum Brain Mapp* 35, 6088–6096.

Kullmann, S., M. Heni, R. Veit, C. Ketterer, F. Schick, H.-U. Häring, A. Fritsche, and H. Preissl, 2012. The obese brain: Association of body mass index and insulin sensitivity with resting state network functional connectivity. *Hum Brain Mapp* 33, 1052–1061.

Kusumoto-Yoshida, I., H. Liu, B.T. Chen, A. Fontanini, and A. Bonci, 2015. Central role for the insular cortex in mediating conditioned responses to anticipatory cues. *Proc Natl Acad Sci U S A* 112, 1190–1195.

Kwong, K.K., J.W. Belliveau, D.A. Chesler, I.E. Goldberg, R.M. Weisskoff, B.P. Poncelet, D.N. Kennedy, B.E. Hoppel, M.S. Cohen, and R. Turner, 1992. Dynamic magnetic resonance imaging of human brain activity during primary sensory stimulation. *Proc Natl Acad Sci* 89, 5675–5679.

Van der Laan, L.N., D.T.D. de Ridder, M. Viergever, and P.M. Smeets, 2011. The first taste is always with the eyes: A meta-analysis on the neural correlates of processing visual food cues. *NeuroImage* 55, 296–303.

Labouebe, G., S. Liu, C. Dias, H. Zou, J.C.Y. Wong, S. Karunakaran, S.M. Clee, A.G. Phillips, B. Boutrel, and S.L. Borgland, 2013. Insulin induces long-term depression of ventral tegmental area dopamine neurons via endocannabinoids. *Nat Neurosci* 16, 300–308.

Lassman, D.J., S. McKie, L.J. Gregory, S. Lal, M. D'Amato, I. Steele, A. Varro, G.J. Dockray, S.C.R. Williams, and D.G. Thompson, 2010. Defining the role of cholecystokinin in the lipid-induced human brain activation matrix. *Gastroenterology* 138, 1514–1524.

Lawrence, N.S., E.C. Hinton, J.A. Parkinson, and A.D. Lawrence, 2012. Nucleus accumbens response to food cues predicts subsequent snack consumption in women and increased body mass index in those with reduced self-control. *NeuroImage* 63, 415–422.

Le, D.S.N.T., K. Chen, N. Pannacciulli, M. Gluck, E.M. Reiman, and J. Krakoff, 2009. Reanalysis of the obesity-related attenuation in the left dorsolateral prefrontal cortex response to a satiating meal using gyral regions-of-interest. *J Am Coll Nutr* 28, 667–673.

Levitsky, D.A. and T. Youn, 2004. The more food young adults are served, the more they overeat. *J Nutr* 134, 2546–2549.

Li, J., An, R., Y. Zhang, X. Li, and S. Wang, 2012. Correlations of macronutrient-induced functional magnetic resonance imaging signal changes in human brain and gut hormone responses. *Am J Clin Nutr* 96, 275–282.

Little, T.J., S. McKie, R.B. Jones, M. D'Amato, C. Smith, O. Kiss, D.G. Thompson, and J.T. McLaughlin, 2014. Mapping glucose-mediated gut-to-brain signalling pathways in humans. *NeuroImage* 96, 1–11.

Lopez, R.B., W. Hofmann, D.D. Wagner, W.M. Kelley, and T.F. Heatherton, 2014. Neural predictors of giving in to temptation in daily life. *Psychol Sci* 25, 1337–1344.

Luo, S., J.R. Monterosso, K. Sarpelleh, and K.A. Page, 2015. Differential effects of fructose versus glucose on brain and appetitive responses to food cues and decisions for food rewards. *Proc Natl Acad Sci* 112, 6509–6514.

Mahler, S.V. and K.C. Berridge, 2011. What and when to "want"? Amygdala-based focusing of incentive salience upon sugar and sex. *Psychopharmacology (Berl)* 221, 407–426.

Malhotra, A., T. Noakes, and S. Phinney, 2015. It is time to bust the myth of physical inactivity and obesity: You cannot outrun a bad diet. *Br J Sports Med* 49:967–968.

Malik, S., F. McGlone, D. Bedrossian, and A. Dagher, 2008. Ghrelin modulates brain activity in areas that control appetitive behavior. *Cell Metab* 7, 400–409.

Mehta, S., S.J. Melhorn, A. Smeraglio, V. Tyagi, T. Grabowski, M.W. Schwartz, and E.A. Schur, 2012. Regional brain response to visual food cues is a marker of satiety that predicts food choice. *Am J Clin Nutr* 96, 989–999.

Mendez, M.F., E.A. Licht, and J.S. Shapira, 2008. Changes in dietary or eating behavior in frontotemporal dementia versus Alzheimer's disease. *Am J Alzheimers Dis Other Demen* 23, 280–285.

Morton, G.J., D.E. Cummings, D.G. Baskin, G.S. Barsh, and M.W. Schwartz, 2006. Central nervous system control of food intake and body weight. *Nature* 443, 289–295.

Morton, G.J., T.H. Meek, and M.W. Schwartz, 2014. Neurobiology of food intake in health and disease. *Nat Rev Neurosci* 15, 367–378.

Müller, T.D., R. Nogueiras, M.L. Andermann, Z.B. Andrews, S.D. Anker, J. Argente, R.L. Batterham, S.C. Benoit, C.Y. Bowers, F. Broglio et al., 2015. Ghrelin. *Mol Metab* 4, 437–460.

Murdaugh, D.L., J.E. Cox, E.W. Cook, and R.E. Weller, 2012. fMRI reactivity to high-calorie food pictures predicts short- and long-term outcome in a weight-loss program. *NeuroImage* 59, 2709–2721.

Nederkoorn, C., K. Houben, W. Hofmann, A. Roefs, and A. Jansen, 2010. Control yourself or just eat what you like? Weight gain over a year is predicted by an interactive effect of response inhibition and implicit preference for snack foods. *Health Psychol* 29, 389–393.

Nitschke, J.B., G.E. Dixon, I. Sarinopoulos, S.J. Short, J.D. Cohen, E.E. Smith, S.M. Kosslyn, R.M. Rose, and R.J. Davidson, 2006. Altering expectancy dampens neural response to aversive taste in primary taste cortex. *Nat Neurosci* 9, 435–442.

Ojemann, J.G., E. Akbudak, A.Z. Snyder, R.C. McKinstry, M.E. Raichle, and T.E. Conturo, 1997. Anatomic localization and quantitative analysis of gradient refocused echo-planar fMRI susceptibility artifacts. *NeuroImage* 6, 156–167.

Pelchat, M.L., A. Johnson, R. Chan, J. Valdez, and J.D. Ragland, 2004. Images of desire: Food-craving activation during fMRI. *NeuroImage* 23, 1486–1493.

Piette, C.E., M.A. Baez-Santiago, E.E. Reid, D.B. Katz, and A. Moran, 2012. Inactivation of basolateral amygdala specifically eliminates palatability-related information in cortical sensory responses. *J Neurosci* 32, 9981–9991.

Piguet, O., 2011. Eating disturbance in behavioural-variant frontotemporal dementia. *J Mol Neurosci* 45, 589–593.

Plassmann, H., J. O'Doherty, and A. Rangel, 2007. Orbitofrontal cortex encodes willingness to pay in everyday economic transactions. *J Neurosci* 27, 9984–9988.

Purnell, J.Q., B.A. Klopfenstein, A.A. Stevens, P.J. Havel, S.H. Adams, T.N. Dunn, C. Krisky, and W.D. Rooney, 2011. Brain functional magnetic resonance imaging response to glucose and fructose infusions in humans. *Diabetes Obes Metab* 13:229–234.

Pursey, K.M., P. Stanwell, R.J. Callister, K. Brain, C.E. Collins, and T.L. Burrows, 2014. Neural responses to visual food cues according to weight status: A systematic review of functional magnetic resonance imaging studies. *Front Nutr* 1, 7.

Rangel, A., 2013. Regulation of dietary choice by the decision-making circuitry. *Nat Neurosci* 16, 1717–1724.

Rothemund, Y., C. Preuschhof, G. Bohner, H.-C. Bauknecht, R. Klingebiel, H. Flor, and B.F. Klapp, 2007. Differential activation of the dorsal striatum by high-calorie visual food stimuli in obese individuals. *NeuroImage* 37, 410–421.

Rudenga, K.J., R. Sinha, and D.M. Small, 2012. Acute stress potentiates brain response to milkshake as a function of body weight and chronic stress. *Int J Obes.* 37, 309–316.

Salem, V. and W.S. Dhillo, 2015. Imaging in endocrinology: The use of functional MRI to study the endocrinology of appetite. *Eur J Endocrinol* 173, R59–R68.

Siep, N., A. Roefs, A. Roebroeck, R. Havermans, M. Bonte, and A. Jansen, 2012. Fighting food temptations: The modulating effects of short-term cognitive reappraisal, suppression and up-regulation on mesocorticolimbic activity related to appetitive motivation. *NeuroImage* 60, 213–220.

Simmons, W.K., K.M. Rapuano, S.J. Kallman, J.E. Ingeholm, B. Miller, S.J. Gotts, J.A. Avery, K.D. Hall, and A. Martin, 2013. Category-specific integration of homeostatic signals in caudal but not rostral human insula. *Nat Neurosci* 16, 1551–1552.

Small, D.M., 2010. Taste representation in the human insula. *Brain Struct Funct* 214, 551–561.

Small, D.M., M.D. Gregory, Y.E. Mak, D. Gitelman, M.M. Mesulam, and T. Parrish, 2003. Dissociation of neural representation of intensity and affective valuation in human gustation. *Neuron* 39, 701–711.

Small, D.M. and J. Prescott, 2005. Odor/taste integration and the perception of flavor. *Exp Brain Res* 166, 345–357.

Small, D.M., R.J. Zatorre, A. Dagher, A.C. Evans, and M. Jones-Gotman, 2001. Changes in brain activity related to eating chocolate: from pleasure to aversion. *Brain J Neurol* 124, 1720–1733.

Smeets, P.A.M., C. de Graaf, A. Stafleu, M.J.P. van Osch, and J. van der Grond, 2005. Functional MRI of human hypothalamic responses following glucose ingestion. *NeuroImage* 24, 363–368.

Smeets, P.A.M., C. de Graaf, A. Stafleu, M.J.P. van Osch, R.A.J. Nievelstein, and J. van der Grond, 2006. Effect of satiety on brain activation during chocolate tasting in men and women. *Am J Clin Nutr* 83, 1297–1305.

Smeets, P.A.M., F.M. Kroese, C. Evers, and D.T.D. de Ridder, 2013. Allured or alarmed: Counteractive control responses to food temptations in the brain. *Behav Brain Res* 248, 41–45.

Smeets, P.A.M., S. Vidarsdottir, C. de Graaf, A. Stafleu, M.J.P. van Osch, M.A. Viergever, H. Pijl, and J. van der Grond, 2007. Oral glucose intake inhibits hypothalamic neuronal activity more effectively than glucose infusion. *Am J Physiol Endocrinol Metab* 293, E754–E758.

Stice, E., S. Yokum, K.S. Burger, L.H. Epstein, and D.M. Small, 2011. Youth at risk for obesity show greater activation of striatal and somatosensory regions to food. *J Neurosci* 31, 4360–4366.

Stoeckel, L.E., R.E. Weller, E.W. Cook, D.B. Twieg, R.C. Knowlton, and J.E. Cox, 2008. Widespread reward-system activation in obese women in response to pictures of high-calorie foods. *NeuroImage* 41, 636–647.

Sun, X., N.B. Kroemer, M.G. Veldhuizen, A.E. Babbs, I.E. de Araujo, D.R. Gitelman, R.S. Sherwin, R. Sinha, and D.M. Small, 2015. Basolateral Amygdala Response to Food Cues in the Absence of Hunger Is Associated with Weight Gain Susceptibility. *J Neurosci* 35, 7964–7976.

Tang, D.W., L.K. Fellows, D.M. Small, and A. Dagher, 2012. Food and drug cues activate similar brain regions: A meta-analysis of functional MRI studies. *Physiol Behav* 106, 317–324.

Tang, D.W., L.K. Fellows, and A. Dagher, 2014. Behavioral and neural valuation of foods is driven by implicit knowledge of caloric content. *Psychol Sci* 25, 2168–2176.

Thomas, J.M., S. Higgs, C.T. Dourish, P.C. Hansen, C.J. Harmer, and C. McCabe, 2015. Satiation attenuates BOLD activity in brain regions involved in reward and increases activity in dorsolateral prefrontal cortex: An fMRI study in healthy volunteers. *Am J Clin Nutr* 101, 697–704.

Tryon, M.S., C.S. Carter, R. Decant, and K.D. Laugero, 2013. Chronic stress exposure may affect the brain's response to high calorie food cues and predispose to obesogenic eating habits. *Physiol Behav* 120, 233–242.

Vainik, U., A. Dagher, L. Dubé, and L.K. Fellows, 2013. Neurobehavioural correlates of body mass index and eating behaviours in adults: A systematic review. *Neurosci Biobehav Rev* 37, 279–299.

Van Opstal, A.M., A.M. Westerink, W.M. Teeuwisse, M.A.M. van der Geest, E.F. van Furth, and J. van der Grond, 2015. Hypothalamic BOLD response to glucose intake and hypothalamic volume are similar in anorexia nervosa and healthy control subjects. *Front Neurosci* 9, 159.

Veldhuizen, M.G., G. Bender, R.T. Constable, and D.M. Small, 2007. Trying to detect taste in a tasteless solution: Modulation of early gustatory cortex by attention to taste. *Chem Senses* 32, 569–581.

Vohs, K.D. and T.F. Heatherton, 2000. Self-regulatory failure: A resource-depletion approach. *Psychol Sci* 11, 249–254.

Wagner, D.D., M. Altman, R.G. Boswell, W.M. Kelley, and T.F. Heatherton, 2013. Self-regulatory depletion enhances neural responses to rewards and impairs top-down control. *Psychol Sci* 24, 2262–2271.

Wallis, J.D., 2012. Cross-species studies of orbitofrontal cortex and value-based decision-making. *Nat Neurosci* 15, 13–19.

Wansink, B. and C.R. Payne, 2008. Eating behavior and obesity at Chinese buffets. *Obesity* 16, 1957–1960.

Wansink, B. and J. Sobal, 2007. Mindless Eating The 200 Daily Food Decisions We Overlook. *Environ Behav* 39, 106–123.

Wansink, B., K. van Ittersum, and J.E. Painter, 2006. Ice cream illusions bowls, spoons, and self-served portion sizes. *Am J Prev Med* 31, 240–243.

Wardle, J., 1990. Conditioning processes and cue exposure in the modification of excessive eating. *Addict Behav* 15, 387–393.

Weygandt, M., K. Mai, E. Dommes, V. Leupelt, K. Hackmack, T. Kahnt, Y. Rothemund, J. Spranger, and J.-D. Haynes, 2013. The role of neural impulse control mechanisms for dietary success in obesity. *NeuroImage* 83, 669–678.

Woods, S., 1991. The eating paradox: How we tolerate food. *Psychol Rev* 98, 488–505.

Woods, S.C., 2009. The control of food intake: Behavioral versus molecular perspectives. *Cell Metab* 9, 489–498.

Yasoshima, Y., H. Yoshizawa, T. Shimura, and T. Miyamoto, 2015. The basolateral nucleus of the amygdala mediates caloric sugar preference over a non-caloric sweetener in mice. *Neuroscience* 291, 203–215.

Yokum, S., J. Ng, and E. Stice, 2011. Attentional bias to food images associated with elevated weight and future weight gain: An FMRI study. *Obesity* 19, 1775–1783.

Zhang, Q., H. Li, and F. Guo, 2011. Amygdala, an important regulator for food intake. *Front Biol* 6, 82–85.

Zheng, H., N.R. Lenard, A.C. Shin, and H.-R. Berthoud, 2009. Appetite control and energy balance regulation in the modern world: Reward-driven brain overrides repletion signals. *Int J Obes* 33 Suppl 2, S8–S13.

7 Development of Hypothalamic Circuits That Control Food Intake and Energy Balance

Sebastien G. Bouret

CONTENTS

7.1   INTRODUCTION

Interest in the importance of early life events in lifelong metabolic regulation has been increasing since the work by Hales and Barker (1992) in the early 1990s. Based on compelling epidemiological evidence, they found a strong association between suboptimal fetal and neonatal nutrition and a number of chronic metabolic conditions later in life, including cardiovascular diseases, hypertension, and diabetes. They proposed that poor nutrition during perinatal development causes a "thrifty phenotype" wherein the individual becomes adapted to an environment with short food supply by growing to a smaller stature, having a lower metabolic rate, and showing less behavioral activity to conserve energy. If such individuals are later exposed to a richer environment, they may instead run a higher risk of developing obesity and type 2 diabetes due to a mismatch between actual and expected nutritional environment. The concept of perinatal programming of obesity and diabetes has then been extended to other nutritional insults, including maternal and/or postnatal overnutrition. It has been suggested that changes in the perinatal environment can affect the structure and function of key metabolically relevant organs such as the pancreas, liver, and adipose tissue. There is also growing appreciation that developmental programming of neural systems involved in energy balance by the perinatal environment represents a potential cause for obesity and diabetes. An important component of this neural system involves neurons located in the hypothalamus. Classic experiments using physical lesions of specific hypothalamic loci and, more recently, studies using conditional, neuron-specific gene targeting strategies have revealed that the hypothalamic regulation of energy homeostasis involves an interconnected neural network that contains specialized neurons located in the arcuate nucleus (ARC), the ventromedial nucleus (VMH), the dorsomedial nucleus (DMH), the paraventricular nucleus (PVN), and the lateral hypothalamic area (LHA) (for review, see Gao and Horvath 2007, Williams and Elmquist 2012) (Figure 7.1). The ARC and VMH appear to be predominant sites for the integration of blood-borne molecules, such as hormones (e.g., leptin, insulin, ghrelin, etc) and nutrients (e.g., glucose, free fatty acids, etc). Within the ARC, primary importance has been given to neurons that coexpress agouti-related peptide (AgRP) and neuropeptide Y (NPY) and the neurons that contain proopiomelanocortin (POMC)-derived peptides. Both NPY/AgRP- and POMC-containing neurons project extensively to other key hypothalamic nuclei, including the PVN, DMH, and LHA, that in turn send projections to intrahypothalamic and extrahypothalamic sites to regulate feeding. Of particular importance are projections to the PVN because it is the most thoroughly characterized hypothalamic interface between the endocrine, autonomic, and somatomotor systems that influence feeding behavior and energy metabolism (Sawchenko 1998, Sawchenko and Swanson 1983, Watts 2000). The complex pattern of neuronal wiring in the adult hypothalamus depends on a series of cellular and endocrine events during development that establish a framework on which functional circuits can be built.

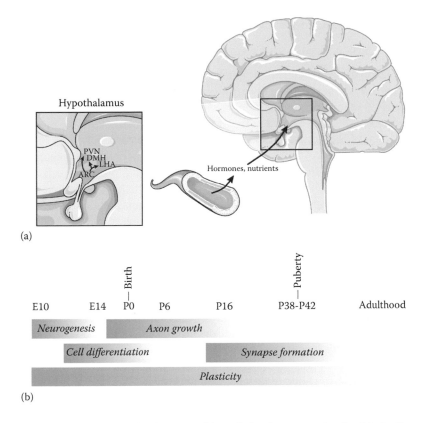

FIGURE 7.1   Anatomy and development of hypothalamic systems involved in feeding and body weight regulation. (a) Circulating hormones that reflect peripheral energy status, such as insulin, leptin, and ghrelin, act directly on metabolically relevant neurons within the arcuate nucleus (ARC) of the hypothalamus to regulate energy balance and glucose homeostasis. ARC neurons in turn send extensive projections to other parts of the hypothalamus, including the paraventricular (PVN) and dorsomedial (DMH) nuclei of the hypothalamus and the lateral hypothalamic area (LHA). These neuronal projections represent important routes for the actions of leptin, insulin, and ghrelin at the hypothalamic level. (b) The hypothalamus undergoes tremendous growth beginning early in gestation and continuing during the postnatal period. During this developmental period, a variety of processes shape the hypothalamic nuclei involved in the control of eating. These include the birth of new cells that populate these areas (neurogenesis) and the development of functional neural connections (axon growth and synaptogenesis). Each of these developmental processes represents an important period of vulnerability during which alterations of the prenatal and early postnatal environments may have long-term and potentially irreversible consequences on hypothalamic development and function. This figure was created in part using illustrations from "Servier Medical Art," with permission.

7.2 MAJOR STAGES OF HYPOTHALAMIC DEVELOPMENT

7.2.1 NEURONAL BIRTH AND CELLULAR SPECIFICATION

The formation of the hypothalamus begins with the proliferation of neural progenitor cells. This developmental event occurs just after the closure of the neural tube at E10 in rats and E9 in mice. Cells that compose hypothalamic nuclei are primarily derived from precursors that are located in the proliferative zone located in the inner and the lower portion of the third ventricle, also known as the neuroepithelium of the third ventricle (Sauer 1935). A key event in the formation of hypothalamic neurons is the terminal mitosis, i.e., the withdrawal of dividing neuronal precursor cells from the mitotic cycle. The birth of cells that compose the hypothalamus was first characterized using empirical approaches, including thymidine incorporation. This assay uses a radioactive nucleoside, [^{3}H]thymidine, which incorporates into the nuclear DNA during the S-phase of the cell cycle. By injecting pregnant rats with [^{3}H]thymidine at various stages of embryonic development, Altman and Bayer (1986) and Ifft (1972) reported more than 30 years ago that the majority of cells located in the hypothalamus were born between embryonic days 13 and 15 in rats. Using a similar approach, Shimada and Nakamura (1973) found that most neurons in the mouse hypothalamus are born between embryonic days 10 and 14 (Figure 7.1). However, the use of radioactive nucleoside presents several disadvantages, including high cost, logistic problems associated with handling of radiolabeled substances, and the lengthy process of exposing and developing autoradiographs (3–12 weeks). In addition, this approach does not allow determination of the chemical phenotype of the generated cells, which is a major limitation considering the phenotypic diversity of hypothalamic neurons. This limitation can be avoided with more contemporary and nonisotopic approaches that use the thymidine analog bromodeoxyuridine BrdU (5-bromo-2′-deoxyuridine) and allow colabeling with various phenotypic markers. BrdU has proven to be useful in determining the birthdate of specific hypothalamic neurons and has revealed, for example, that the majority of leptin-responsive neurons in the adult mouse hypothalamus are born during a developmental period that is largely restricted to embryonic day 12 (Ishii and Bouret 2012) (Table 7.1). In contrast, neurons expressing melanin-concentrating hormone (MCH) have a relatively long neurogenic period. The majority

---

TABLE 7.1
Birthdate of Hypothalamic Neurons Involved in Metabolic Regulation

	Birthdate	Reference
POMC neurons	E10 (mice)	Padilla, Carmody, and Zeltser 2010
MCH neurons	E10–E14 (mice); E12–E16 (rats)	Brischoux, Fellmann, and Risold 2001, Croizier et al. 2010
Leptin-sensitive neurons	E12 (mice)	Ishii and Bouret 2012
VMH neurons	E12–E16 (mice); E13–E15 (rats)	Ishii and Bouret 2012, McClellana, Parker, and Tobet 2006
SF1 neurons	E10 (mice)	Cheung et al. 2013

of MCH neurons are born at embryonic days 12–13 in rats and embryonic day 10 in mice, but some as late as embryonic day 16 in rats and embryonic day 14 in mice (Brischoux, Fellmann, and Risold 2001, Croizier et al. 2010) (Table 7.1). MCH neurons are generated in two waves showing an outside–in gradient, with MCH neurons located next to the third ventricle generated after those located close to the cerebral peduncle (Brischoux, Fellman, and Risold 2001, Croizier et al. 2011, Risold et al. 2009). In addition, *pro-MCH* mRNA as well as MCH immunoreactivity is detected in the LHA as early as embryonic day 13 in rats and embryonic day 11 in mice. VMH neurons are also born during a relatively long neurogenic period. Many neurons in these nuclei are born on embryonic day 12 in mice and embryonic day 13 in rats, but some neurons are generated as late as embryonic day 16 in mice and embryonic day 15 in rats (Ishii and Bouret 2012, McClellana, Parker, and Tobet 2006) (Table 7.1). Within the VMH, the first SF-1 neurons are observed as early as embryonic day 10 (Cheung et al. 2013) (Table 7.1). In the mouse ARC, Padilla, Carmody, and Zeltser (2010) recently reported that the majority of POMC neurons are born as early as embryonic day 10 and acquire their terminal peptidergic phenotype during midgestation (Table 7.1). Notably, cell lineage experiments also reveal that a subpopulation of embryonic *Pomc*-expressing precursors subsequently adopt a mature NPY phenotype (Padilla, Carmody, and Zeltser 2010). The expression of *Npy* and *Pomc* mRNAs continues to increase in the ARC during the postnatal period, reaching maximal expression levels by postnatal day 15 (PD15) in rats (Cottrell et al. 2009).

7.2.2 Axon Growth

Differentiated neurons send out axonal processes that carry information to target cells. Some hypothalamic neurons, such as ARC neurons, have relatively short axons and make connections primarily to neurons within the hypothalamus. Other hypothalamic neurons, such as LHA neurons, send long axons to distant targets that include the brainstem and the cortex. In part because of their importance for appetite regulation, the first systematic studies that examined the development of hypothalamic feeding projections defined the ontogeny of projection pathways from ARC AgRP/NPY neurons. Using immunohistochemistry, Grove et al. (2013) reported that projections immunopositive for AgRP/NPY are immature at birth and develop mainly during the second week of postnatal life in rats. The same temporal pattern was observed for the development of POMC projections in mice (Nilsson et al. 2005) (Figure 7.1). The fact that microinjection of NPY in the area comprising the PVN at P2 resulted in increased milk and water intakes raises the hypothesis that NPY receptors may be present and functional in the PVN before innervation of this nucleus by ARC AgRP/NPY fibers (Capuano, Leibowitz, and Barr 1993). However, the use of immunohistochemistry to study the development pattern of axonal projections should be used with caution. For example, changes in the density of AgRP/NPY immunoreactivity may be due to alterations in the density of axon terminals and reflect a true change in the organization of brain circuitry, but it may also simply reflect alterations in neuropeptide synthesis and transport or changes in local processing and release. Axonal tracing remains the gold standard to study neuronal connections. Studies using the fluorescent tracer DiI have demonstrated that ARC axons that are found in the DMH, and PVN of mouse neonates develop in a pattern that mirrors that of the innervation of terminals containing AgRP/NPY (Bouret, Draper, and Simerly 2004a). By P6, ARC projections extend through the periventricular zone of the hypothalamus to provide inputs to the DMH, followed by inputs to the PVN between P8 and P10. ARC projections to LHA develop significantly later, with the mature pattern of innervation first apparent on P12. Not until P18 does the pattern of ARC axonal projections achieve a distribution resembling that seen in the adult (Figure 7.1). The sequential innervation of ARC targets also suggests that leptin signaling may differentially activate neurons in these target nuclei during development. Consistent with this idea, peripheral leptin-injection-induced c-Fos-immunoreactivity (a marker of neuronal activation) was observed in the ARC as early as postnatal day 6, whereas leptin-induced c-Fos was not observed in the PVN before postnatal day 10 (Bouret, Draper, and Simerly 2004a). Notably, the PVN does not express leptin receptors at this age, suggesting that leptin induces cFos activation in the PVN indirectly (Caron et al. 2010); thus, the development of leptin-induced neuronal activation in target nuclei of the ARC coincides with their innervation by ARC axons.

In contrast to the development of projections from the ARC, efferent projections from the DMH to the PVN and LHA are fully established by P6 (Bouret, Draper, and Simerly 2004a). Also, projections from the VMH develop prior to those from the ARC. By P10, VMH axons provide strong inputs to the LHA, whereas, at this age, the LHA is almost devoid of fibers from the ARC (Bouret, Draper, and Simerly 2004a). Similarly, MCH neurons in the LHA begin to send axonal projections around embryonic days 11–12 (Croizier et al. 2011). Together, these anatomical observations indicate that hypothalamic axon growth is a dynamic and relative long developmental process that starts during midgestation and continues well past the second week of postnatal life (Figure 7.1).

7.2.3 Synapse Formation

The formation of synapses follows the development of axon projections. There are several ways to quantify synapses. The gold standard is electron microscopy, as this is the only way to see synaptic vesicles and thereby say definitively that a synapse is truly present. This technique was used very effectively by Matsumoto and colleagues in the 1970s, who reported a gradual increase in the number of synapses in the ARC from birth to adulthood (Matsumoto and Arai 1976). Ultrastructural analysis of synapses in the rat ARC reveals very few axodendritic or axosomatic synapses on P5, whereas by P20 (periweaning), about one-half of the synapses found in adult animals are already formed. The number of synapses found in the ARC continues to increase after weaning to reach an adult-like pattern by P45 (Matsumoto and Arai 1976) (Figure 7.1). Electrophysiology can also be used to study when functional synapses are forming. Using this approach, Colmers and colleagues showed that there is an age-dependent increase in the electrophysiological response to melanocortin by specific sets of PVN neurons, with a maximal response observed at P28–P35 (Melnick et al. 2007), suggesting that synapses between POMC axons and PVN target neurons are not structurally and functionally mature until puberty.

7.3 DEVELOPMENTAL ASPECTS OF THE HYPOTHALAMIC RESPONSE TO METABOLIC HORMONES

7.3.1 DEVELOPMENTAL REGULATION OF METABOLIC HORMONE SECRETION

Before assessing the ontogeny of the hypothalamic response to metabolic hormones, it is critical that we have a good understanding of the secretion profile of these hormones during development. Leptin is one of the first major metabolic hormones to appear during development. In adults, leptin is primarily secreted by adipocytes, but a variety of tissues produce leptin during embryonic development. On embryonic day 13, high levels of leptin gene expression are found in the fetal liver and cartilage-bone structures, followed by cardiac expression between embryonic days 16 and 18 (Hoggard et al. 1997). In addition to being produced by the embryo itself, dams also secrete high levels of leptin during pregnancy, but whether maternal leptin crosses the placenta remains controversial. Circulating leptin levels increase markedly during the postnatal period and exhibit a distinct surge between P8 and P12 in mice (Ahima, Prabakaran, and Flier 1998). These significantly higher levels of postnatal circulating leptin are associated with greater expression of leptin mRNA in both white (abdominal) and brown (interscapular) adipose tissue (Devaskar et al. 1997). There is a coordinated decrease in levels of leptin mRNA and leptin peptide after weaning, i.e., when pups switch from maternal milk to an adult diet (Devaskar et al. 1997).

Similar to leptin, ghrelin is also developmentally regulated during perinatal life. In rodents, high levels of *ghrelin* mRNA are detected in the fetus at embryonic day 12, and by embryonic day 17, detectable levels of acylated (the "active" form) and desacylated (the "inactive" form) ghrelin are present in blood (Nakahara et al. 2006, Torsello et al. 2003). The pancreas appears to be a major source of ghrelin expression during perinatal life. *Ghrelin* mRNA and protein are found at high levels in fetal pancreatic islets, whereas low levels of ghrelin are detected in the fetal stomach (Chanoine and Wong 2004, Lee et al. 2002, Wierup et al. 2002). These observations suggest that, in contrast to the adult, the source of circulating fetal ghrelin may be the pancreas, not the stomach. However, stomach ghrelin expression increases gradually after birth to reach adult-like levels by 3–5 weeks of life (Hayashida et al. 2002, Lee et al. 2002, Torsello et al. 2003). Simultaneously, pancreatic ghrelin expression declines progressively from birth to weaning and becomes barely detectable in the adult pancreas (Wierup et al. 2002).

Measurable levels of insulin are also detected in whole embryos as early as embryonic day 8 (Spaventi, Antica, and Pavelic 1990). The earliest time point for insulin immunodetection in the pancreas is embryonic day 9, which also coincides with a period of elevated levels of insulin (Teitelman et al. 1993, Spaventi, Antica, and Pavelic 1990), which returns to basal levels at embryonic day 12 (Spaventi, Antica, and Pavelic 1990). However, the number of insulin-positive cells in the pancreas at embryonic days 9 is relatively low, suggesting that the insulin detected at this early stage may also be extra-pancreatic. Supporting this hypothesis, insulin expression is detected in tissues other than the pancreas during early embryonic life. Notably, insulin expression is observed in the central nervous system of mouse embryos at embryonic day 9, which corresponds with the elevated levels of insulin found in embryonic tissues (Deltour et al. 1993). It is also important to note that maternal insulin cannot cross the placental barrier. However, maternal glucose is actively transported to the fetus, where it can stimulate insulin secretion early during fetal development (Baumann, Deborde, and Illsley 2002). Pathological conditions, such maternal insulin deficiency and maternal hyperinsulinemia, cause maternal hyperglycemia, which in turn triggers compensatory perinatal hyperinsulinemia (Desoye, Gauster, and Wadsack 2011). This developmental hyperinsulinemia is thought to be a major contributor to the perinatal programming for obesity and diabetes (Martin-Gronert and Ozanne 2005, Paderson 1971, Paderson and Osler 1961). During postnatal life, insulin and glucose levels remain relatively stable and do not exhibit major developmental regulation (Bouret et al. unpublished data, Srinivasan et al. 2008), unlike other metabolic hormones such as leptin and ghrelin.

7.3.2 ONTOGENY OF THE RESPONSE OF HYPOTHALAMIC NEURONS TO METABOLIC HORMONES

Accumulating evidence suggests that there are differences in the biological actions of metabolic hormones between adults and neonates. For example, in sharp contrast to the potent anorexigenic and orexigenic effects of leptin and ghrelin, respectively, in adults, acute injection of those hormones does not significantly influence milk intake or body weight in neonatal rats or mice (Piao et al. 2008, Steculorum and Bouret 2011a). A possible explanation for this lack of response is that the neonatal brain is relatively insensitive to leptin and ghrelin and may present hormonal resistance. However, leptin and ghrelin receptors are expressed in nuclei known to regulate feeding, including the ARC, and acute peripheral leptin or ghrelin treatment activates ARC neurons during early postnatal life (Baquero et al. 2014, Bouret et al. 2012, Caron et al. 2010, Steculorum and Bouret 2011a). Furthermore, the observation that the short form of the leptin receptor, which is considered to be one of the main leptin transporters, is expressed in brain microvessels as early as at birth suggests that leptin can cross the blood–brain barrier and reach the brain at an early age (Pan et al. 2008). Further supporting the functional role of leptin in the postnatal ARC, acute leptin administration in rat neonates causes changes in *Pomc* and *Npy* gene expression (Proulx, Richard, and Walker 2002). In addition, acute ghrelin injection to mouse pups on P10 decreases and increases *Pomc* and *Npy* mRNA, respectively, in the ARC (Steculorum and Bouret 2011a). Collectively, these results support the hypothesis that metabolic hormone receptors are present and functional in the developing hypothalamus but that the roles of leptin and ghrelin during neonatal life may differ from those in adults.

7.4 HORMONAL CONTROL OF HYPOTHALAMIC DEVELOPMENT

7.4.1 LEPTIN

An important number of developmental signals control the ultimate architecture of hypothalamic feeding pathways. These signals can influence one or multiple components of hypothalamic development, including neurogenesis and axon growth. Among this array of signals, significant attention has been given to the importance of metabolic hormones in hypothalamic development. A particularly salient example is the neurotrophic role of leptin during development. Axonal labeling of ARC axons with the anterograde tracer DiI showed that mice genetically deficient in leptin (ob/ob) display a marked disruption in the development of ARC axonal projections during early postnatal life (Bouret, Draper, and Simerly 2004b) (Figure 7.2). Another important observation is that the disruption of ARC pathways in ob/ob mice is permanent because fewer ARC fibers are also found in the hypothalamus of adult ob/ob mice. But perhaps the most important discovery was that leptin acts primarily during a restricted neonatal period to exert its developmental effects on ARC neural projections. Peripheral leptin injections during the first two weeks of postnatal life restore a normal pattern of ARC projections in ob/ob mice (Bouret, Draper, and Simerly 2004b). However, the treatment of adult ob/ob mice with leptin is ineffective and does not increase the density of ARC projections. Notably, neonatal leptin exposure selectively restores ARC projections onto preautonomic, but not onto neuroendocrine, neurons (Bouyer and Simerly 2013). Together, these findings demonstrate that leptin is required for normal postnatal development of ARC projections and suggest

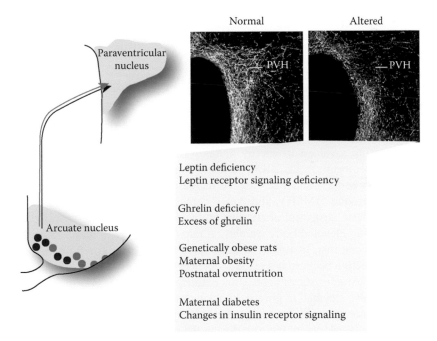

FIGURE 7.2 Developmental programming of hypothalamic feeding pathways. The developmental programming of hypothalamic neural systems by the perinatal hormonal environment represents a possible mechanism by which alterations in maternal and/or postnatal nutrition predispose the offspring to obesity. The development axonal projections from the arcuate nucleus to the paraventicular nucleus of the hypothalamus appears to be highly sensitive to changes in the nutritional environment. Excess of nutrition during prenatal and/or postnatal life are associated with structural defects in the hypothalamus. These effects appear to be mediated, to some extent, by abnormal leptin, ghrelin, and insulin secretion and/or signaling during critical periods of fetal and/or postnatal development.

that the postnatal leptin surge is a key developmental signal that shapes the architecture of hypothalamic circuits that control energy balance.

A likely molecular mechanism underlying the developmental effects of leptin on hypothalamic circuits is the expression of leptin receptors (LepRb) by ARC neurons. As described previously, the developing ARC contains high levels of *Leprb* mRNA (Baquero et al. 2014, Caron et al. 2010), and administration of leptin to mouse neonates results in the activation of major LepRb signaling pathways, including pSTAT3, pERK, and pAKT (Bouret et al. 2012). Moreover, the development of ARC projections is disrupted in LepRb-deficient mice (db/db) and rats (fa/fa) as well as in mouse neonates that lack LepRb → pSTAT3 and LepRb → pERK signaling (Bouret and Simerly 2007, Bouret et al. 2012). The observation that direct exposure of ARC explants to leptin induces neurite outgrowth and that this effect is blocked if the explants are derived from db/db mice further supports the idea that leptin acts directly on LepRb-containing ARC neurons to promote axon growth (Bouret, Draper, and Simerly 2004b, Bouret et al. 2012). However, not all hypothalamic sites that express LepRb respond to the trophic action of leptin. For example, the DMH contains relatively high levels of LepRb during postnatal life (Caron et al. 2010), yet its projections to the PVN appear normal in ob/ob mice (Bouret, Draper, and Simerly 2004b).

7.4.2 GHRELIN

Although the potent orexigenic efficacy of ghrelin is not present in the initial 2–3 postnatal weeks in mice or rats (Piao et al. 2008, Steculorum and Bouret 2011a), ghrelin in early postnatal life does have a lasting developmental effect on hypothalamic circuits involved in energy homeostasis and influences body weight in adulthood (Steculorum et al. 2015). Mouse neonates injected with an antighrelin compound between P4 and P22 display increased densities of alpha-melanocyte stimulating hormone (αMSH)- and AgRP-containing axons innervating the PVN (Figure 7.2). These structural alterations are accompanied by long-term metabolic defects, including elevated body weight, fat mass, and hyperglycemia (Steculorum et al. 2015). In contrast, treatment of adult mice with the antighrelin compound is relatively ineffective because it does not increase the density of ARC projections to levels that are characteristic of control mice. Intriguingly, the density of ARC axonal projections is also elevated in ghrelin knockout mouse pups, but it becomes normal in adult knockout animals, indicating that ARC projections continue to be plastic not just early in development but also during the postweaning period in response to genetically programmed events.

Not only the correct timing but also the correct amplitude of ghrelin appears important for normal development of hypothalamic feeding pathways because neonatal hyperghrelinemia causes permanent alterations in the development of ARC neural projections (Figure 7.2). Chronic injection of exogenous ghrelin to wild-type mouse neonates between P4 and P12 results in a marked reduction in the density of ARC fibers innervating the PVN. Similar to leptin, the site of action for the developmental effects of ghrelin likely includes direct actions on ARC neurons: direct exposure of isolated explants from the ARC to ghrelin blunts neurite extension (Steculorum et al. 2015). Therefore, during neonatal life, ghrelin appears to act as an inhibitory signal influencing key developmental events in the same hypothalamic pathways that will convey ghrelin signals in mature mice (Steculorum et al. 2015).

7.4.3 INSULIN

Insulin has long been associated with growth and development. Maternal injections of insulin between gestational day 15 and 20 induce obesity in the offspring (Jones et al. 1995), which is accompanied by increased hypothalamic norepinephrine levels (Jones et al. 1995) and increased density of norepinephrine-containing fibers innervating the PVN (Jones, Olster, and States 1996). In addition, intra-hypothalamic injection of insulin on P8 is associated with morphological alterations of hypothalamic nuclei (including the ARC and VMH) and lifelong metabolic disturbances (Plagemann et al. 1992, 1999b). The manipulation of maternal insulin levels can also be achieved experimentally by injecting streptozotocin (STZ), a pancreatic beta cell toxin, during gestation. Maternal hypoinsulinemia caused by STZ injections is associated with a reduced density of POMC- and NPY-containing fibers in the offspring (Steculorum and Bouret 2011b). Moreover, pups born to STZ-treated dams display an increased number of NPY-, POMC- and galanin-containing neurons in the ARC (Franke et al. 2005, Plagemann et al. 1998, 1999a, Steculorum and Bouret 2011b). This change in ARC cell number is prevented by normalization of glycemia using pancreatic islet transplantation (Franke et al. 2005). These observations suggest that maternal insulin and/or glucose levels are critical for the proper determination of neuronal cell number and axonal connectivity in the hypothalamus (Figure 7.2). However, because insulin injection often results in a marked decrease in circulating glucose levels, it makes it difficult to study the effects of insulin independently of glucose. Nevertheless, the observation that direct exposure of isolated organotypic hypothalamic explants to insulin promotes axon growth supports the hypothesis that insulin alone represents a powerful neurotrophic agent (Toran-Allerand, Ellis, and Pfenninger 1988).

7.5 DEVELOPMENT OF HYPOTHALAMIC CIRCUITS IN THE CONTEXT OF PERINATAL OBESITY

As described earlier, the rodent hypothalamus develops during a relatively long period, beginning early in gestation and continuing during the postnatal period. The developing hypothalamus is therefore exposed to two distinct environments: one in utero and the other extra utero. These developmental windows represent important intervals of vulnerability during which alterations in the nutritional environment may lead to abnormal hypothalamic development and subsequent function. Because maternal obesity and childhood obesity contribute to many negative outcomes in the infant, including lifelong obesity and diabetes, a number of studies have specifically attempted to evaluate the consequences of perinatal obesity on hypothalamic development.

7.5.1 Animal Models of Perinatal Obesity

Maternal high-fat diet (HFD) feeding during pregnancy is probably the most widely used approach for studying the consequences of maternal obesity in rodents. Offspring born to obese females fed a HFD (45% to 60% of calories from fat) during gestation only or during both gestation and lactation become progressively overweight (Chen, Simar, and Morris 2009, Kirk et al. 2009). In addition, the offspring of HFD-induced obese females become hyperphagic and glucose intolerant and display an increase in adiposity (Chen, Simar, and Morris 2009, Kirk et al. 2009). The model of diet-induced obesity (DIO) developed by Levin et al. (1997) is particularly well suited for the study of the underlying biological processes that contribute to the development of obesity in humans because Levin's DIO rats share several features with human obesity, including polygenic inheritance. This animal model is also useful for the study of the relative contribution of genetic versus environmental factors in metabolic programming. Similar to the animals that are born to HFD dams, the offspring of mothers that are genetically predisposed to DIO are obese, hyperphagic, and glucose intolerant when fed a high-energy diet, whereas the offspring that are born to diet-resistant dams do not show these effects (Levin et al. 2003, Ricci and Levin 2003).

Because of the importance of postnatal organ development, including the hypothalamus, animal models of postnatal metabolic programming have been developed to specifically target this developmental period. An approach that has proven extremely fruitful for the study of postnatal overfeeding is the reduction of litter size. Raising pups in small litters (SLs) increases milk availability and markedly accelerates preweaning growth. Pups raised in SL remain heavier throughout life (Bouret et al. 2007, Davidowa and Plagemann 2000, Glavas et al. 2010) and postnatally overfed animals show accelerated and exacerbated weight gain and impaired glucose homeostasis when fed a HFD (Glavas et al. 2010).

7.5.2 Perinatal Obesity and Hypothalamic Hormonal Resistance

Resistance to the regulatory action of metabolic hormones is a hallmark of obesity in adult individuals. For example, most forms of obesity are associated with a diminished response of the hypothalamus to the appetite-suppressing effects of leptin (Enriori et al. 2006, Myers, Cowley, and Munzberg 2008). Interestingly, animals exposed to perinatal obesogenic conditions also exhibit leptin resistance. Adult offspring born to obese (HFD and DIO) dams display a blunted response to the anorectic effects of leptin (Kirk et al. 2009, Levin and Dunn-Meynell 2002, Yura et al. 2005). Moreover, this diminished response to leptin is associated with a reduced ability of leptin to induce LepRb signaling in ARC neurons, which demonstrates that it is a centrally mediated phenomenon (Kirk et al. 2009, Bouret et al. 2008, Yura et al. 2005). Insulin sensitivity also appears to be affected in rats selectively bred to develop DIO (Clegg et al. 2005). Importantly, the development of leptin resistance occurs before the animals become obese, suggesting that this hormonal resistance may initiate the development and maintenance of obesity. A likely mechanism underlying the hormonal resistance is the abnormally elevated levels of leptin and/or an alteration in receptor expression and/or signaling during neonatal life. For example, maternal obesity/diabetes and postnatal overnutrition cause marked increases in leptin levels during postnatal life and reduce the ability of leptin to induce phosphorylation of STAT3 in the ARC during critical periods of hypothalamic development (Bouret et al. 2007, 2008, Glavas et al. 2010, Kirk et al. 2009, Steculorum and Bouret 2011b). Also, down-regulation of hypothalamic LepR mRNA has been described in several animal models of nutritional programming, including SL, DIO, and maternal malnutrition, and inhibition of leptin binding has been reported in the hypothalamus of DIO rats (Chen, Simar, and Morris 2009, Cripps et al. 2009, Irani, Dunn-Meynell, and Levin 2007, Levin et al. 2003, Levin, Dunn-Meynell, and Banks 2004).

Nutritionally induced hormonal resistance is not limited to leptin. Ghrelin resistance is also observed in the SL model: postnatally overfed mouse pups exhibit elevated ghrelin levels between P16 and P22. Surprisingly, normalization of neonatal hyperghrelinemia in neonates raised in SL did not ameliorate metabolic outcomes, suggesting that neonatally overfed mice are relatively insensitive to neonatal ghrelin and may present ghrelin resistance. Consistent with this hypothesis, the ability of peripheral ghrelin to induce c-Fos in the ARC is markedly attenuated in overnourished pups (Collden et al. 2015). However, SL pups display a normal response to central ghrelin, raising the possibility that the mechanisms underlying early ghrelin resistance include defective transport of the hormone across the blood–brain barrier to the cerebrospinal fluid or to its sites of action within the brain. The cellular mechanisms involved in attenuated ghrelin transport likely involve decreased ghrelin uptake by tanycytes. These specialized ependymoglial cells located in the median eminence have recently emerged as critical regulators of hormone transport into the brain, including into the hypothalamus, and neonatal overnutrition alters the ability of tanycytes to transport ghrelin into the ARC (Collden et al. 2015).

7.5.3 MOLECULAR CHANGES OBSERVED IN THE HYPOTHALAMUS DURING PERINATAL OBESITY

A variety of regulatory processes are perturbed in animals born in an obesogenic environment, including an imbalance in the hypothalamic expression of appetite regulators. In most cases, programmed overweight is associated with an elevated ratio of orexigenic to anorexigenic neuropeptide expression in the hypothalamus. For example, maternal obesity, as well as postnatal overnutrition, causes an overall increase in the expression of orexigenic neuropeptides, such as NPY and AgRP, and a decrease in the expression of anorexigenic neuropeptides, such as POMC and cocaine and amphetamine-regulated transcript peptide (CART) (Chen, Simar, and Morris 2009, Coupe et al. 2010, Cripps et al. 2009, López et al. 2005, Remmers et al. 2010, Srinivasan et al. 2008). It has been postulated that the increased ratio of orexigenic to anorexigenic neuropeptides may explain the increased drive to eat in perinatally malprogrammed animals. It appears that the observed changes in neuropeptide gene expression reflect an acquired mechanism that originates from a malprogramming of hypothalamic neuropeptidergic systems during early life, rather than being a consequence of metabolic dysfunction, such as overweight and hyperphagia. Consistent with this idea, changes in neuropeptide gene expression are often observed as early as embryonic life and/or during the first postnatal weeks, i.e., prior to the development of overweight and hyperphagia (Chen, Simar, and Morris 2009, Cripps et al. 2009, Gupta et al. 2009, Morris and Chen 2008, Remmers et al. 2010, Srinivasan et al. 2008, Terroni et al. 2005). In addition to its adverse effects on the expression of appetite-regulating genes, postnatal overfeeding affects neuronal response to neuropeptides. For example, PVN neurons of chronically overfed pups display reduced electrophysiological responses to ARC neuropeptides such as NPY, AgRP, aMSH, and CART (Davidowa, Li, and Plagemann 2003).

7.5.4 Neurodevelopmental Changes Associated with Perinatal Obesity

The capacity of diet to alter proliferation in the developing hypothalamus has been demonstrated in a rodent model of maternal obesity. Maternal high-fat feeding increases hypothalamic cell proliferation in rat embryos, resulting in higher numbers of neurons containing orexigenic neuropeptides (i.e., galanin, enkephalin, dynorphin, MCH, and orexin) in the PVN and LHA (Chang et al. 2008). In general, rodent studies indicate that the adverse effects of a maternal obesogenic environment on hypothalamic cell numbers are similar whether they occur during gestation or during gestation and lactation. For example, offspring of HFD mothers crossfostered with control mothers during lactation exhibit similar changes in orexigenic cell number and metabolic outcomes compared with pups raised by HFD mothers during pregnancy and lactation (Chang et al. 2008). Increased nutrition and growth, specifically during early postnatal life, also influence neural cell numbers in the hypothalamus and increase the number of neurons that produce orexigenic neuropeptides (Plagemann et al. 1999c).

Impaired organization of hypothalamic circuits is also a common feature of nutritional malprogramming. In particular, perturbations in the establishment of ARC neural projections have been reported in virtually all animals subjected to nutritional insults during perinatal life. However, the degree of disruption may differ according to the nature of the nutritional insult. Chronic consumption of an HFD during pregnancy and lactation reduces the density of ARC AgRP fibers that innervate the PVN (Grayson et al. 2010, Kirk et al. 2009) (Figure 7.2). Maternal consumption of HFD during lactation (but not during pregnancy) appears sufficient to cause obesity and diabetes and to alter the development of POMC projections (Vogt et al. 2014). The precise biological mechanisms that underlie the perinatal nutritionally induced alterations in hypothalamic organization and function remain largely unknown. However, recent evidence has indicated that abnormal leptin and insulin signaling during postnatal development may represent a likely cause for the HFD-induced alterations in hypothalamic development. For example, obesity-prone DIO rats display an abnormal organization of projections derived from the ARC (Figure 7.2) and in vitro experiments indicate that this may result from diminished responsiveness of ARC neurons to the trophic actions of leptin during critical periods of postnatal development. Furthermore, Vogt et al. (2014) elegantly demonstrated that abrogation of insulin receptors in POMC neurons improves ARC projection and glucose metabolism in pups raised by obese dams (Figure 7.2).

7.6 PERSPECTIVES

It is now clear from several different fields of research that the disruption of neurodevelopmental processes can lead to diseases later in life. The hypothalamus develops during a relatively long period, beginning early in gestation and continuing during the postnatal period. These developmental windows represent important periods of vulnerability during which alterations in the perinatal environment may lead to abnormal hypothalamic development and subsequent function. A comprehensive understanding of perinatally acquired obesity will require a developmental map of the feeding neural system's intricate wiring diagram, the breakdown of which will ultimately be responsible for the emergence of a particular metabolic phenotype. For example, much attention has focused on the effect of perinatal factors on the development of hypothalamic neural circuits. However, we now know that the central systems regulating energy homeostasis contain a distributed and interconnected neural network involving multiple regions of the brain. It will therefore be critical to have a better understanding of how changes in perinatal nutrition and hormones impact the development and function of other nonhypothalamic circuits, such as midbrain and hindbrain circuits.

LITERATURE CITED

Ahima, R.S., D. Prabakaran, and J.S. Flier. 1998. Postnatal leptin surge and regulation of circadian rhythm of leptin by feeding. Implications for energy homeostasis and neuroendocrine function. *J Clin Invest* 101 (5):1020–1027.

Altman, J., and S.A. Bayer. 1986. The development of the rat hypothalamus. *Adv Anat. Embryol Cell Biol* 100 (1–178).

Baquero, A.F., A.J. de Solis, S.R. Lindsley, M.A. Kirigiti, M.S. Smith, M.A. Cowley, L.M. Zeltser, and K.L. Grove. 2014. Developmental switch of leptin signaling in arcuate nucleus neurons. *J Neurosci* 34 (30):9982–9994.

Baumann, M.U., S. Deborde, and N.P. Illsley. 2002. Placental glucose transfer and fetal growth. *Endocrine* 19 (1):13–22.

Bouret, S.G., S.H. Bates, S. Chen, M.G. Myers, and R.B. Simerly. 2012. Distinct roles for specific leptin receptor signals in the development of hypothalamic feeding circuits. *J Neurosci* 32 (4):1244–1252.

Bouret, S.G., C. Burt-Solorzano, C.-H. Wang, and R.B. Simerly. 2007. Impact of neonatal nutrition on development of brain metabolic circuits in mice. *Proc 37th Ann Mtg Soc Neurosci, San Diego, CA.*

Bouret, S.G., S.J. Draper, and R.B. Simerly. 2004a. Formation of projection pathways from the arcuate nucleus of the hypothalamus to hypothalamic regions implicated in the neural control of feeding behavior in mice. *J Neurosci* 24 (11):2797–2805.

Bouret, S.G., S.J. Draper, and R.B. Simerly. 2004b. Trophic action of leptin on hypothalamic neurons that regulate feeding. *Science* 304 (5667):108–110.

Bouret, S.G., J.N. Gorski, C.M. Patterson, S. Chen, B.E. Levin, and Richard B. Simerly. 2008. Hypothalamic neural projections are permanently disrupted in diet-induced obese rats. *Cell Metab* 7 (2):179–185.

Bouret, S.G., and R.B. Simerly. 2007. Development of leptin-sensitive circuits. *J Neuroendocrinol* 19 (8):575–582.

Bouyer, K., and R.B. Simerly. 2013. Neonatal leptin exposure specifies innervation of presympathetic hypothalamic neurons and improves the metabolic status of leptin-deficient mice. *J Neurosci* 33 (2):840–851.

Brischoux, F., D. Fellman, and P.-Y. Risold. 2001. Ontogenetic development of the dien-cephalic MCH neurons: A hypothalamic 'MCH area' hypothesis. *Eur J Neurosci* 13:1733–1744.

Capuano, C.A., S.F. Leibowitz, and G.A. Barr. 1993. Effect of paraventricular injection of neuropeptide Y on milk and water intake of preweanling rat. *Neuropeptides* 24:177–182.

Caron, E., C. Sachot, V. Prevot, and S.G. Bouret. 2010. Distribution of leptin-sensitive cells in the postnatal and adult mouse brain. *J Comp Neurol* 518 (4):459–476.

Chang, G.-Q., V. Gaysinskaya, O. Karatayev, and S.F. Leibowitz. 2008. Maternal High-fat diet and fetal programming: Increased proliferation of hypothalamic peptide-producing neurons that increase risk for overeating and obesity. *J Neurosci* 28 (46):12107–12119.

Chanoine, J.-P., and A.C.K. Wong. 2004. Ghrelin gene expression is markedly higher in fetal pancreas compared with fetal stomach: Effect of maternal fasting. *Endocrinology* 145 (8):3813–3820.

Chen, H., D. Simar, and M.J. Morris. 2009. Hypothalamic neuroendocrine circuitry is pro-grammed by maternal obesity: Interaction with postnatal nutritional environment. *PLoS ONE* 4 (7):e6259.

Cheung, C.C., D.M. Kurrasch, J.K. Liang, and H.A. Ingraham. 2013. Genetic labeling of steroidogenic factor-1 (SF-1) neurons in mice reveals ventromedial nucleus of the hypo-thalamus (VMH) circuitry beginning at neurogenesis and development of a separate non-SF-1 neuronal cluster in the ventrolateral VMH. *J Comp Neurol* 521:1268–1288.

Clegg, D.J., S.C. Benoit, J.A. Reed, S.C. Woods, Ambrose Dunn-Meynell, and Barry E. Levin. 2005. Reduced anorexic effects of insulin in obesity-prone rats fed a moderate-fat diet. *Am J Physiol Regul Integr Comp Physiol* 288 (4):R981–R986.

Collden, G., E. Balland, J. Parkash, E. Caron, F. Langlet, V. Prevot, and S.G. Bouret. 2015. Neonatal overnutrition causes early alterations in the central response to peripheral ghrelin. *Mol Metab* 4 (1):15–24.

Cottrell, E.C., R.L. Cripps, J.S. Duncan, P. Barrett, J.G. Mercer, A. Herwig, and S.E. Ozanne. 2009. Developmental changes in hypothalamic leptin receptor: Relationship with the postnatal leptin surge and energy balance neuropeptides in the postnatal rat. *Am J Physiol Regul Integr Comp Physiol* 296:R631–639.

Coupe, B., V. Amarger, I. Grit, A. Benani, and P. Parnet. 2010. Nutritional programming affects hypothalamic organization and early response to leptin. *Endocrinology* 151: 702–713.

Cripps, R.L., M.S.M. ÄëGronert, Z.A. Archer, C.N. Hales, J.G. Mercer, and S.E. Ozanne. 2009. Programming of hypothalamic neuropeptide gene expression in rats by maternal dietary protein content during pregnancy and lactation. *Clin Sci* 117 (2):85–93.

Croizier, S., C. Amiot, X. Chen, F. Presse, J.-L. Nahon, J.Y. Wu, D. Fellmann, and P.-Y. Risold. 2011. Development of posterior hypothalamic neurons enlightens a switch in the prosencephalic basic plan. *PLoS ONE* 6 (12):e28574.

Croizier, S., G. Franchi-Bernard, C. Colard, F. Poncet, A. La Roche, and P.-Y. Risold. 2010. A comparative analysis shows morphofunctional differences between the rat and mouse melanin-concentrating hormone systems. *PLoS ONE* 5 (11):e15471.

Davidowa, H., Y. Li, and A. Plagemann. 2003. Altered responses to orexigenic (AGRP, MCH) and anorexigenic (a-MSH, CART) neuropeptides of paraventricular hypothalamic neu-rons in early postnatally overfed rats. *Eur. J Neurosci* 18 (3):613–621.

Davidowa, H., and A. Plagemann. 2000. Decreased inhibition by leptin of hypothalamic arcuate neurons in neonatally overfed young rats. *Neuroreport* 11 (12):2795–2798.

Deltour, L., P. Leduque, N. Blume, O. Madsen, P. Dubois, J. Jami, and D. Bucchini. 1993. Differential expression of the two nonallelic proinsulin genes in the developing mouse embryo. *Proc Natl Acad Sci* 90 (2):527–531.

Desoye, G., M. Gauster, and C. Wadsack. 2011. Placental transport in pregnancy pathologies. *Am J Clin Nutr* 94:1896S–1902S.

Devaskar, S.U., C. Ollesch, R.A. Rajakumar, and P.A. Rajakumar. 1997. Developmental changes in ob gene expression and circulating leptin peptide concentration. *Biochem Biophys Res Commun* 238:44–47.

Enriori, P.J., A.E. Evans, P. Sinnayah, and M.A. Cowley. 2006. Leptin resistance and obesity. *Obesity* 14 (suppl 5):254S–258S.

Franke, K., T. Harder, L. Aerts, K. Melchior, S. Fahrenkrog, E. Rodekamp, T. Ziska, F.A. Van Assche, J.W. Dudenhausen, and A. Plagemann. 2005. Programming of orexigenic and anorexigenic hypothalamic neurons in offspring of treated and untreated diabetic mother rats. *Brain Res* 1031 (2):276–283.

Gao, Q., and T.L. Horvath. 2007. Neurobiology of feeding and energy expenditure. *Annu Rev Neurosci* 30 (1):367–398.

Glavas, M.M., M.A. Kirigiti, X.Q. Xiao, P.J. Enriori, S.K. Fisher, A.E. Evans, B.E. Grayson, M.A. Cowley, M.S. Smith, and K.L. Grove. 2010. Early overnutrition results in early-onset arcuate leptin resistance and increased sensitivity to high-fat diet. *Endocrinology* 151 (4):1598–1610.

Grayson, B.E., P.R. Levasseur, S.M. Williams, M.S. Smith, D.L. Marks, and K.L. Grove. 2010. Changes in melanocortin expression and inflammatory pathways in fetal offspring of nonhuman primates fed a high-fat diet. *Endocrinology* 151 (4):1622–1632.

Grove, K.L., S. Allen, B.E. Grayson, and M.S. Smith. 2003. Postnatal development of the hypothalamic neuropeptide Y system. *Neuroscience* 116 (2):393–406.

Gupta, A., M. Srinivasan, S. Thamadilok, and M.S. Patel. 2009. Hypothalamic alterations in fetuses of high fat diet-fed obese female rats. *J Endocrinol* 200 (3):293–300.

Hales, C.N., and D.J.P. Barker. 1992. Type 2 (non-insulin-dependent) diabetes mellitus: The thrifty phenotype hypothesis. *Diabetologia* 35 (7):595–601.

Hayashida, T., K. Nakahara, M.S. Mondal, Y. Date, M. Nakazato, M. Kojima, K. Kangawa, and N. Murakami. 2002. Ghrelin in neonatal rats: Distribution in stomach and its possible role. *J Endocrinol* 173 (2):239–245.

Hoggard, N., L. Hunter, J.S. Duncan, L.M. Williams, P. Trayhurn, and J.G. Mercer. 1997. Leptin and leptin receptor mRNA and protein expression in the murine fetus and placenta. *PNAS* 94 (20):11073–11078.

Ifft, J.D. 1972. An autoradiographic study of the time of final division of neurons in rat hypothalamic nuclei. *J Comp Neurol* 144:193–204.

Irani, B.G., A.A. Dunn-Meynell, and B.E. Levin. 2007. Altered hypothalamic leptin, insulin, and melanocortin binding associated with moderate-fat diet and predisposition to obesity. *Endocrinology* 148 (1):310–316.

Ishii, Y., and S.G. Bouret. 2012. Embryonic birthdate of hypothalamic leptin-activated neurons in mice. *Endocrinology* 153 (8):3657–3667.

Jones, A.P., E.N. Pothos, P. Rada, D.H. Olster, and B.G. Hoebel. 1995. Maternal hormonal manipulations in rats cause obesity and increase medial hypothalamic norepinephrine release in male offspring. *Develop Brain Res* 88 (2):127–131.

Jones, A.P., D.H. Olster, and B. States. 1996. Maternal insulin manipulations in rats organize body weight and noradrenergic innervation of the hypothalamus in gonadally intact male offspring. *Dev Brain Res* 97 (1):16–21.

Kirk, S.L., A.-M. Samuelsson, M. Argenton, H. Dhonye, T. Kalamatianos, L. Poston, P.D. Taylor, and C.W. Coen. 2009. Maternal obesity induced by diet in rats permanently influences central processes regulating food intake in offspring. *PLoS ONE* 4 (6):e5870.

Lee, H.M., G. Wang, E.W. Englander, M. Kojima, and G.H. Greeley Jr. 2002. Ghrelin, a new gastrointestinal endocrine peptide that stimulates insulin secretion: Enteric distribution, ontogeny, influence of endocrine, and dietary manipulations. *Endocrinology* 143:185–90.

Levin, B.E., and A.A. Dunn-Meynell. 2002. Reduced central leptin sensitivity in rats with diet-induced obesity. *Am J Physiol Regul Integr Comp Physiol* 283 (4):R941–R948.

Levin, B.E., A.A. Dunn-Meynell, B. Balkan, and R.E. Keesey. 1997. Selective breeding for diet-induced obesity and resistance in Sprague-Dawley rats. *Am J Physiol Regul Integr Comp Physiol* 273 (2):R725–R730.

Levin, B.E., A.A. Dunn-Meynell, and W.A. Banks. 2004. Obesity-prone rats have normal blood-brain barrier transport but defective central leptin signaling before obesity onset. *Am J Physiol Regul Integr Comp Physiol* 286 (1):R143–R150.

Levin, B.E., A.A. Dunn-Meynell, M.R. Ricci, and D.E. Cummings. 2003. Abnormalities of leptin and ghrelin regulation in obesity-prone juvenile rats. *Am J Physiol Endocrinol Metab* 285 (5):E949–E957.

López, M., L.M. Seoane, S. Tovar, M.C. García, R. Nogueiras, C. Diéguez, and R.M. Señarís. 2005. A possible role of neuropeptide Y, agouti-related protein and leptin receptor isoforms in hypothalamic programming by perinatal feeding in the rat. *Diabetologia* 48 (1):140–148.

Martin-Gronert, M.S., and S.E. Ozanne. 2005. Programming of appetite and type 2 diabetes. *Early Human Dev* 81 (12):981–988.

Matsumoto, A., and Y. Arai. 1976. Developmental changes in synaptic formation in the hypothalamic arcuate nucleus of female rats. *Cell Tissue Res* 14 (169):143–156.

McClellana, K.M., K.L. Parker, and S.A. Tobet. 2006. Development of the ventromedial nucleus of the hypothalamus. *Front Neuroendocrinol* 27 (2):193–209.

Melnick, I., N. Pronchuck, M.A. Cowley, K.L. Grove, and W.F. Colmers. 2007. Developmental switch in neuropeptide Y and melanocortin effects in the paraventricular nucleus of the hypothalamus *Neuron* 56 (6):1103–1115.

Morris, M.J., and H. Chen. 2008. Established maternal obesity in the rat reprograms hypothalamic appetite regulators and leptin signaling at birth. *Int J Obes* 33 (1):115–122.

Myers, M.G., M.A. Cowley, and H. Munzberg. 2008. Mechanisms of leptin action and leptin resistance. *Annu Rev Physiol* 70:537–556.

Nakahara, K., M. Nakagawa, Y. Baba, M. Sato, K. Toshinai, Y. Date, M. Nakazato, M. Kojima, M. Miyazato, H. Kaiya, H. Hosoda, K. Kangawa, and N. Murakami. 2006. Maternal ghrelin plays an important role in rat fetal development during pregnancy. *Endocrinology* 147 (3):1333–1342.

Nilsson, I., J.E. Johansen, M. Schalling, T. Hokfelt, and S.O. Fetissov. 2005. Maturation of the hypothalamic arcuate agouti-related protein system during postnatal development in the mouse. *Dev Brain Res* 155 (2):147–154.

Paderson, J. 1971. Diabetes mellitus and pregnancy: Present status of the hyperglycaemia–hyperinsulinism theory and the weight of the newborn baby. *Postgrad Med J* Suppl: 66–67.

Paderson, J., and M. Osler. 1961. Hyperglycemia as the cause of characteristic features of the foetus and newborn of diabetic mothers. *Dan Med Bull* (8):78–83.

Padilla, S.L., J.S. Carmody, and L.M. Zeltser. 2010. POMC-expressing progenitors give rise to antagonistic neuronal populations in hypothalamic feeding circuits. *Nat Med* 16 (4):403–405.

Pan, W., H. Hsuchou, T. Hong, and A.J. Kastin. 2008. Developmental changes of leptin receptors in cerebral microvessels: Unexpected relation to leptin transport. *Endocrinology* 149 (3):877–885.

Piao, H., H. Hosoda, K. Kangawa, T. Murata, K. Narita, and T. Higuchi. 2008. Ghrelin stimulates milk intake by affecting adult type feeding behaviour in postnatal rats. *J Neuroendocrinol* 20 (3):330–334.

Plagemann, A., T. Harder, U. Janert, A. Rake, F. Rittel, W. Rohde, and G. Dörner. 1999a. malformations of hypothalamic nuclei in hyperinsulinemic offspring of rats with gestational diabetes. *Develop Neurosci* 21 (1):58–67.

Plagemann, A., T. Harder, K. Melchior, A. Rake, W. Rohde, and G. Dörner. 1998. Elevation of hypothalamic neuropeptide Y-neurons in adult offspring of diabetic mother rats. *Neuroreport* 10 (15):3211–3216.

Plagemann, A., T. Harder, A. Rake, U. Janert, K. Melchior, W. Rohde, and G. Dorner. 1999b. Morphological alterations of hypothalamic nuclei due to intrahypothalamic hyperinsulinism in newborn rats. *Int J Develop Neurosci* 17 (1):37–44.

Plagemann, A., T. Harder, A. Rake, T. Waas, K. Melchior, T. Ziska, W. Rohde and G. Dorner. 1999c. Observations on the orexigenic hypothalamic neuropeptide Y-system in neonatally overfed weanling rats. *J Neuroendocrinol* 11:541–546.

Plagemann A., I. Heidrich, F. Götz, W. Rohde, and G. Dörner. 1992. Lifelong enhanced diabetes susceptibility and obesity after temporary intrahypothalamic hyperinsulinism during brain organization. *Exp Clin Endocrinol* 99 (2):91–95.

Proulx, K., D. Richard, and C.-D. Walker. 2002. Leptin regulates appetite-related neuropeptides in the hypothalamus of developing rats without affecting food intake. *Endocrinology* 143 (12):4683–4692.

Remmers, F., L.A. Verhagen, R.A. Adan, and H.A. Delemarre-van de Waal. 2010. Hypothalamic neuropeptide expression of juvenile and middle-aged rats after early postnatal food restriction. *Endocrinology* 149 (7):3617–3625.

Ricci, M.R., and B.E. Levin. 2003. Ontogeny of diet-induced obesity in selectively bred Sprague-Dawley rats. *Am J Physiol Regul Integr Comp Physiol* 285 (3):R610–R618.

Risold, P.Y., S. Croizier, K. Legagneux, F. Brischoux, D. Fellmann, and B. Griffond. 2009. The development of the MCH system. *Peptides* 30 (11):1969–1972.

Sauer, F.C. 1935. Mitosis in the neural tube. *J Comp Neurol* 62 (2):377–405.

Sawchenko, P.E. 1998. Toward a new neurobiology of energy balance, appetite, and obesity: The anatomists weigh in. *J Comp Neurol* 402:435–441.

Sawchenko, P.E., and L.W. Swanson. 1983. The organization of forebrain afferents to the paraventricular and supraoptic nuclei of the rat. *J Comp Neurol* 218 (2):121–44.

Shimada, M., and T. Nakamura. 1973. Time of neuron origin in mouse hypothalamic nuclei. *Exp Neurol* 41 (1):163–173.

Spaventi, R., M. Antica, and K. Pavelic. 1990. Insulin and insulin-like growth factor I (IGF I) in early mouse embryogenesis. *Development* 108 (3):491–495.

Srinivasan, M., P. Mitrani, G. Sadhanandan, C. Dodds, S. Shbeir-ElDika, S. Thamotharan, H. Ghanim, P. Dandona, S.U. Devaskar, and M.S. Patel. 2008. A high-carbohydrate diet in the immediate postnatal life of rats induces adaptations predisposing to adult-onset obesity. *J Endocrinol* 197 (3):565–574.

Steculorum, S.M., and S.G. Bouret. 2011a. Developmental effects of ghrelin. *Peptides* 32 (11):2362–2366.

Steculorum, S.M., and S.G. Bouret. 2011b. Maternal Diabetes Compromises the Organization of Hypothalamic Feeding Circuits and Impairs Leptin Sensitivity in Offspring. *Endocrinology* 152 (11):4171–4179.

Steculorum S.M., G. Collden, B. Coupe, S. Croizier, S. Lockie, Z.B. Andrews, F. Jarosch, S. Klussmann, and S.G. Bouret. 2015. Neonatal ghrelin programs development of hypothalamic feeding circuits *J Clin Invest* 125 (2):846–858.

Teitelman, G., S. Alpert, J.M. Polak, A. Martinez, and D. Hanahan. 1993. Precursor cells of mouse endocrine pancreas coexpress insulin, glucagon and the neuronal proteins tyrosine hydroxylase and neuropeptide Y, but not pancreatic polypeptide. *Development* 118:1031–1039.

Terroni, P.L., F.W. Anthony, M.A. Hanson, and F.R. Cagampang. 2005. Expression of agouti-related peptide, neuropeptide Y, pro-opiomelanocortin and the leptin receptor isoforms in fetal mouse brain from pregnant dams on a protein-restricted diet. *Brain Res* 140 (1–2):111–115.

Toran-Allerand, C.D., L. Ellis, and K.H. Pfenninger. 1988. Estrogen and insulin synergism in neurite growth enhancement in vitro: Mediation of steroid effects by interactions with growth factors? *Dev Brain Res.* 41:87–100.

Torsello, A., B. Scibona, G. Leo, E. Bresciani, R. Avallone, I. Bulgarelli, M. Luoni, M. Zoli, G. Rindi, D. Cocchi, and V. Locatelli. 2003. Ontogeny and tissue-specific regulation of ghrelin mRNA expression suggest that ghrelin is primarily involved in the control of extraendocrine functions in the rat. *Neuroendocrinology* 77 (2):91–99.

Vogt, M.C., L. Paeger, S. Hess, S.M. Steculorum, M. Awazawa, B. Hampel, S. Neupert, H.T. Nicholls, J. Mauer, A.C. Hausen, R. Predel, P. Kloppenburg, T.L. Horvath, and J.C. Bruning. 2014. Neonatal insulin action impairs hypothalamic neurocircuit formation in response to maternal high-fat feeding. *Cell* 156:495–509.

Watts, A.G. 2000. Understanding the neural control of ingestive behaviors: Helping to separate cause from effect with dehydration-associated anorexia. *Horm Behav* 37 (4):261–283.

Wierup, N., H. Svensson, H. Mulder, and F. Sundler. 2002. The ghrelin cell: A novel developmentally regulated islet cell in the human pancreas. *Reg Pep* 107 (1–3):63–69.

Williams, K.W., and J.K. Elmquist. 2012. From neuroanatomy to behavior: Central integration of peripheral signals regulating feeding behavior. *Nat Neurosci* 15:1350–1355.

Yura, S., H. Itoh, N. Sagawa, H. Yamamoto, H. Masuzaki, K. Nakao, M. Kawamura, M. Takemura, K. Kakui, Y. Ogawa, and S. Fujii. 2005. Role of premature leptin surge in obesity resulting from intrauterine undernutrition. *Cell Metab* 1 (6):371–378.

8 Maternal and Epigenetic Factors That Influence Food Intake and Energy Balance in Offspring

Lin Song, Miranda D. Johnson,
and Kellie L.K. Tamashiro

CONTENTS

8.1 INTRODUCTION

It is well documented that maternal environment is a key regulator of offspring development. The thrifty phenotype hypothesis put forth by Hales and Barker in 1992 states that suboptimal nutrition in early life leads to adverse metabolic consequences in adulthood (Hales and Barker 1992, Locke et al. 2015). They went on to show that fetal nutrient restriction results in increased cardiovascular risk, type 2 diabetes mellitus, and elevated cholesterol (Barker et al. 1993, Fall et al. 1995, Hales et al. 1991). These studies resulted in the broader developmental origins of health and disease hypothesis, which encompasses the idea that early life environment can result in long-term changes to the offspring (Gluckman and Hanson 2004), independent of genetics.

A long-standing example of early life programming is the Dutch hunger winter of 1944. Ravelli et al. (1998) found that in utero exposure to severe maternal caloric restriction (~600–800 kcal/d) resulted in maladaptive consequences for offspring later in life. Furthermore, the time of exposure during gestation resulted in alternate outcomes, such that exposure during the first half of pregnancy increased the risk for obesity, while restriction during the third trimester into early life had a reduced risk for obesity but higher incidence of late-life type 2 diabetes mellitus (Ravelli, Stein, and Susser 1976).

Rodent studies utilizing prenatal and postnatal environmental alterations such as dietary manipulations to dams and/or offspring and large litter rearing are sufficient to increase the offspring's likelihood of becoming obese (Faust, Johnson, and Hirsch 1980, Guo and Jen 1995, Levin and Govek 1998, Ozanne and Hales 2004, Patterson et al. 2010, Sun et al. 2012, 2014, Wu et al. 1998). While several obese rat and mouse models were identified based on spontaneously occurring single gene mutations (Coleman 1973, Lee et al. 1996, Yeo et al. 1998, Zhang et al. 1994), they do not account for most severe obese patients. Twin studies report heritability of obesity between 40% to 70% and a recent meta-analysis of nearly 340,000 individuals identified 97 genome-wide significant loci that were associated with body mass index (BMI), of which 56 genes were novel (Locke et al. 2015). Those loci together account for only ~2.7% of BMI variation. Therefore, it is clear that obesity is the result of interactions between multiple genetic and environmental influences suggesting involvement of epigenetic factors which will be discussed later in this chapter.

8.2 MATERNAL BEHAVIOR INFLUENCES OFFSPRING DEVELOPMENT

The perinatal environment supports the development and health of offspring. Perturbations to this environment can have detrimental effects on the developing fetus and neonate that have persistent pathological consequences through adolescence and adulthood. Despite the wealth of evidence that the perinatal period is very sensitive to environmental stressors, such as altered nutrition, stress, and infection, the mechanisms through which these disruptions influence development remain poorly understood. One area of active investigation is the effect of maternal care behavior on offspring hypothalamic–pituitary–adrenal (HPA) axis function and regulation of the stress response. The offspring of rat dams that exhibit the high maternal care profile (high amount of licking and grooming and nursing with an arched back posture toward their pups) exhibit an attenuated glucocorticoid response when challenged by an acute stressor such as restraint stress (Weaver et al. 2004). These offspring have a greater amount of glucocorticoid receptor ("GR", *Nr3c1*) expression in the hippocampus, a critical brain region that controls the HPA axis and stress response. Since the GR is a key receptor involved in negative feedback of the HPA axis, alterations in its levels in the brain have direct consequences on stress reactivity of the HPA axis. Changes in epigenetic marks on DNA have been identified as one potential molecular mechanism linking maternal care behavior to altered GR expression and stress response in the offspring.

This chapter will focus on the effect of maternal diet and metabolic status, both prenatal and postnatal, on offspring ingestive behavior and metabolic outcomes. Mechanistically, alterations in neurodevelopment associated with changes in endocrine milieu perinatally have been documented and likely contribute to long-term changes in offspring. Epigenetic modifications have also emerged as potential molecular mediators for altered long-term outcomes for offspring due to perturbations during development.

8.3   MATERNAL NUTRITION

8.3.1   MATERNAL UNDERNUTRITION OR PROTEIN RESTRICTION

Maternal undernutrition via caloric restriction, macronutrient restriction (low protein diet), or uterine artery ligation has for several decades been a focus in the field due to epidemiological evidence that famine exposure during gestation has long-term consequences on the metabolic health of offspring (Ravelli et al. 1998). In fact, small for gestational age offspring are prone to similar metabolic outcome as offspring born to obese mothers and effects are further exacerbated by subsequent postnatal overnutrition. Several longitudinal studies in humans have found that caloric restriction in utero, followed by "catch-up" growth due to increased nutrient abundance during the postnatal period, results in a greater risk for developing obesity and type 2 diabetes as adults (Eriksson et al. 2006, Hales et al. 1991). Ozanne et al. (2004) demonstrated that offspring of mouse dams fed a low protein diet (8%) *prenatally* followed by cross-fostering to control dams to support catch-up growth, weighed more by postnatal day 7 (P7) than controls and *postnatal* protein restricted pups. Furthermore, offspring that were exposed to this paradigm and weaned on an obesity-inducing diet were more susceptible to obesity's negative effects on longevity (Ozanne and Hales 2004). Intrauterine growth restricted offspring of dams that underwent caloric restriction in utero then nursed by ad lib fed dams had increased adiposity and plasma leptin levels and were hyperphagic as adults (Desai et al. 2005). However, it is clear that a greater public health concern in developed countries currently surrounds the effects of maternal overnutrition (increased caloric consumption and greater fat/sugar intake) or obesity and diabetes on offspring rather than undernutrition. More women are overweight and obese prior to conception, and the prevalence of overweight/obese mothers has risen dramatically over the last 15 years. In 2003–2004, about 28.5% of US women aged 20–39 years were obese (Ogden et al. 2006). By 2013–2014, the prevalence of obesity increased to 37.0% (Flegal et al. 2016), emphasizing the urgency of this public health issue.

8.3.2 Maternal Overnutrition or High-Fat/High-Sugar Diets

8.3.2.1 Feeding Behavior Consequences

The effects of maternal high-fat (HF) diet during early life are also apparent in offspring food intake during postnatal life. Prior to P9, gastric load serves as the primary regulator of pup ingestive behavior (Swithers and Hall 1989). During the early postnatal period until the beginning of the third week of life, pups primarily engage in suckling behavior, rather that independent ingestion (Hall 1985). Offspring of HF-fed dams weigh significantly more at P7, but not at birth, suggesting several possibilities such that either maternal milk may be higher in fat and overall energy content or HF-offspring might be consuming more due to increased suckling (Purcell et al. 2011). The increase in pup body weight is likely due to increased hyperphagia at P7 shown by increased consumption of warm, sweetened milk from filter paper in an independent ingestion test, rather than differences in dam milk fat content as differences in fat content were only significantly higher toward the end of the preweaning period. While food intake in the home cage is not an accurate measure of caloric consumption due to the inability to dissociate dam and pup food intake, recent data indicate that HF-fed offspring spend more time engaging in independent feeding after a nursing bout compared to chow-fed offspring (Kojima, Catavero, and Rinaman 2016). The authors concluded that this increase in HF diet consumption, rather than nursing as chow and HF offspring spent similar amounts of time nursing, attributed to the increase in body weight seen in HF-fed offspring. With respect to food choice, HF offspring preferred diets higher in fat content, compared to sugar, as they had an increased number of operant responses compared to control offspring (Naef et al. 2011). In addition, increased preference for fat appears to be sex-specific as HF female offspring do not show an increase in preference compared to males (Carlin, George, and Reyes 2013). In nonhuman primates, offspring exposed to both maternal obesity and HF diet show an increased intake of food that is high in fat and sugar (Rivera et al. 2015). These studies suggest that the increased body weight displayed by HF offspring initially, as well as sustained through adulthood, could be due to a greater intake of and preference for palatable foods.

8.3.2.2 Obesity/Excess Adiposity

Most rodent studies report that offspring exposed to HF diet during gestation and lactation have an increased body weight at weaning (Desai et al. 2014, Howie et al. 2013, Sun et al. 2012). However, there are studies that report low birth weight (Dudley et al. 2011, Howie et al. 2009, McCurdy et al. 2009), which may be due to differences in the duration of HF exposure and fat composition of the diets. Nevertheless, the offspring from HF mothers display rapid catch-up growth. The increased body weight of offspring from HF dams is paralleled by increased fat mass and elevated plasma leptin (Bouanane et al. 2009, Howie et al. 2009, Sun et al. 2012). When perinatal maternal HF exposure was combined with postnatal HF consumption by the adult offspring of maternal HF-fed dams, an additive adverse effect of increased body weight was shown when compared to HF fed offspring of lean dams (Howie et al. 2009, Shankar et al. 2008).

8.3.2.3   Insulin Resistance

Offspring of maternal obese or overnutrition dams showed glucose intolerance at weaning and postnatal HF diet continued to impair glucose tolerance in adulthood (Chen, Simar, and Morris 2009, Desai et al. 2014, Sun et al. 2012). Hyperinsulinemia has been reported in rodent offspring of obese dams (Buckley et al. 2005, Fernandez-Twinn et al. 2012, Howie et al. 2013). Taylor et al. (2005) also demonstrated in rodents that prenatal and suckling exposure to a fat-rich diet leads to whole body insulin resistance and pancreatic ß-cell dysfunction in adulthood. The endocrine pancreas development is also programmed by early nutritional environment (Reusens and Remacle 2006). It is possible that maternal insulin resistance during pregnancy is one of the important factors driving the development of insulin resistance in the offspring. Studies also found that maternal insulin resistance alone, without maternal obesity or hyperglycemia, can promote glucose intolerance, hyperinsulinemia, and hyperglycemia in male offspring (Isganaitis et al. 2014). In the liver-specific insulin receptor knockout (LIRKO) mouse model, which exhibits sustained hyperinsulinemia and transient hyperglycemia during pregnancy, the control offspring born to LIRKO mothers display higher blood glucose and plasma insulin concentration in early postnatal days, and reduced pancreas ß-cell area is also observed shortly after birth (Kahraman et al. 2014). These results suggest that maternal obesity and insulin resistance during pregnancy programs to reduce whole body insulin sensitivity of the offspring and may be due in part to impaired endocrine pancreas development in early postnatal life.

8.3.2.4   Cardiovascular Disease

Offspring that are exposed to maternal obesity and diabetes are at increased risk of premature death from cardiovascular disease (Reynolds et al. 2013). Blackmore et al. (2014) showed that offspring from obese dams develop pathologic cardiac hypertrophy, severe systolic, and diastolic dysfunction. These changes are independent of current body weight and develop despite the offspring eating a healthy diet after weaning. Maternal HF exposure also predisposes offspring to postnatal dietary-induced cardiac hypertrophy and contractile defect (Turdi et al. 2013). Young adult offspring (3 to 8 weeks of age) of maternal obesity dams show increased heart weight, left ventricular volume, heart weight to body weight, and heart weight to tibial length (Fernandez-Twinn et al. 2012). However, by 12 weeks, heart weights are similar between groups (Blackmore et al. 2014). In humans, fetal myocardial dysfunction with reduced left and right ventricle global rate and strain was detected during the first trimester of gestation in obese pregnant women (Bjork Ingul et al. 2015). Collectively, maternal diet-induced obesity during pregnancy and lactation leads to cardiac hypertrophy and dysfunction at an early stage, independent of offspring body weight and adiposity.

8.3.2.5   Liver Dysfunction

The development of obesity in maternal HF exposed offspring often results in the onset of metabolic syndrome, including insulin resistance and cardiovascular disease. Nonalcoholic fatty liver disease (NAFLD) is considered an additional feature of the metabolic syndrome (Marchesini et al. 2001). The prevalence of NAFLD has increased in the past few decades and become one of the most common causes of adult chronic liver disease in the United States (Younossi et al. 2011).

In a number of animal models, maternal obesity or overnutrition is found to result in elevated triglyceride levels, increased inflammatory markers, and fatty liver in offspring (Bouanane et al. 2010, Buckley et al. 2005, Chen et al. 2014). In rodents, offspring fed HF diets during gestation and lactation showed greater hepatic lipid content, increased levels of peroxisome proliferator-activated receptor gamma (PPARγ), and reduced triglyceride lipase (Alfaradhi et al. 2014, Chen et al. 2014), which program the development of offspring NAFLD (Oben et al. 2010). Studies found that fostering lean offspring by HF-fed dams caused hepatic steatosis in 3-month-old offspring, whereas fostering HF offspring to low-fat fed dams prevented hepatic steatosis (Oben et al. 2010). There are also studies in mice showing that offspring exposed to HF diet during only gestation, only lactation, or both developed hepatic steatosis even when the moms were not obese (Gregorio et al. 2010). In nonhuman primates, offspring that had been exposed to excess lipids, independent of maternal obesity and/or diabetes, exhibited elevated hepatic expression of gluconeogenic enzymes, transcription factors, and increased evidence of hepatic oxidative stress. The fetal glycerol levels and hepatic triglyceride levels were increased and persisted at P180 (McCurdy et al. 2009). These signs are consistent with the development of NAFLD. Reversing the maternal HF diet to a low-fat diet during a subsequent pregnancy improved fetal hepatic phenotype without changing maternal body weight (McCurdy et al. 2009). These results indicate that gestation and lactation periods are critical in the development of liver metabolism.

8.4   MECHANISTIC PATHWAYS LINKING MATERNAL BEHAVIOR TO OFFSPRING PHENOTYPE

8.4.1   Hormones as Trophic Factors during Hypothalamic Development

Key hormones play critical roles during development, specifically leptin, insulin, and ghrelin. Leptin circulates as a 16-kDa peptide hormone released primarily from adipocytes (Zhang et al. 1994). In the developing rodent fetus, where little adipose tissue is present, leptin can be produced by the placenta to increase cord blood levels of leptin (Hoggard et al. 1997, Masuzaki et al. 1997, Senaris et al. 1997). During postnatal life, pups have very little adipose tissue, with a major source of leptin coming from the maternal milk during lactation (Casabiell et al. 1997). In the human fetus, leptin levels increase during the last trimester as a significant amount of subcutaneous adipose tissue is present during this time (Smith and Waddell 2003, Widdowson 1950, Widdowson and Spray 1951).

Studies measuring independent ingestion have shown that exogenous treatment of rat pups with leptin, administered either acutely or chronically, does not affect food intake or body weight during the postnatal period (Proulx, Richard, and Walker 2002). Furthermore, while endogenous levels of leptin peak at P10, this is not associated with a subsequent decrease in body weight (Ahima, Prabakaran, and Flier 1998). Therefore, since the rise in leptin levels during postnatal life does not serve as an indicator of metabolic need or energy status, this led to a series of experiments investigating leptin's function as a neurotrophic factor. While it was known that the arcuate nucleus (ARC) sent neuronal projections to other hypothalamic nuclei involved in body weight regulation, such as the dorsomedial nucleus (DMN), lateral hypothalamus (LH), and the paraventricular nucleus (PVN), it was not yet known when those projections developed. Utilizing DiI axonal labeling, it was shown that projections from the ARC to other intrahypothalamic nuclei develop during the postnatal period (Bouret, Draper, and Simerly 2004c). In addition, the leptin deficient *ob/ob* mouse has disrupted ARC to PVN and ARC to LH projections, indicating that leptin may play a role in the development of these pathways (Bouret, Draper, and Simerly 2004d). Interestingly, ARC to DMN projections in *ob/ob* mice are indistinguishable from wild-type littermates, suggesting that this neural projection pathway is not leptin dependent. Additional studies using *ob/ob* mice demonstrated that ARC to PVN and LH projections can be rescued if leptin is given during postnatal development, but not adulthood, and treatment of wild-type mouse ARC explants with leptin-induced neurite outgrowth. Therefore, the postnatal peak in leptin levels is critical for the development of the hypothalamus and intervention strategies can correct insufficiencies only if administered during this critical period.

Maternal glucose, but not insulin, is actively transported across the placenta and results in production and secretion of insulin from the fetal pancreas (Pedersen, Bojsen-Moller, and Poulsen 1954, Pedersen and Osler 1961). In mice, maternal HF diet during lactation resulted in hyperinsulinemia and impaired development of alpha-melanocyte stimulating hormone (αMSH) and agouti-related protein (AgRP) ARC neuronal projections to intrahypothalmic sites (Vogt et al. 2014). In addition, the offspring had increased body weight, adiposity, leptin levels, and insulin resistance. Insulin deficiency during pregnancy, as shown in mouse models of streptozotocin (STZ)-induced diabetes, also results in offspring with increased body weight and decreased leptin signaling (Steculorum and Bouret 2011). Not surprisingly, mice born to STZ dams have reduced αMSH and AgRP ARC projections, due to reduced outgrowth of proopiomelanocortin (POMC) and neuropeptide Y (NPY)/AgRP neurons rather a reduction in neuronal number.

Recently, ghrelin, a potent orexigenic hormone released primarily from gastric P/D1 cells (Kojima et al. 1999), has been shown to play a role in hypothalamic development (Steculorum et al. 2015). Ghrelin levels are low until P14, after ARC–PVN pathway projections are developed. In mice treated with a ghrelin inhibitor or in ghrelin knockout mouse, there are an increased number of ARC-PVN pathway projections, but only pharmacological inhibition of ghrelin increases body weight, adiposity, and leptin levels. As adults, ghrelin knockout mice have comparable ARC-PVN pathway development to wild-type mice, suggesting that compensatory mechanisms are involved in plasticity. Furthermore, administration of ghrelin during early life at a time when ghrelin levels are typically low results in fewer ARC–PVN pathway projections and increased body weight postweaning. Collectively, these results indicate that ghrelin acts during a discrete period of time during postnatal life to aid in hypothalamic development. Thus, metabolic hormones that are important for regulation of energy balance in later life also have a significant role during critical periods of neurodevelopment.

8.4.2 HYPOTHALAMIC DEVELOPMENT

Although clear evidence from both rodents and nonhuman primates shows that maternal HF diet consumption predisposes offspring to increased risk for obesity and metabolic diseases, the underlying mechanisms are still not clear. Recent studies indicate that maternal HF diet consumption impairs the formation of hypothalamic neural circuitry that regulates physiology and behavior (Vogt et al. 2014). As discussed previously, circulating hormones such as leptin, insulin, and ghrelin play important roles in the development of hypothalamic feeding circuits (Bouret, Draper, and Simerly 2004b, Steculorum et al. 2015, Vogt et al. 2014). Intrahypothalamic insulin injection during the time that hypothalamic projections are forming results in elevated body weight and insulin level, impaired glucose tolerance, and increased diabetes susceptibility in rat pups (Plagemann et al. 1992). Perinatal leptin level is also a critical factor for the proper formation of neural pathways in the hypothalamus (Bouret, Draper, and Simerly 2004b, Valleau and Sullivan 2014). Offspring that were exposed to maternal HF diet during lactation had increased plasma leptin and insulin at weaning (Desai et al. 2014, Sun et al. 2012), which may alter the development of the brain circuitry regulating energy and behavior.

In the ARC, orexigenic neurons expressing NPY/AgRP are inhibited by rising glucose levels, while anorexigenic neurons expressing POMC are excited by glucose abundance (Muroya et al. 1999, Stefater and Seeley 2010). Studies in rodents showed that ARC NPY, AgRP, and POMC mRNA expression at 9 weeks of age were not affected by maternal obesity. However, PVN NPY Y1 receptor, Y2 receptor, and melanocortin 4 receptor (MC4R) mRNA expression was lower in offspring from obese dams (Chen et al. 2014). Maternal obesity also dampened in vivo stimulation of hypothalamic NPY mRNA expression in response to acute hyperglycemia and lowered in vitro hypothalamic glucose uptake and lactate release (Chen, Simar, and Morris 2014). In nonhuman primates, fetuses from maternal HF diet moms had increased hypothalamic POMC and MC4R and decreased AgRP mRNA expression in the early-third trimester, and because projections from the ARC to the PVN develop during the third trimester, AgRP-immunoreactive fibers were also found to be decreased in the PVN of fetuses from HF diet moms (Grayson et al. 2010b). However, fetal plasma leptin levels do not rise until after hypothalamic development is mostly complete in nonhuman primates (Grayson et al. 2006); therefore, although leptin plays critical role in rodent brain development, there is limited evidence supporting the importance of leptin in primate brain development (Grayson et al. 2010a).

8.4.3 INFLAMMATORY MECHANISMS

The immune system also plays an important role in brain development. Communication between the brain and the immune system have gained greater attention as potential mechanisms mediating the effects of maternal diet and obesity on brain development and behavior in offspring. Prenatal cytokine exposure alone is sufficient to induce later-life obesity (Dahlgren et al. 2001), and acute and chronic inflammation has been found to affect function of the melanocortin signaling system in adult rodents (Scarlett et al. 2007, 2008). Animal models have shown that maternal obesity and consumption of a HF diet during pregnancy result in increased maternal inflammation and oxidative stress and are associated with greater adiposity and adverse metabolic outcomes in offspring (Sen and Simmons 2010). In the nonhuman primate, maternal HF diet consumption was associated with increased proinflammatory cytokine interleukin 1β (IL-1β), IL-1 receptor, and markers of activated microglia in the hypothalamus of third trimester fetuses, suggesting an inflammatory state in brains of exposed offspring (Grayson et al. 2010a). The consequences of perinatal maternal HF diet consumption on hypothalamic development in offspring has not been as well studied as that on the hippocampus. In a series of studies using rodent models, Bilbo and Tsang (2010) have demonstrated that markers of microglial activation and inflammation are increased in the hippocampus of offspring of pregnant dams fed a HF diet within one day after birth, resembling immune activation seen following early-life infection. These offspring also have greater anxiety and cognitive deficits in adulthood, indicating that perinatal inflammation associated with maternal HF diet consumption can have long-term consequences on brain development and behavior (Bilbo and Tsang 2010). Additional studies are required to determine whether fetal and neonatal inflammation resulting from maternal HF diet consumption has similar consequences for the development of the hypothalamus and associated brain regions that regulate body weight and control feeding behavior.

8.4.4 EPIGENETIC MECHANISMS

Another mechanism by which environmental factors such as maternal diet or behavior during the prenatal and neonatal periods can have long-term phenotypic influences may involve epigenetic modifications. The term "epigenetic" literally translates to "above the genome" and was first coined by developmental biologist Conrad Waddington in the 1940s (Waddington 1942, 2012). Epigenetic regulation of gene expression is achieved via modifications that are made to the DNA without changing the DNA sequence itself (reviewed in Jaenisch and Bird 2003). Epigenetic regulation of gene expression is a normal biological process that leads to long-lasting changes involved in embryonic development and organogenesis. Changes in epigenetic markers are associated with a variety of diseases, including many cancers and neurological disorders.

Epigenetic modifications include posttranslational histone modifications (acetylation, methylation, phosphorylation, sumoylation, ubiquitination, and biotinylation), noncoding small RNAs such as microRNAs, and DNA methylation. Cytosine DNA methylation is a covalent modification of DNA in which a methyl group is transferred from S-adenosylmethionine to the C-5 position of cytosine by a family of cytosine (DNA-5)-methyltransferases. DNA methylation is considered to be the most stable of epigenetic processes because of the strong covalent bond that connects the methyl (CH_3)-group to the cytosine of cytosine-guanine (CpG) dinucleotides in the DNA sequence. DNA methylation typically occurs at "CpG islands," or regions rich in CpG dinucleotides (formally defined as G + C content ≥ 0.5 and $CpG_{obs}/CpG_{exp} \geq 0.6$) (Bird 1986). It was initially thought that epigenetic modifications were laid down during early embryogenesis and remained stable throughout life. However, increasing evidence shows that is not the case and it is clear that epigenetic processes can be dynamic across the lifespan and respond to a variety of environmental cues to influence gene expression and impact physiology and behavior.

Maternal health and behavior clearly influence fetal development and have long-term health consequences. Gene expression changes occurring early in development impact brain maturation and function throughout adulthood. Increasing attention has been directed toward epigenetic processes as molecular mediators through which early life environmental experiences can have persistent effects on behavior, independent of genetic sequences. The role of epigenetic modifications in fetal metabolic programming is in its infancy compared to, for example, the more developed field of cancer biology. Recent studies have found that epigenetic regulatory mechanisms are associated with energy balance pathways including those involved with the controls of food intake, energy expenditure and adiposity (Chango and Pogribny 2015, Waterland 2014).

8.4.4.1   Epigenetic Influences on Energy Homeostasis

Food intake, energy expenditure, and body fat content are under the control of an intricate network of neural and hormonal signals (Schwartz et al. 2000, Woods et al. 1998). The hormones leptin and insulin are central to communications within key neuronal circuits in the brain containing target receptors that initiate responses to control food intake and energy expenditure and regulate body weight (reviewed in Ahima et al. 2000, Cone et al. 2001, Elmquist, Elias, and Saper 1999, Niswender and Schwartz 2003, Woods et al. 2003).

Regulation of genes involved in leptin and insulin signaling pathways is epigenetically mediated and may be influenced by the early life environment. The leptin gene promoter includes a CpG island that contains putative binding sites for transcription factors, including AP2, SP1, and C/EBP-alpha. These regulatory sites play an important role in leptin expression (Melzner et al. 2002, Stoger 2006). Recent studies suggest that DNA methylation of the leptin gene could be part of the cascade of events leading to fetal metabolic programming. Maternal obesity and diabetes before and during pregnancy in humans can alter leptin gene promoter DNA methylation in the placenta, potentially leading to a differential supply of leptin to the fetus and contributing to metabolic programming of offspring causing obesity and related conditions (Lesseur et al. 2014). As discussed in previous sections of this chapter, leptin has a critical trophic role during neurodevelopment, and disruption of its expression and availability could have serious consequences by impairing neural circuit development and maturation during early life (Bouret et al. 2012, Bouret, Draper, and Simerly 2004a,b). The hypothalamic insulin receptor (IR) promoter is also regulated by DNA methylation in its promoter region and has been found to be hypermethylated with overfeeding during neonatal life (Plagemann et al. 2010), potentially leading to altered expression of the IR. Together, both the leptin and insulin signaling pathways are epigenetically regulated to some extent and have been found to be altered with changes in perinatal nutrition, which has widespread effects on downstream effectors and significant behavioral and metabolic consequences.

Leptin and insulin influence the expression of numerous targets in the hypothalamus and in other regions of the brain to affect feeding behavior, energy expenditure, and energy homeostasis. One hypothalamic target gene that has received increasing attention recently is POMC. There is growing evidence that hypothalamic POMC is a target for metabolic programming as its regulation is controlled by DNA methylation of its promoter (Newell-Price, King, and Clark 2001). In a rat model, overnutrition during the neonatal period is associated with hypermethylation of POMC near an Sp1 transcription factor binding site (Plagemann et al. 2009), which is necessary for leptin- and insulin-mediated regulation of hypothalamic expression of POMC. The metabolic phenotype of the overnourished rats included obesity, hyperleptinemia, hyperinsulinemia, and hyperglycemia (Plagemann et al. 2009). In humans, obese children had increased methylation of several CpG sites of POMC in peripheral blood cells (PBCs) compared to normal-weight control children (Kuehnen et al. 2012). It is unknown how DNA methylation of POMC in PBCs relate to that in the hypothalamus or any other brain area, and this is a focus of preclinical studies to determine whether PBC DNA methylation may serve as a peripheral biomarker for molecular changes in the brain.

8.4.4.2 Epigenetic Influences on Reward Signaling and Diet Preference

Altered energy homeostasis resulting in obesity arises out of an imbalance between energy intake and expenditure. Ingestion of palatable, energy-dense foods can contribute to accelerated weight gain and obesity. The dopamine and opioid neural circuits are associated with reward behavior that can affect an individual's preference for and consumption of palatable foods. Maternal obesity has been shown to influence the development and function of offspring's reward systems. Mice that are maintained on a HF diet for 3 months prior to pregnancy have offspring that show a preference for palatable foods. These offspring have lower global and gene-specific (dopamine transporter, mu-opioid receptor, and preproenkephalin) promoter DNA methylation and concurrent overexpression of these genes in brain regions associated with reward behavior (Vucetic, Kimmel, and Reyes 2011, Vucetic et al. 2010).

8.4.4.3 Mechanisms Responsible for Epigenetic Alterations in Response to Maternal Behavior and Diet

How early exposure to alterations in maternal behavior and diet translates to differences in epigenetic modifications to affect gene expression is largely unknown and is a growing area of active research. Changes in the environment may be communicated to the developing fetus or neonate via endocrine signals (e.g., leptin, insulin, glucocorticoids) or nutrient supply (e.g., glucose, amino acids, fatty acids). In addition, micronutrients could play a role particularly in dietary alterations because folate, choline, methionine, and vitamins ultimately affect methyl donor supply through one-carbon metabolism. Direct influences on the expression of epigenetic enzymes such as DNA methyltransferases (DNMTs) and DNA demethylases, which add and remove methyl groups from DNA, respectively, could ultimately affect DNA methylation levels. The epigenetic machinery themselves (DNMT1, DNMT3a, and methyl CpG binding proteins) are also susceptible to changes in diet (Ghoshal et al. 2006, Lillycrop et al. 2007).

Together, these data suggest that alterations in nutrition during sensitive periods of development can have persistent effects on epigenetic regulation of genes that control food intake and energy expenditure leading to changes in body weight and risk of developing obesity and other metabolic disorders. Human studies indicate that DNA methylation patterns can be affected by maternal obesity and diet, and these epigenetic modifications can persist for decades (Ahmed 2010, Stein et al. 2007), and possibly be inherited by future generations (Lange and Schneider 2010, Painter et al. 2008). These data further support the notion that epigenetic mechanisms may contribute to the long-lasting effects of maternal behavior and metabolic status prior to and during pregnancy and could represent novel therapeutic targets.

8.4.4.4 Reversibility of Epigenetic Changes

While accumulating evidence suggests that maternal factors prior to and during pregnancy, including diet, obesity, and diabetes, can influence the epigenetic state of the genome and bias offspring toward obesity and metabolic disorders, an important question arises about whether the reverse is also true. Can maternal diet manipulations be used to prevent or reverse the adverse consequences of an unbalanced maternal diet or unhealthy lifestyle (i.e., maternal diabetes or obesity) on offspring? Studies using a genetic model, the *Agouti* mouse, suggest that it may indeed be possible to alter offspring phenotype by changing maternal diet composition. Normally, brown mice can become yellow and obese when the *Agouti* gene spontaneously has a retroviral element inserted into it. When this element is methylated, *Agouti* gene expression is decreased and the mice maintain a normal phenotype (brown coat color and lean). Only when *Agouti* is *unmethylated* do the mice increase expression of *Agouti* and manifest the yellow and obese phenotype (Michaud et al. 1994). If mouse dams are fed a diet containing high levels of methyl donors during pregnancy, they produce a higher than expected number of offspring with normal phenotype, suggesting that the high-methyl-group-containing diet may lead to increased DNA methylation in the offspring (Wolff et al. 1998). In a follow-up study using heterozygous viable yellow agouti (A^{vy}/a) mice, maternal dietary genistein (major phytoestrogen in soy) supplementation during gestation resulted in A^{vy}/a offspring with brown coat color and decreased incidence of obesity. This phenotype was significantly associated with greater methylation at six CpG sites in the A^{vy} intracisternal A particle retrotransposon (Dolinoy et al. 2006), leading to less expression of *Agouti* and a normal phenotype.

Additional work using a maternal HF diet mouse model also supports the notion that dietary methyl donor supplements may have beneficial effects for offspring. Feeding pregnant mice a 60% HF diet results in offspring who have an increased propensity to develop obesity. Decreased metabolic rate and increased fat preference were associated with alterations in brain gene expression in reward neural circuitry, which may have resulted, in part, from global hypomethylation of DNA in the prefrontal cortex and nucleus accumbens but not in the ventral tegmental area. Methyl donor supplementation to maternal diet during pregnancy attenuated or reversed some of the behaviors that biased offspring toward obesity. Together, the data suggest that dietary methyl donor supplementation during gestation may be beneficial in preventing adverse consequences of maternal HF diet consumption during pregnancy (Carlin, George, and Reyes 2013). There are, however, some caveats to these findings. Perhaps most important is the fact that methyl donors are not specifically targeted to regions of DNA that show deficient methylation. It remains to be determined whether an excess supply of methyl donors during pregnancy, a sensitive developmental period, has unintended negative effects on other genes that are not affected by maternal HF diet. Overall, however, these findings support the potential for dietary interventions in reversing epigenetic changes.

8.4.4.5   Perspectives and Future Directions

While progress has been made in identifying epigenetic modifications that are associated with adverse consequences resulting from changes in maternal behavior or diet during pregnancy, there is very little evidence to support a *causal* role for epigenetic modifications in changing gene expression and phenotypes in those models. In fact, a majority of studies report the *correlation* of DNA methylation with gene transcription in heterogeneous cell populations, particularly in the brain, where it is difficult to obtain a sufficient quantity of homogeneous cells from a specific brain nucleus to do epigenetic assays. Thus, it is unclear whether variations in gene expression at the single-cell level can be explained by differential methylation in individual genes. New technologies that allow measurement of DNA methylation and gene expression in a single cell may help the field begin to move in that direction.

The field is also limited by the tools available to manipulate DNA methylation at the single nucleotide level, particularly in vivo, in order to determine relationships between DNA methylation and physiology and behavior. As new tools are developed to manipulate epigenetic marks on specific genes in specific cell types, we will learn more about whether epigenetic processes directly result in phenotypic traits.

Finally, the move toward individualized medicine and personalized health care has ignited the search for disease markers, including epigenetic profiles in easily accessible tissues and fluids such as blood or saliva. For example, DNA methylation of the leptin promoter varies with obesity, and, in humans, peripheral blood samples from obese adolescents show a negative relationship between methylation of the leptin promoter and BMI (Garcia-Cardona et al. 2014). A biomarker such as this might serve as a tool to predict degree of success in weight loss under specific therapeutic conditions and would be beneficial for clinical use. The degree to which epigenetic profiles in blood cells or saliva reflect that in different organs, particularly the brain, remains to be determined.

LITERATURE CITED

Ahima, R. S., D. Prabakaran, and J. S. Flier. 1998. Postnatal leptin surge and regulation of circadian rhythm of leptin by feeding. Implications for energy homeostasis and neuroendocrine function. *J Clin Invest* 101 (5):1020–7.

Ahima, R. S., C. B. Saper, J. S. Flier, and J. K. Elmquist. 2000. Leptin regulation of neuroendocrine systems. *Front Neuroendocrinol* 21 (3):263–307.

Ahmed, F. 2010. Epigenetics: Tales of adversity. *Nature* 468 (7327):S20.

Alfaradhi, M. Z., D. S. Fernandez-Twinn, M. S. Martin-Gronert, B. Musial, A. Fowden, and S. E. Ozanne. 2014. Oxidative stress and altered lipid homeostasis in the programming of offspring fatty liver by maternal obesity. *Am J Physiol Regul Integr Comp Physiol* 307 (1):R26–34.

Barker, D. J., C. N. Martyn, C. Osmond, C. N. Hales, and C. H. Fall. 1993. Growth in utero and serum cholesterol concentrations in adult life. *BMJ* 307 (6918):1524–7.

Bilbo, S. D., and V. Tsang. 2010. Enduring consequences of maternal obesity for brain inflammation and behavior of offspring. *FASEB J* 24 (6):2104–15.

Bird, A. P. 1986. CpG-rich islands and the function of DNA methylation. *Nature* 321 (6067): 209–13.

Bjork Ingul, C., L. Loras, E. Tegnander, S. H. Eik-Nes, and A. Brantberg. 2015. Maternal obesity affects foetal myocardial function already in first trimester. *Ultrasound Obstet Gynecol* 47:433–442.

Blackmore, H. L., Y. Niu, D. S. Fernandez-Twinn, J. L. Tarry-Adkins, D. A. Giussani, and S. E. Ozanne. 2014. Maternal diet-induced obesity programs cardiovascular dysfunction in adult male mouse offspring independent of current body weight. *Endocrinology* 155 (10):3970–80.

Bouanane, S., N. B. Benkalfat, F. Z. Baba Ahmed, H. Merzouk, N. S. Mokhtari, S. A. Merzouk, J. Gresti, C. Tessier, and M. Narce. 2009. Time course of changes in serum oxidant/antioxidant status in overfed obese rats and their offspring. *Clin Sci (Lond)* 116 (8):669–80.

Bouanane, S., H. Merzouk, N. B. Benkalfat, N. Soulimane, S. A. Merzouk, J. Gresti, C. Tessier, and M. Narce. 2010. Hepatic and very low-density lipoprotein fatty acids in obese offspring of overfed dams. *Metabolism* 59 (12):1701–9.

Bouret, S. G., S. H. Bates, S. Chen, M. G. Myers, Jr., and R. B. Simerly. 2012. Distinct roles for specific leptin receptor signals in the development of hypothalamic feeding circuits. *J Neurosci* 32 (4):1244–52.

Bouret, S. G., S. J. Draper, and R. B. Simerly. 2004a. Formation of projection pathways from the arcuate nucleus of the hypothalamus to hypothalamic regions implicated in the neural control of feeding behavior in mice. *J Neurosci* 24 (11):2797–805.

Bouret, S. G., S. J. Draper, and R. B. Simerly. 2004b. Trophic action of leptin on hypothalamic neurons that regulate feeding. *Science* 304 (5667):108–10.

Bouret, S. G., S. J. Draper, and R. B. Simerly. 2004c. Formation of projection pathways from the arcuate nucleus of the hypothalamus to hypothalamic regions implicated in the neural control of feeding behavior in mice. *J Neurosci* (11):2797–805.

Bouret, S. G., S. J. Draper, and R. B. Simerly. 2004d. Trophic action of leptin on hypothalamic neurons that regulate feeding. *Science* 304 (5667):108–10.

Buckley, A. J., B. Keseru, J. Briody, M. Thompson, S. E. Ozanne, and C. H. Thompson. 2005. Altered body composition and metabolism in the male offspring of high fat-fed rats. *Metabolism* 54 (4):500–7.

Carlin, J., R. George, and T. M. Reyes. 2013. Methyl donor supplementation blocks the adverse effects of maternal high fat diet on offspring physiology. *PLoS One* 8 (5):e63549.

Casabiell, X., V. Pineiro, M. A. Tome, R. Peino, C. Dieguez, and F. F. Casanueva. 1997. Presence of leptin in colostrum and/or breast milk from lactating mothers: A potential role in the regulation of neonatal food intake. *J Clin Endocrinol Metab* 82 (12):4270–3.

Chango, A., and I. P. Pogribny. 2015. Considering maternal dietary modulators for epigenetic regulation and programming of the fetal epigenome *Nutrients* 7 (4):2748–70.

Chen, H., D. Simar, and M. J. Morris. 2009. Hypothalamic neuroendocrine circuitry is programmed by maternal obesity: Interaction with postnatal nutritional environment. *PLoS One* 4 (7):e6259.

Chen, H., D. Simar, and M. J. Morris. 2014. Maternal obesity impairs brain glucose metabolism and neural response to hyperglycemia in male rat offspring. *J Neurochem* 129 (2):297–303.

Chen, H., D. Simar, K. Pegg, S. Saad, C. Palmer, and M. J. Morris. 2014. Exendin-4 is effective against metabolic disorders induced by intrauterine and postnatal overnutrition in rodents. *Diabetologia* 57 (3):614–22.

Coleman, D. L. 1973. Effects of parabiosis of obese with diabetes and normal mice. *Diabetologia* 9 (4):294–8.

Cone, R. D., M. A. Cowley, A. A. Butler, W. Fan, D. L. Marks, and M. J. Low. 2001. The arcuate nucleus as a conduit for diverse signals relevant to energy homeostasis. *Int J Obes Relat Metab Disord* 25 Suppl 5:S63–7.

Dahlgren, J., C. Nilsson, E. Jennische, H. P. Ho, E. Eriksson, A. Niklasson, P. Bjorntorp, K. Albertsson Wikland, and A. Holmang. 2001. Prenatal cytokine exposure results in obesity and gender-specific programming. *Am J Physiol Endocrinol Metab* 281 (2):E326–34.

Desai, M., D. Gayle, J. Babu, and M. G. Ross. 2005. Programmed obesity in intrauterine growth-restricted newborns: Modulation by newborn nutrition. *Am J Physiol Regul Integr Comp Physiol* 288 (1):R91–6.

Desai, M., J. K. Jellyman, G. Han, M. Beall, R. H. Lane, and M. G. Ross. 2014. Maternal obesity and high-fat diet program offspring metabolic syndrome. *Am J Obstet Gynecol* 211 (3):237.

Dolinoy, D. C., J. R. Weidman, R. A. Waterland, and R. L. Jirtle. 2006. Maternal genistein alters coat color and protects Avy mouse offspring from obesity by modifying the fetal epigenome. *Environ Health Perspect* 114 (4):567–72.

Dudley, K. J., D. M. Sloboda, K. L. Connor, J. Beltrand, and M. H. Vickers. 2011. Offspring of mothers fed a high fat diet display hepatic cell cycle inhibition and associated changes in gene expression and DNA methylation. *PLoS One* 6 (7):e21662.

Elmquist, J. K., C. F. Elias, and C. B. Saper. 1999. From lesions to leptin: Hypothalamic control of food intake and body weight. *Neuron* 22 (2):221–32.

Eriksson, J. G., C. Osmond, E. Kajantie, T. J. Forsen, and D. J. Barker. 2006. Patterns of growth among children who later develop type 2 diabetes or its risk factors *Diabetologia* 49 (12):2853–8.

Fall, C. H., C. Osmond, D. J. Barker, P. M. Clark, C. N. Hales, Y. Stirling, and T. W. Meade. 1995. Fetal and infant growth and cardiovascular risk factors in women. *BMJ* 310 (6977):428–32.

Faust, I. M., P. R. Johnson, and J. Hirsch. 1980. Long-term effects of early nutritional experience on the development of obesity in the rat. *J Nutr* 110 (10):2027–34.

Fernandez-Twinn, D. S., H. L. Blackmore, L. Siggens, D. A. Giussani, C. M. Cross, R. Foo, and S. E. Ozanne. 2012. The programming of cardiac hypertrophy in the offspring by maternal obesity is associated with hyperinsulinemia, AKT, ERK, and mTOR activation. *Endocrinology* 153 (12):5961–71.

Flegal, K. M., D. Kruszon-Moran, M. D. Carroll, C. D. Fryar, and C. L. Ogden. 2016. Trends in obesity among adults in the United States, 2005 to 2014. *JAMA* 315 (21):2284–91.

Garcia-Cardona, M. C., F. Huang, J. M. Garcia-Vivas, C. Lopez-Camarillo, B. E. Del Rio Navarro, E. Navarro Olivos, E. Hong-Chong, F. Bolanos-Jimenez, and L. A. Marchat. 2014. DNA methylation of leptin and adiponectin promoters in children is reduced by the combined presence of obesity and insulin resistance. *Int J Obes (Lond)* 38 (11):1457–65.

Ghoshal, K., X. Li, J. Datta, S. Bai, I. Pogribny, M. Pogribny, Y. Huang, D. Young, and S. T. Jacob. 2006. A folate- and methyl-deficient diet alters the expression of DNA methyltransferases and methyl CpG binding proteins involved in epigenetic gene silencing in livers of F344 rats. *J Nutr* 136 (6):1522–7.

Gluckman, P. D., and M. A. Hanson. 2004. The developmental origins of the metabolic syndrome. *Trends Endocrinol Metab* 15 (4):183–7.

Grayson, B. E., S. E. Allen, S. K. Billes, S. M. Williams, M. S. Smith, and K. L. Grove. 2006. Prenatal development of hypothalamic neuropeptide systems in the nonhuman primate. *Neurosci* 143 (4):975–86.

Grayson, B. E., P. Kievit, M. S. Smith, and K. L. Grove. 2010a. Critical determinants of hypothalamic appetitive neuropeptide development and expression: Species considerations. *Front Neuroendocrinol* 31 (1):16–31.

Grayson, B. E., P. R. Levasseur, S. M. Williams, M. S. Smith, D. L. Marks, and K. L. Grove. 2010b. Changes in melanocortin expression and inflammatory pathways in fetal offspring of nonhuman primates fed a high-fat diet. *Endocrinology* 151 (4):1622–32.

Gregorio, B. M., V. Souza-Mello, J. J. Carvalho, C. A. Mandarim-de-Lacerda, and M. B. Aguila. 2010. Maternal high-fat intake predisposes nonalcoholic fatty liver disease in C57BL/6 offspring. *Am J Obstet Gynecol* 203 (5):495e1–8.

Guo, F., and K.-L. Jen. 1995. High-fat feeding during pregnancy and lactation affects offspring metabolism in rats. *Physiol Behav* 57:681–6.

Hales, C. N., and D. J. Barker. 1992. Type 2 (non-insulin-dependent) diabetes mellitus: The thrifty phenotype hypothesis. *Diabetologia* 35 (7):595–601.

Hales, C. N., D. J. Barker, P. M. Clark, L. J. Cox, C. Fall, C. Osmond, and P. D. Winter. 1991. Fetal and infant growth and impaired glucose tolerance at age 64. *BMJ* 303 (6809):1019–22.

Hall, W. G. 1985. What we know and don't know about the development of independent ingestion in rats. *Appetite* 6 (4):333–56.

Hoggard, N., L. Hunter, J. S. Duncan, L. M. Williams, P. Trayhurn, and J. G. Mercer. 1997. Leptin and leptin receptor mRNA and protein expression in the murine fetus and placenta. *Proc Natl Acad Sci USA* 94 (20):11073–8.

Howie, G. J., D. M. Sloboda, T. Kamal, and M. H. Vickers. 2009. Maternal nutritional history predicts obesity in adult offspring independent of postnatal diet. *J Physiol* 587 (Pt 4):905–15.

Howie, G. J., D. M. Sloboda, C. M. Reynolds, and M. H. Vickers. 2013. Timing of maternal exposure to a high fat diet and development of obesity and hyperinsulinemia in male rat offspring: Same metabolic phenotype, different developmental pathways? *J Nutr Metab* 2013:517384.

Isganaitis, E., M. Woo, H. Ma, M. Chen, W. Kong, A. Lytras, V. Sales, J. Decoste-Lopez, K. J. Lee, C. Leatherwood, D. Lee, C. Fitzpatrick, W. Gall, S. Watkins, and M. E. Patti. 2014. Developmental programming by maternal insulin resistance: Hyperinsulinemia, glucose intolerance, and dysregulated lipid metabolism in male offspring of insulin-resistant mice. *Diabetes* 63 (2):688–700.

Jaenisch, R., and A. Bird. 2003. Epigenetic regulation of gene expression: How the genome integrates intrinsic and environmental signals. *Nat Genet* 33 Suppl:245–54.

Kahraman, S., E. Dirice, D. F. De Jesus, J. Hu, and R. N. Kulkarni. 2014. Maternal insulin resistance and transient hyperglycemia impact the metabolic and endocrine phenotypes of offspring. *Am J Physiol Endocrinol Metab* 307 (10):E906–18.

Kojima, S., C. Catavero, and L. Rinaman. 2016. Maternal high-fat diet increases independent feeding in pre-weanling rat pups. *Physiol Behav* 157:237–45.

Kojima, M., H. Hosoda, Y. Date, M. Nakazato, H. Matsuo, and K. Kangawa. 1999. Ghrelin is a growth-hormone-releasing acylated peptide from stomach. *Nature* 402 (6762):656–60.

Kuehnen, P., M. Mischke, S. Wiegand, C. Sers, B. Horsthemke, S. Lau, T. Keil, Y. A. Lee, A. Grueters, and H. Krude. 2012. An Alu element-associated hypermethylation variant of the POMC gene is associated with childhood obesity. *PLoS Genet* 8 (3):e1002543.

Lange, U. C., and R. Schneider. 2010. What an epigenome remembers. *Bioessays* 32 (8):659–68.

Lee, G. H., R. Proenca, J. M. Montez, K. M. Carroll, J. G. Darvishzadeh, J. I. Lee, and J. M. Friedman. 1996. Abnormal splicing of the leptin receptor in diabetic mice. *Nature* 379 (6566):632–5.

Lesseur, C., D. A. Armstrong, A. G. Paquette, Z. Li, J. F. Padbury, and C. J. Marsit. 2014. Maternal obesity and gestational diabetes are associated with placental leptin DNA methylation. *Am J Obstet Gynecol* 211 (6):654e1–9.

Levin, B. E., and E. Govek. 1998. Gestational obesity accentuates obesity in obesity-prone progeny. *Am J Physiol* 275 (4 Pt 2):R1374–9.

Lillycrop, K. A., J. L. Slater-Jefferies, M. A. Hanson, K. M. Godfrey, A. A. Jackson, and G. C. Burdge. 2007. Induction of altered epigenetic regulation of the hepatic glucocorticoid receptor in the offspring of rats fed a protein-restricted diet during pregnancy suggests that reduced DNA methyltransferase-1 expression is involved in impaired DNA methylation and changes in histone modifications. *Br J Nutr* 97 (6):1064–73.

Locke, A. E., B. Kahali, S. I. Berndt, A. E. Justice, T. H. Pers, F. R. Day, C. Powell, S. Vedantam, M. L. Buchkovich, J. Yang, D. C. Croteau-Chonka, T. Esko, T. Fall, T. Ferreira, S. Gustafsson, Z. Kutalik, J. Luan, R. Magi, J. C. Randall, T. W. Winkler, A. R. Wood, T. Workalemahu, J. D. Faul, J. A. Smith, J. Hua Zhao, W. Zhao, J. Chen, R. Fehrmann, A. K. Hedman, J. Karjalainen, E. M. Schmidt, D. Absher, N. Amin, D. Anderson, M. Beekman, J. L. Bolton, J. L. Bragg-Gresham, S. Buyske, A. Demirkan, G. Deng, G. B. Ehret, B. Feenstra, M. F. Feitosa, K. Fischer, A. Goel, J. Gong, A. U. Jackson, S. Kanoni, M. E. Kleber, K. Kristiansson, U. Lim, V. Lotay, M. Mangino, I. Mateo Leach, C. Medina-Gomez, S. E. Medland, M. A. Nalls, C. D. Palmer, D. Pasko, S. Pechlivanis, M. J. Peters, I. Prokopenko, D. Shungin, A. Stancakova, R. J. Strawbridge, Y. Ju Sung, T. Tanaka, A. Teumer, S. Trompet, S. W. van der Laan, J. van Setten, J. V. Van Vliet-Ostaptchouk, Z. Wang, L. Yengo, W. Zhang, A. Isaacs, E. Albrecht, J. Arnlov, G. M. Arscott, A. P. Attwood, S. Bandinelli, A. Barrett, I. N. Bas, C. Bellis, A. J. Bennett, C. Berne, R. Blagieva, M. Bluher, S. Bohringer, L. L. Bonnycastle, Y. Bottcher, H. A. Boyd, M. Bruinenberg, I. H. Caspersen, Y. D. Ida Chen, R. Clarke, E. W. Daw, A. J. de Craen, G. Delgado, M. Dimitriou, A. S. Doney, N. Eklund, K. Estrada, E. Eury, L. Folkersen, R. M. Fraser, M. E. Garcia, F. Geller, V. Giedraitis, B. Gigante, A. S. Go, A. Golay, A. H. Goodall, S. D. Gordon, M. Gorski, H. J. Grabe, H. Grallert, T. B. Grammer, J. Grassler, H. Gronberg, C. J. Groves, G. Gusto, J. Haessler, P. Hall, T. Haller, G. Hallmans, C. A. Hartman, M. Hassinen, C. Hayward, N. L. Heard-Costa, Q. Helmer, C. Hengstenberg, O. Holmen, J. J. Hottenga, A. L. James, J. M. Jeff, A. Johansson, J. Jolley, T. Juliusdottir, L. Kinnunen, W. Koenig, M. Koskenvuo, W. Kratzer, J. Laitinen, C. Lamina, K. Leander, N. R. Lee, P. Lichtner, L. Lind, J. Lindstrom, K. Sin Lo, S. Lobbens, R. Lorbeer, Y. Lu, F. Mach, P. K. Magnusson, A. Mahajan, W. L. McArdle, S. McLachlan, C. Menni, S. Merger, E. Mihailov, L. Milani, A. Moayyeri, K. L. Monda, M. A. Morken, A. Mulas, G. Muller, M. Muller-Nurasyid, A. W. Musk, R. Nagaraja, M. M. Nothen, I. M. Nolte, S. Pilz, N. W. Rayner, F. Renstrom, R. Rettig, J. S. Ried, S. Ripke, N. R. Robertson, L. M. Rose, S. Sanna, H. Scharnagl, S. Scholtens, F. R. Schumacher, W. R. Scott, T. Seufferlein, J. Shi, A. Vernon Smith, J. Smolonska, A. V. Stanton, V. Steinthorsdottir, K. Stirrups, H. M. Stringham, J. Sundstrom, M. A. Swertz, A. J. Swift, A. C. Syvanen, S. T. Tan, B. O. Tayo, B. Thorand, G. Thorleifsson, J. P. Tyrer, H. W. Uh, L. Vandenput, F. C. Verhulst, S. H. Vermeulen, N. Verweij, J. M. Vonk, L. L. Waite, H. R. Warren, D. Waterworth, M. N. Weedon, L. R. Wilkens, C. Willenborg, T. Wilsgaard, M. K. Wojczynski, A. Wong, A. F. Wright, Q. Zhang, Study LifeLines Cohort, E. P. Brennan, M. Choi, Z. Dastani, A. W. Drong, P. Eriksson, A. Franco-Cereceda, J. R. Gadin, A. G. Gharavi, M. E. Goddard, R. E. Handsaker, J. Huang, F. Karpe, S. Kathiresan, S. Keildson, K. Kiryluk, M. Kubo, J. Y. Lee, L. Liang, R. P. Lifton, B. Ma, S. A. McCarroll, A. J. McKnight, J. L. Min, M. F. Moffatt, G. W. Montgomery, J. M. Murabito, G. Nicholson, D. R. Nyholt,

Y. Okada, J. R. Perry, R. Dorajoo, E. Reinmaa, R. M. Salem, N. Sandholm, R. A.
Scott, L. Stolk, A. Takahashi, T. Tanaka, F. M. Van't Hooft, A. A. Vinkhuyzen, H. J.
Westra, W. Zheng, K. T. Zondervan, A. DIPOGen Consortium, Agen-Bmi Working
Group, C. ARDIOGRAMplusC4D Consortium, C. KDGen Consortium, Glgc, Icbp,
Magic Investigators, Ther Consortium Mu, M. IGen Consortium, Page Consortium,
Consortium ReproGen, Genie Consortium, Consortium International Endogene, A. C.
Heath, D. Arveiler, S. J. Bakker, J. Beilby, R. N. Bergman, J. Blangero, P. Bovet, H.
Campbell, M. J. Caulfield, G. Cesana, A. Chakravarti, D. I. Chasman, P. S. Chines,
F. S. Collins, D. C. Crawford, L. A. Cupples, D. Cusi, J. Danesh, U. de Faire, H. M.
den Ruijter, A. F. Dominiczak, R. Erbel, J. Erdmann, J. G. Eriksson, M. Farrall, S. B.
Felix, E. Ferrannini, J. Ferrieres, I. Ford, N. G. Forouhi, T. Forrester, O. H. Franco,
R. T. Gansevoort, P. V. Gejman, C. Gieger, O. Gottesman, V. Gudnason, U. Gyllensten,
A. S. Hall, T. B. Harris, A. T. Hattersley, A. A. Hicks, L. A. Hindorff, A. D. Hingorani,
A. Hofman, G. Homuth, G. K. Hovingh, S. E. Humphries, S. C. Hunt, E. Hypponen,
T. Illig, K. B. Jacobs, M. R. Jarvelin, K. H. Jockel, B. Johansen, P. Jousilahti, J. W.
Jukema, A. M. Jula, J. Kaprio, J. J. Kastelein, S. M. Keinanen-Kiukaanniemi, L. A.
Kiemeney, P. Knekt, J. S. Kooner, C. Kooperberg, P. Kovacs, A. T. Kraja, M. Kumari,
J. Kuusisto, T. A. Lakka, C. Langenberg, L. Le Marchand, T. Lehtimaki, V. Lyssenko,
S. Mannisto, A. Marette, T. C. Matise, C. A. McKenzie, B. McKnight, F. L. Moll, A. D.
Morris, A. P. Morris, J. C. Murray, C. Nelis, C. Ohlsson, A. J. Oldehinkel, K. K. Ong,
P. A. Madden, G. Pasterkamp, J. F. Peden, A. Peters, D. S. Postma, P. P. Pramstaller,
J. F. Price, L. Qi, O. T. Raitakari, T. Rankinen, D. C. Rao, T. K. Rice, P. M. Ridker,
J. D. Rioux, M. D. Ritchie, I. Rudan, V. Salomaa, N. J. Samani, J. Saramies, M. A.
Sarzynski, H. Schunkert, P. E. Schwarz, P. Sever, A. R. Shuldiner, J. Sinisalo, R. P.
Stolk, K. Strauch, A. Tonjes, D. A. Tregouet, A. Tremblay, E. Tremoli, J. Virtamo,
M. C. Vohl, U. Volker, G. Waeber, G. Willemsen, J. C. Witteman, M. C. Zillikens,
L. S. Adair, P. Amouyel, F. W. Asselbergs, T. L. Assimes, M. Bochud, B. O. Boehm, E.
Boerwinkle, S. R. Bornstein, E. P. Bottinger, C. Bouchard, S. Cauchi, J. C. Chambers,
S. J. Chanock, R. S. Cooper, P. I. de Bakker, G. Dedoussis, L. Ferrucci, P. W. Franks, P.
Froguel, L. C. Groop, C. A. Haiman, A. Hamsten, J. Hui, D. J. Hunter, K. Hveem, R. C.
Kaplan, M. Kivimaki, D. Kuh, M. Laakso, Y. Liu, N. G. Martin, W. Marz, M. Melbye,
A. Metspalu, S. Moebus, P. B. Munroe, I. Njolstad, B. A. Oostra, C. N. Palmer, N. L.
Pedersen, M. Perola, L. Perusse, U. Peters, C. Power, T. Quertermous, R. Rauramaa, F.
Rivadeneira, T. E. Saaristo, D. Saleheen, N. Sattar, E. E. Schadt, D. Schlessinger, P. E.
Slagboom, H. Snieder, T. D. Spector, U. Thorsteinsdottir, M. Stumvoll, J. Tuomilehto,
A. G. Uitterlinden, M. Uusitupa, P. van der Harst, M. Walker, H. Wallaschofski, N. J.
Wareham, H. Watkins, D. R. Weir, H. E. Wichmann, J. F. Wilson, P. Zanen, I. B. Borecki,
P. Deloukas, C. S. Fox, I. M. Heid, J. R. O'Connell, D. P. Strachan, K. Stefansson, C. M.
van Duijn, G. R. Abecasis, L. Franke, T. M. Frayling, M. I. McCarthy, P. M. Visscher,
A. Scherag, C. J. Willer, M. Boehnke, K. L. Mohlke, C. M. Lindgren, J. S. Beckmann,
I. Barroso, K. E. North, E. Ingelsson, J. N. Hirschhorn, R. J. Loos, and E. K. Speliotes.
2015. Genetic studies of body mass index yield new insights for obesity biology. *Nature*
518 (7538):197–206. doi: 10.1038/nature14177.
Marchesini, G., M. Brizi, G. Bianchi, S. Tomassetti, E. Bugianesi, M. Lenzi, A. J. McCullough,
S. Natale, G. Forlani, and N. Melchionda. 2001. Nonalcoholic fatty liver disease: A fea-
ture of the metabolic syndrome. *Diabetes* 50 (8):1844–50.
Masuzaki, H., Y. Ogawa, N. Sagawa, K. Hosoda, T. Matsumoto, H. Mise, H. Nishimura, Y.
Yoshimasa, I. Tanaka, T. Mori, and K. Nakao. 1997. Nonadipose tissue production of
leptin: Leptin as a novel placenta-derived hormone in humans. *Nat Med* 3 (9):1029–33.
McCurdy, C. E., J. M. Bishop, S. M. Williams, B. E. Grayson, M. S. Smith, J. E. Friedman,
and K. L. Grove. 2009. Maternal high-fat diet triggers lipotoxicity in the fetal livers of
nonhuman primates. *J Clin Invest* 119 (2):323–35.

Melzner, I., V. Scott, K. Dorsch, P. Fischer, M. Wabitsch, S. Bruderlein, C. Hasel, and P. Moller. 2002. Leptin gene expression in human preadipocytes is switched on by maturation-induced demethylation of distinct CpGs in its proximal promoter. *J Biol Chem* 277 (47):45420–7.

Michaud, E. J., M. J. van Vugt, S. J. Bultman, H. O. Sweet, M. T. Davisson, and R. P. Woychik. 1994. Differential expression of a new dominant agouti allele (Aiapy) is correlated with methylation state and is influenced by parental lineage. *Genes Dev* 8 (12):1463–72.

Muroya, S., T. Yada, S. Shioda, and M. Takigawa. 1999. Glucose-sensitive neurons in the rat arcuate nucleus contain neuropeptide Y. *Neurosci Lett* 264 (1–3):113–6.

Naef, L., L. Moquin, G. Dal Bo, B. Giros, A. Gratton, and C. D. Walker. 2011. Maternal high-fat intake alters presynaptic regulation of dopamine in the nucleus accumbens and increases motivation for fat rewards in the offspring. *Neuroscience* 176:225–36.

Newell-Price, J., P. King, and A. J. Clark. 2001. The CpG island promoter of the human proopiomelanocortin gene is methylated in nonexpressing normal tissue and tumors and represses expression. *Mol Endocrinol* 15 (2):338–48.

Niswender, K. D., and M. W. Schwartz. 2003. Insulin and leptin revisited: Adiposity signals with overlapping physiological and intracellular signaling capabilities. *Front Neuroendocrinol* 24 (1):1–10.

Oben, J. A., A. Mouralidarane, A. M. Samuelsson, P. J. Matthews, M. L. Morgan, C. McKee, J. Soeda, D. S. Fernandez-Twinn, M. S. Martin-Gronert, S. E. Ozanne, B. Sigala, M. Novelli, L. Poston, and P. D. Taylor. 2010. Maternal obesity during pregnancy and lactation programs the development of offspring non-alcoholic fatty liver disease in mice. *J Hepatol* 52 (6):913–20.

Ogden, C. L., M. D. Carroll, L. R. Curtin, M. A. McDowell, C. J. Tabak, and K. M. Flegal. 2006. Prevalence of overweight and obesity in the United States, 1999–2004. *JAMA* 295 (13):1549–55.

Ozanne, S. E., and C. N. Hales. 2004. Lifespan: Catch-up growth and obesity in male mice. *Nature* 427 (6973):411–2.

Ozanne, S. E., R. Lewis, B. J. Jennings, and C. N. Hales. 2004. Early programming of weight gain in mice prevents the induction of obesity by a highly palatable diet. *Clin Sci* 106 (2):141–5.

Painter, R. C., C. Osmond, P. Gluckman, M. Hanson, D. I. Phillips, and T. J. Roseboom. 2008. Transgenerational effects of prenatal exposure to the Dutch famine on neonatal adiposity and health in later life. *BJOG* 115 (10):1243–9.

Patterson, C. M., S. G. Bouret, S. Park, B. G. Irani, A. A. Dunn-Meynell, and B. E. Levin. 2010. Large Litter rearing enhances leptin sensitivity and protects selectively bred diet-induced obese (DIO) rats from becoming obese. *Endocrinology* 151:4270–9.

Pedersen, J., B. Bojsen-Moller, and H. Poulsen. 1954. Blood sugar in newborn infants of diabetic mothers. *Acta Endocrinol (Copenhagen)* 15 (1):33–52.

Pedersen, J., and M. Osler. 1961. Hyperglycemia as the cause of characteristic features of the foetus and newborn of diabetic mothers. *Dan Med Bull* 8:78–83.

Plagemann, A., T. Harder, M. Brunn, A. Harder, K. Roepke, M. Wittrock-Staar, T. Ziska, K. Schellong, E. Rodekamp, K. Melchior, and J. W. Dudenhausen. 2009. Hypothalamic proopiomelanocortin promoter methylation becomes altered by early overfeeding: An epigenetic model of obesity and the metabolic syndrome. *J Physiol* 587 (Pt 20):4963–76.

Plagemann, A., I. Heidrich, F. Gotz, W. Rohde, and G. Dorner. 1992. Lifelong enhanced diabetes susceptibility and obesity after temporary intrahypothalamic hyperinsulinism during brain organization. *Exp Clin Endocrinol* 99 (2):91–5.

Plagemann, A., K. Roepke, T. Harder, M. Brunn, A. Harder, M. Wittrock-Staar, T. Ziska, K. Schellong, E. Rodekamp, K. Melchior, and J. W. Dudenhausen. 2010. Epigenetic malprogramming of the insulin receptor promoter due to developmental overfeeding. *J Perinat Med* 38 (4):393–400.

Proulx, K., D. Richard, and C. D. Walker. 2002. Leptin regulates appetite-related neuropeptides in the hypothalamus of developing rats without affecting food intake. *Endocrinology* 143 (12):4683–92.

Purcell, R. H., Bo Sun, L. L. Pass, M. L. Power, T. H. Moran, and K. L. K. Tamashiro. 2011. Maternal stress and high-fat diet effect on maternal behavior, milk composition, and pup ingestive behavior. *Physiol Behav* 104 (3):474–9.

Ravelli, A. C., J. H. van der Meulen, R. P. Michels, C. Osmond, D. J. Barker, C. N. Hales, and O. P. Bleker. 1998. Glucose tolerance in adults after prenatal exposure to famine. *Lancet* 351 (9097):173–7.

Ravelli, G. P., Z. A. Stein, and M. W. Susser. 1976. Obesity in young men after famine exposure in utero and early infancy. *N Engl J Med* 295 (7):349–53.

Reusens, B., and C. Remacle. 2006. Programming of the endocrine pancreas by the early nutritional environment. *Int J Biochem Cell Biol* 38 (5–6):913–22.

Reynolds, R. M., K. M. Allan, E. A. Raja, S. Bhattacharya, G. McNeill, P. C. Hannaford, N. Sarwar, A. J. Lee, and J. E. Norman. 2013. Maternal obesity during pregnancy and premature mortality from cardiovascular event in adult offspring: Follow-up of 1 323 275 person years. *BMJ* 347:f4539.

Rivera, H. M., P. Kievit, M. A. Kirigiti, L. A. Bauman, K. Baquero, P. Blundell, T. A. Dean, J. C. Valleau, D. L. Takahashi, T. Frazee, L. Douville, J. Majer, M. S. Smith, K. L. Grove, and E. L. Sullivan. 2015. Maternal high-fat diet and obesity impact palatable food intake and dopamine signaling in nonhuman primate offspring. *Obesity (Silver Spring)* 23 (11):2157–64.

Scarlett, J. M., E. E. Jobst, P. J. Enriori, D. D. Bowe, A. K. Batra, W. F. Grant, M. A. Cowley, and D. L. Marks. 2007. Regulation of central melanocortin signaling by interleukin-1 beta. *Endocrinology* 148 (9):4217–25.

Scarlett, J. M., X. Zhu, P. J. Enriori, D. D. Bowe, A. K. Batra, P. R. Levasseur, W. F. Grant, M. M. Meguid, M. A. Cowley, and D. L. Marks. 2008. Regulation of agouti-related protein messenger ribonucleic acid transcription and peptide secretion by acute and chronic inflammation. *Endocrinology* 149 (10):4837–45.

Schwartz, M. W., S. C. Woods, D. Porte, Jr., R. J. Seeley, and D. G. Baskin. 2000. Central nervous system control of food intake. *Nature* 404 (6778):661–71.

Sen, S., and R. A. Simmons. 2010. Maternal antioxidant supplementation prevents adiposity in the offspring of Western diet-fed rats. *Diabetes* 59 (12):3058–65.

Senaris, R., T. Garcia-Caballero, X. Casabiell, R. Gallego, R. Castro, R. V. Considine, C. Dieguez, and F. F. Casanueva. 1997. Synthesis of leptin in human placenta. *Endocrinology* 138 (10):4501–4.

Shankar, K., A. Harrell, X. Liu, J. M. Gilchrist, M. J. Ronis, and T. M. Badger. 2008. Maternal obesity at conception programs obesity in the offspring. *Am J Physiol Regul Integr Comp Physiol* 294 (2):R528–38.

Smith, J. T., and B. J. Waddell. 2003. Leptin distribution and metabolism in the pregnant rat: Transplacental leptin passage increases in late gestation but is reduced by excess glucocorticoids. *Endocrinology* 144 (7):3024–30.

Steculorum, S. M., and S. G. Bouret. 2011. Maternal diabetes compromises the organization of hypothalamic feeding circuits and impairs leptin sensitivity in offspring. *Endocrinology* 152 (11):4171–9.

Steculorum, S. M., G. Collden, B. Coupe, S. Croizier, S. Lockie, Z. B. Andrews, F. Jarosch, S. Klussmann, and S. G. Bouret. 2015. Neonatal ghrelin programs development of hypothalamic feeding circuits. *J Clin Invest* 125 (2):846–58.

Stefater, M. A., and R. J. Seeley. 2010. Central nervous system nutrient signaling: The regulation of energy balance and the future of dietary therapies. *Annu Rev Nutr* 30:219–35.

Stein, A. D., H. S. Kahn, A. Rundle, P. A. Zybert, K. van der Pal-de Bruin, and L. H. Lumey. 2007. Anthropometric measures in middle age after exposure to famine during gestation: Evidence from the Dutch famine. *Am J Clin Nutr* 85 (3):869–76.

Stoger, R. 2006. In vivo methylation patterns of the leptin promoter in human and mouse. *Epigenetics* 1 (4):155–62.

Sun, B., R. H. Purcell, C. E. Terrillion, J. Yan, T. H. Moran, and K. L. Tamashiro. 2012. Maternal high-fat diet during gestation or suckling differentially affects offspring leptin sensitivity and obesity. *Diabetes* 61 (11):2833–41.

Sun, B., L. Song, K. L. Tamashiro, T. H. Moran, and J. Yan. 2014. Large litter rearing improves leptin sensitivity and hypothalamic appetite markers in offspring of rat dams fed high-fat diet during pregnancy and lactation. *Endocrinology* 155 (9):3421–33.

Swithers, S. E., and W. G. Hall. 1989. A nutritive control of independent ingestion in rat pups emerges by nine days of age. *Physiol Behav* 46 (5):873–9.

Taylor, P. D., J. McConnell, I. Y. Khan, K. Holemans, K. M. Lawrence, H. Asare-Anane, S. J. Persaud, P. M. Jones, L. Petrie, M. A. Hanson, and L. Poston. 2005. Impaired glucose homeostasis and mitochondrial abnormalities in offspring of rats fed a fat-rich diet in pregnancy. *Am J Physiol Regul Integr Comp Physiol* 288 (1):R134–9.

Turdi, S., W. Ge, N. Hu, K. M. Bradley, X. Wang, and J. Ren. 2013. Interaction between maternal and postnatal high fat diet leads to a greater risk of myocardial dysfunction in offspring via enhanced lipotoxicity, IRS-1 serine phosphorylation and mitochondrial defects. *J Mol Cell Cardiol* 55:117–29.

Valleau, J. C., and E. L. Sullivan. 2014. The impact of leptin on perinatal development and psychopathology. *J Chem Neuroanat* 61–62:221–32.

Vogt, M. C., L. Paeger, S. Hess, S. M. Steculorum, M. Awazawa, B. Hampel, S. Neupert, H. T. Nicholls, J. Mauer, A. C. Hausen, R. Predel, P. Kloppenburg, T. L. Horvath, and J. C. Bruning. 2014. Neonatal insulin action impairs hypothalamic neurocircuit formation in response to maternal high-fat feeding. *Cell* 156 (3):495–509.

Vucetic, Z., J. Kimmel, and T. M. Reyes. 2011. Chronic high-fat diet drives postnatal epigenetic regulation of mu-opioid receptor in the brain. *Neuropsychopharmacology* 36 (6):1199–206.

Vucetic, Z., J. Kimmel, K. Totoki, E. Hollenbeck, and T. M. Reyes. 2010. Maternal high-fat diet alters methylation and gene expression of dopamine and opioid-related genes. *Endocrinology* 151 (10):4756–64.

Waddington, C. H. 1942. The epigenotype. *Endeavour*:18–20.

Waddington, C. H. 2012. The epigenotype. 1942. *Int J Epidemiol* 41 (1):10–3.

Waterland, R. A. 2014. Epigenetic mechanisms affecting regulation of energy balance: Many questions, few answers. *Annu Rev Nutr* 34:337–55.

Weaver, I. C., N. Cervoni, F. A. Champagne, A. C. D'Alessio, S. Sharma, J. R. Seckl, S. Dymov, M. Szyf, and M. J. Meaney. 2004. Epigenetic programming by maternal behavior. *Nat Neurosci* 7 (8):847–54.

Widdowson, E. M. 1950. Chemical composition of newly born mammals *Nature* 166 (4224): 626–8.

Widdowson, E. M., and C. M. Spray. 1951. Chemical development in utero. *Arch Dis Child* 26 (127):205–14.

Wolff, G. L., R. L. Kodell, S. R. Moore, and C. A. Cooney. 1998. Maternal epigenetics and methyl supplements affect agouti gene expression in Avy/a mice. *FASEB J* 12 (11):949–57.

Woods, S. C., R. J. Seeley, D. G. Baskin, and M. W. Schwartz. 2003. Insulin and the blood–brain barrier. *Curr Pharm Des* 9 (10):795–800.

Woods, S. C., R. J. Seeley, D. Porte, Jr., and M. W. Schwartz. 1998. Signals that regulate food intake and energy homeostasis. *Science* 280 (5368):1378–83.

Wu, Q., Y. Mizushima, M. Komiya, T. Matsuo, and M. Suzuki. 1998. Body fat accumulation in the male offspring of rats fed high-fat diets. *J Clin Biochem Nutr* 25:71–9.

Yeo, G. S., I. S. Farooqi, S. Aminian, D. J. Halsall, R. G. Stanhope, and S. O'Rahilly. 1998. A frameshift mutation in MC4R associated with dominantly inherited human obesity. *Nat Genet* 20 (2):111–2.

Younossi, Z. M., M. Stepanova, M. Afendy, Y. Fang, Y. Younossi, H. Mir, and M. Srishord. 2011. Changes in the prevalence of the most common causes of chronic liver diseases in the United States from 1988 to 2008. *Clin Gastroenterol Hepatol* 9 (6):524–30 e1; quiz e60.

Zhang, Y., R. Proenca, M. Maffei, M. Barone, L. Leopold, and J. M. Friedman. 1994. Positional cloning of the mouse obese gene and its human homologue. *Nature* 372 (6505):425–32.

9 Monitoring and Maintenance of Brain Glucose Supply
Importance of Hindbrain Catecholamine Neurons in This Multifaceted Task

Sue Ritter

CONTENTS

9.1 IMPORTANCE OF GLUCOSE MONITORING FOR NORMAL BRAIN FUNCTION

Glucose is the essential metabolic fuel for the brain. Acute and severe reduction of brain glucose leads quickly to impairment of cognitive and reflex function, autonomic failure, seizures, loss of consciousness, and permanent and irreversible brain damage and, if not rapidly corrected, can be lethal. Because of its importance to survival and brain function, maintenance of adequate blood glucose for brain metabolism is an urgent and continuous physiological priority. Survival depends on the fact that reduced brain glucose availability (glucoprivation) evokes highly coordinated glucoregulatory responses adapted to conserve and restore this essential fuel. These responses include increased food intake, mobilization of stored glucose, increased gastric motility, corticosterone secretion, suppression of reproductive responses, and others. Despite these protective responses to glucose deficit, diabetic patients on insulin therapy are faced with a constant threat of glucoprivic crisis due to inadvertent mismatch of prevailing glucose levels and insulin dose that results in a fall in blood glucose concentrations (iatrogenic hypoglycemia). In the aftermath of a severe hypoglycemic episode or after repeated hypoglycemic bouts, the responsiveness of central mechanisms to glucose deficit is reduced, resulting in a condition known as hypoglycemia associated autonomic failure (HAAF) and hypoglycemia unawareness (Cryer 2001, Dagogo-Jack, Craft, and Cryer 1993). In this condition, both the cognitive awareness of hypoglycemia and the normally elicited glucoregulatory responses (known as counterregulatory responses [CRRs]) are diminished or absent, greatly increasing the threat of death or injury resulting from a subsequent hypoglycemic episode. The prevalence of diabetes for all age groups worldwide was estimated to be 2.8% (171 million) in 2000 and is projected to rise to 4.4% (366 million) by 2030 (Wild et al. 2004). The number of diabetics worldwide threatened with iatrogenic hypoglycemia and HAAF will therefore rise during the coming years. Hypoglycemia is not limited to diabetics, however, but can be associated with stomach removal or gastric bypass surgery, diseases of liver or kidneys, heart attack, stroke, alcohol addiction, and other metabolic problems. These medical problems reveal the impact of glucose deficit on brain function and survival, providing a strong incentive to understand the physiology and mechanisms of the brain's glucoregulatory circuitry.

Carbohydrates are the most abundant nutrient on the planet, but they are costly in terms of their required storage space, and glycogen storage within the brain itself is minimal. Rather than storing glycogen, the brain relies on delivery of glucose by the blood from peripheral sources. Even in the periphery, however, the amount of stored glucose is minimal. George Bray (1994) calculated that in a normal-weight adult human body, stored nutrients amount to approximately 140,000 kcal fat, 24,000 kcal protein, but only 800 kcal total as glucose, including both glycogen and circulating glucose. On a 2000 kcal/day diet of 40% carb, 40% fat, and 20% protein, daily intake of fat and protein amount to about 0.57% and 1.67% of body stores, respectively, whereas daily intake of carbohydrates would be comparable to total body carbohydrate stores. Add to this the fact that the brain is highly active, accounting for about 20% of ongoing whole body energy metabolism at rest, despite its small size

(2% of body weight) (Clark and Sokoloff 1999). In addition, brain glucose levels are significantly lower than in peripheral blood under all conditions, as shown by results of microdialysis studies (Silver and Erecinska 1994). During euglycemic conditions (about 5 mM glucose peripherally), brain glucose concentrations range between 1 and 2.5 mM and may vary depending on local activity levels. During severe hypoglycemia (2–3 mM glucose peripherally), brain concentrations as low as 0.5 have been measured, and during hyperglycemia (up to 20 mM glucose peripherally), brain concentrations may rise to only about 5 mM. CRRs are elicited when blood glucose levels fall to 3.6–3.8 mM (Cryer 1997). From these considerations, it is clear not only that glucose availability must be effectively monitored by the brain, but also that glucose must be monitored separately from other nutrient sources (fat and protein) that cannot be utilized by the brain. Caloric monitoring of overall nutrient availability, although important for other reasons, is not appropriate or sufficient to protect brain function in the face of glucose deficit.

9.2 GLUCOSE-SENSING MECHANISMS

Although it is clear that the brain monitors glucose availability in order to ensure overall neurological function and survival, it also is likely that glucose monitoring mechanisms exist to provide for local regional and cellular energy requirements that vary across the brain depending on local activity levels. In addition, there may be glucose monitoring mechanisms that contribute to maintenance of overall energy homeostasis through control of daily food intake and energy expenditure. A significant body of research also suggests that the sensitivity of some central glucose-sensing mechanisms is gender related and modifiable by ambient hormonal conditions (Briski, Ibrahim, and Tamrakar 2014, Cersosimo et al. 2000, Cherian and Briski 2012, Tamrakar et al. 2015). Indeed, glucose sensitivity has been detected in numerous central and peripheral neurons, as well as in nonneuronal cell populations. Nonneural brain cells that appear to have glucose-sensing capability include ependymocytes (Maekawa et al. 2000, Moriyama et al. 2004) and astrocytes (Marty et al. 2005). For a review of astrocyte participation in glucose monitoring, see Rogers et al. in this volume (Chapter 10). Peripheral nonneural glucose-sensing cell types include, for example, pancreatic alpha and beta cells, glucagon-like 1-secreting enteroendocrine cells in the intestinal mucosa, and taste cells in the oral cavity. In addition to these, a glucose-sensing capability with impact on central control of CRRs has been convincingly demonstrated in the portal mesenteric vein (PMV) (Bohland et al. 2014, Donovan and Watts 2014, Jokiaho, Donovan, and Watts 2014, Saberi, Bohland, and Donovan 2008), although the cellular phenotype(s) of the PMV glucose sensors has not been identified.

Neurons with glucose-sensing capability have been categorized as being either glucose excited (gE) or glucose inhibited (gI) (Song et al. 2001). gE neurons are activated by high glucose and gI neurons are inhibited by high glucose. Both gE and gI neurons have been identified in brain sites of recognized importance for control of metabolism and food intake, including the ventromedial and lateral hypothalamus (Aou et al. 1984) and the caudal hindbrain (Adachi et al. 1984, Mizuno and Oomura 1984), as well as in structures less directly associated with feeding and metabolism, such as the amygdala (Nakano et al. 1986) and subfornical organ (Medeiros, Dai, and Ferguson 2012).

Mechanisms contributing to the glucose-sensing capabilities of gE and gI neurons include sensors directly linked to and dependent upon intracellular glucose metabolism. Many, but not all, gE neurons utilize adenosine triphosphate (ATP)-gated potassium channels (KATP channels). KATP channels are directly controlled by glucose metabolism. ATP generated by glucose metabolism closes these inhibitory K+ channels, leading to depolarization and thus linking fuel availability directly to membrane polarity. These channels were first described as the mechanism responsible for glucose sensing in the pancreatic beta cell. Subsequently, they have been investigated extensively in the ventromedial hypothalamus (Ashford, Boden, and Treherne 1990a, 1990b, Dunn-Meynell, Rawson, and Levin 1998, Kang et al. 2004, Levin et al. 2004), where inactivation of this channel reduces glucose-induced alteration of neuronal firing (Miki et al. 2001), as well as in the nucleus of the solitary tract (NTS) (Dallaporta, Perrin, and Orsini 2000). Although highly suited for glucose sensing, ATP-gated channels are also found ubiquitously in non-glucose-sensing cells in brain and periphery (Dunn-Meynell, Rawson, and Levin 1998).

The best characterized of the gI cell type are the neuropeptide Y (NPY)/agouti-related peptide (AGRP) neurons in the ventromedial hypothalamus and orexin neurons in the lateral hypothalamus (Burdakov and Gonzalez 2009, Oomura et al. 1969), but they have also been studied in the dorsal hindbrain (Adachi, Kobashi, and Funahashi 1995, Balfour, Hansen, and Trapp 2006). The mechanisms utilized for glucose sensing by gI neurons are still unclear, but glucose-stimulated K+ and Cl− channels have been implicated (Song et al. 2001).

5′ adenosine monophosphate-activated protein kinase (AMPK) is also considered to be a sensor of cellular energy status and is present in some gE neurons, for example, gonadotropin releasing hormone neurons (Roland and Moenter 2011). AMPK is activated (phosphorylated) by a decrease in the cellular ATP/AMP ratio (Kahn et al. 2005). Phosphorylation promotes cellular metabolism, resulting in generation of ATP. AMPK is not exclusively located in glucose-sensing neurons but is important in maintaining cellular energy levels in a variety of cell types.

In contrast to KATP channels and AMPK, glucokinase (GK), a hexokinase IV isoform, is thought to be present only in cells that are glucose sensing. Hexokinases mediate phosphorylation of glucose to glucose-6-phosphate (G6P), the first step in glycolysis (and glycogen synthesis). GK differs importantly from the hexokinase isoforms that initiate glycolysis in most cells in that it selectively phosphorylates only glucose, has a low affinity for glucose, and is not inhibited by its product, G6P (Dunn-Meynell et al. 2002, Iynedjian 2009). Peripherally, GK plays a major role in stimulating beta cell insulin secretion in response to elevation of blood glucose levels. Although GK is distributed sparsely in the brain, it has been detected in areas important for control of food intake (Dunn-Meynell et al. 2002, Kang et al. 2006, Lynch et al. 2000), including in hypothalamic gE and gI neurons and NTS (Balfour, Hansen, and Trapp 2006).

Glucose transporters (GLUTs) 1–4 are critical for glucose homeostasis, and some isoforms may contribute to glucose sensing (Mueckler and Thorens 2013, Thorens 1996, Thorens and Mueckler 2010). GLUT1 transports glucose into the brain across the capillary endothelium that forms the blood–brain barrier. It is also expressed in astrocytes and red blood cells. GLUT1 is upregulated by hypoglycemia but not altered by hyperglycemia. GLUT2 is strongly associated with glucose-sensing cells in the brain and periphery but is not found exclusively in such cells. Peripherally, GLUT2 is expressed in pancreatic beta cells, hepatic and intestinal endothelial cells, and the kidney. Centrally, GLUT2 is expressed in some neurons (including neurons in feeding-related areas of the hypothalamus and hindbrain), in astrocytes, and endothelial cells, including tanycytes in the ventricular lining. GLUT2 has a uniquely high Km for glucose (approximately 17 mM), providing for fast and efficient transport of glucose into brain cells under all physiological brain glucose concentrations (1–2.5 mM), except during extreme hypoglycemic conditions. Because of the strong association of GLUT2 with glucose sensitive cells in the brain and periphery, astrocytic cells expressing GLUT2 have been proposed to be glucoreceptors involved in elicitation of CRRs. The proposed roles of GLUT2 and astrocytes in central glucose monitoring have been discussed extensively in this volume (R.C. Rogers et al.) and will not be discussed further here. GLUT3 is the predominant GLUT in most, possibly all, neurons. GLUT4 is insulin regulated and primarily expressed by peripheral tissues, where insulin is required for glucose uptake. All of these transporters contribute in some way, directly or indirectly, to the availability and distribution of glucose within the brain, but their specific involvement in CRRs remains to be convincingly demonstrated and depends largely on whether the cells that express them actually communicate with neurons involved in executing glucoregulatory responses. The functions of GLUT5–14 largely remain to be determined.

The sodium-linked GLUT 1 and 2 (SGLT1 and 2) also are of interest as glucose sensors (Mueckler and Thorens 2013, Thorens 1996, Thorens and Mueckler 2010, Yu et al. 2010, 2013). These membrane proteins are capable of transporting glucose into cells against the glucose concentration gradient by coupling glucose transport to inward depolarizing sodium current that, in neurons, contributes to glucose-induced depolarization. They are found in both neural and nonneural cell types. Peripherally, SGLT1 and 2 are present in the proximal tubule of the kidney and in enterocytes of the small intestine. SGLTs have been identified centrally in the hippocampus, amygdala, hypothalamus, cerebral cortex, and striatum but appear to have little or no expression in the hindbrain (Yu et al. 2010, 2013). They are present in both gE and gI neurons (Burdakov and Gonzalez 2009, Gonzalez, Reimann, and Burdakov 2009, O'Malley et al. 2006). SGLT1 and 2 have been described as "nonmetabolic glucose sensors" in part because neurons that express SGLTs, glucose-induced excitation or inhibition (respectively), are mimicked, rather than blocked, by antimetabolic glucose analogues, alpha-methylglucopyranoside (alpha-MDG), and 2-deoxy-D-glucose (2DG) (Gonzalez, Reimann, and Burdakov 2009). These effects are dependent on SGLT (they are abolished by elimination of sodium and by SGLT inhibitors) and are independent of GK (they are not altered by glucosamine). It has been proposed that the nonmetabolic glucose sensing mediated by these receptors enables cells to monitor glucose availability in the extracellular space independently of cellular metabolism, possibly allowing such cells to serve a predictive function, sensing extracellular glucose decline prior to intracellular metabolic deficit. Hypothalamic orexin neurons are examples of gI neurons that respond to ambient glucose via SGLTs (Burdakov and Gonzalez 2009, Burdakov and Lesage 2010, Gonzalez, Reimann, and Burdakov 2009). SGLT3 is also suggested to be a glucose-sensing element but does not have a transport function (Diez-Sampedro et al. 2003). The possible contribution of SGLT3 to neuronal glucose monitoring requires further study.

9.3 PERIPHERAL RESPONSES TO GLUCOSE DEFICIT

Control of blood glucose concentration begins with the opposing actions of pancreatic hormones, glucagon, and insulin, secretion of which are directly responsive to blood glucose levels. Insulin is required for glucose uptake and utilization by most peripheral tissues. However, when glucose levels fall, pancreatic beta cells are inhibited and insulin secretion is reduced, thereby limiting glucose uptake by peripheral tissues and conserving circulating glucose to the benefit of the brain. Low glucose and insulin levels also activate glucagon secretion. Glucagon acts on the liver to stimulate glycogenolysis, gluconeogenesis, and entry of glucose into the blood. Glucagon secretion is also under strong autonomic (Havel et al. 1994) and central control by both hypothalamic and hindbrain sites (Andrew, Dinh, and Ritter 2007, Borg et al. 1995, Marty et al. 2005).

In addition to affecting blood glucose concentrations via direct effects on pancreatic alpha and beta cells, peripheral glucose deficit also alerts the central nervous system by activating receptors in the PMV (Saberi, Bohland, and Donovan 2008). These glucose sensors project to neurons in the dorsomedial hindbrain that transmit messages to more rostral brain sites (Fujita et al. 2007, Hevener, Bergman, and Donovan 2000, Matveyenko et al. 2007). These signals from the PMV appear to be transmitted to the brain via spinal afferents, as sectioning the celiac–superior mesenteric ganglion and T5 spinal transection, but not vagotomy (Fujita and Donovan 2005, Jackson et al. 1997, 2000), significantly reduces the sympathoadrenal response to hypoglycemia. Dennervation of the portal and superior mesenteric vein reduces the adrenal epinephrine (E) response to graded onset of hypoglycemic conditions by 91% (Saberi, Bohland, and Donovan 2008). Interestingly, the PMV glucose sensors are most responsive to gradual, rather than abrupt, declines in blood glucose, and portal-mesenteric denervation eliminates the response to slow-onset hypoglycemia (Saberi, Bohland, and Donovan 2008). Hence, these are not the receptors that respond to precipitous drops in blood glucose, as occurs with insulin overdose.

The PMV responsiveness to gradual-onset hypoglycemia may serve a preventative function, rather than a restorative function, since denervation of the PMV eliminates the response to gradual-onset hypoglycemia but does not eliminate the response to acute glucose deficit. A mechanism such as this may be important to the maintenance of glucose levels in the brain under normal conditions, such as during the intermeal interval or during brief periods of food deprivation, where adequate fuel reserves are available, but may require gradual mobilization. This mechanism, in addition to maintaining glucose levels, would also serve to avoid premature and excessive mobilization of metabolic fuels. As noted, the glucoreceptive mechanism in the PMV has not been systematically investigated. However, GLUT2 knockout mice do not detect glucose changes in the PMV

(Burcelin and Thorens 2001), suggesting a critical contribution of this GLUT to the sensing mechanism.

Vagal afferents also appear to be glucose sensing. Elevated glucose activates K(ATP) channels in a subpopulation of gastric afferents, resulting in activation of the afferent neuron (Grabauskas et al. 2010, 2013). Other work has shown that glucose modulates the responsiveness of gastric vagal afferents to serotonin (Troy et al. 2016).

9.4 CENTRAL RESPONSES TO GLUCOSE DEFICIT

Key responses to acute glucoprivic challenge are initiated by receptors within the brain. These include increased appetite, the sole mechanism for restoration of deficient glucose supplies (Miselis and Epstein 1975, Smith and Epstein 1969), and increased gastric motility, which facilitates absorption of ingested nutrients within the digestive tract (Cryer 1999, Hermann, Viard, and Rogers 2014). Glucoprivation also triggers secretion of corticosteroid releasing hormone (CRH), with a consequent increase in downstream corticotropin secretion that, among other actions, facilitates peripheral fatty acid metabolism, thereby conserving available glucose for brain utilization. Glucoprivation also stimulates adrenal medullary epinephrine (E) secretion (Cannon, McIver, and Bliss 1924), which complements the adrenal cortical response by stimulating lipolysis and mobilizing glycogen release from storage sites. Glucose deficit also suppresses estrous cycles (I'Anson, Starer, and Bonnema 2003, I'Anson et al. 2003, Nagatani et al. 1996), a response that conserves fuel over the long-term by preventing pregnancy.

9.5 IMPORTANCE OF HINDBRAIN CATECHOLAMINE NEURONS IN SYSTEMIC GLUCOREGULATION

Because glucose monitoring likely contributes to a variety of physiological processes, and because biochemical mechanisms involved in glucose monitoring may differ depending on the specific functions served, determining the mechanisms and cellular populations in brain and periphery that detect, avert, and repair hypoglycemic conditions is a complex task. Nevertheless, current evidence has begun to define a system of catecholamine (CA) neurons in the hindbrain that responds immediately to acute and urgent glucose deficit by enlisting widespread behavioral, endocrine, and autonomic systems to restore brain glucose levels (Ritter et al. 2011). The remainder of this review will focus primarily on hindbrain CA neurons and their connections and functional interactions with forebrain and spinal sites involved in mediation of glucose restorative and glucose protective responses. Evidence implicating glucodetection mechanisms potentially capable of activating CA neurons during glucose deficit also will be discussed briefly.

9.5.1 BRIEF OVERVIEW OF HINDBRAIN CA NEUROANATOMY

Given the array of CRRs evoked by glucose deficit, it is apparent that glucoregulation involves circuitry and mechanisms that extend throughout the longitudinal axis of the central nervous system and into the periphery. Nevertheless, it is incontrovertible that all of the CRRs can be elicited by inducing glucoprivic conditions selectively at specific hindbrain sites (Andrew, Dinh, and Ritter 2007, Ritter, Dinh, and Zhang 2000). In addition, glucoprivically evoked feeding, corticosteroid secretion, adrenal medullary secretion, and suppression of reproductive responses all require intact hindbrain CA neurons (Ritter, Bugarith, and Dinh 2001, Ritter, Dinh, and Li 2006, Ritter et al. 2003). The diverse projections and high degree of collateralization of hindbrain CA neurons are ideally suited to triggering rapid and coordinated mobilization of physiologically diverse glucoregulatory responses. That said, it appears that not all CA neurons are involved in glucoregulatory function, but rather that subgroups of these neurons are functionally heterogeneous (Guyenet et al. 2013), with select subpopulations of CA neurons being specialized to mediate CRR, while other subpopulations are involved in non-CRR functions. An ongoing challenge, therefore, is to determine which specific CA neurons mediate glucoregulatory functions, thus enabling a productive analysis of the circuitry and glucose-sensing mechanisms that enable them to perform their critical glucoprotective functions.

As a prologue to further discussion of hindbrain CA neurons implicated in glucoregulatory function, a simplified diagram showing the distribution of E and norepinephrine (NE) subgroups, designated as C and A groups, respectively, is presented in Figure 9.1. For more detailed neuroanatomy of these cell groups, refer to Paxinos and Watson (1997). Both C and A groups synthesize NE and can be identified by the presence of the biosynthetic enzymes, tyrosine hydroxylase (TH) and dopamine-β-hydroxylase (DBH). E neurons can be distinguished from NE neurons by their unique expression of phenethanolamine-N-methyltransferase (PNMT), which converts NE to E. Together, these E and NE neurons are referred to as "'hindbrain CA'" neurons to distinguish them from the dopaminergic neurons in the midbrain and hypothalamus.

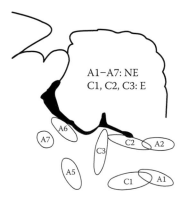

FIGURE 9.1 Diagramatic view showing anatomical relationship between hindbrain catecholamine cell groups. "A" groups are noradrenergic. "C" groups are adrenergic. The dorsal groups are situated in the dorsomedial medulla. Group A2 is roughly coextensive with the area postrema. The ventral groups are located in the ventrolateral medulla and are distributed over a similar rostrocaudal extent. Noradrenergic cell groups A5–A7, located more rostrally in the hindbrain, are not shown here.

9.5.2   EVIDENCE FOR HINDBRAIN PARTICIPATION
IN GLUCOSE COUNTERREGULATION

The hindbrain was identified by very early studies as a site where stimulation produced mobilization of peripheral glucose stores. Subsequently, in the 1980s, experiments by Harvey Grill and his students definitively showed that two crucial glucoprivic responses—increased consummatory feeding and hyperglycemia—could be elicited by systemic glucoprivation in chronic decerebrate rats in which the brain was completely transected at the supracollicular level (DiRocco and Grill 1979, Flynn and Grill 1983). These results indicated that receptors and reflex circuitry capable of mediating these responses are present in the hindbrain. Robert Ritter (Ritter, Slusser, and Stone 1981) demonstrated that the anti-glycolytic agent, 5-thio-D-glucose (5TG), stimulated food intake and blood glucose responses when injected into either the lateral or fourth cerebroventricle (LV or 4V). However, if the cerebral aqueduct, connecting the forebrain ventricles with the fourth ventricle, was acutely occluded, feeding in response to LV 5TG was abolished and the adrenomedullary hyperglycemic response was severely impaired. In contrast, 4V 5TG continued to be effective in stimulating robust feeding and blood glucose responses in the aqueduct occluded rat.

The presence of hindbrain glucoreceptors controlling these and other glucoregulatory responses was confirmed by experiments revealing that nanoinjections of 5TG directly into specific hindbrain tissue sites evoked increased feeding, hyperglycemia, glucagon, and corticosterone secretion (Andrew, Dinh, and Ritter 2007, Ritter, Dinh, and Zhang 2000). Figure 9.2 shows hindbrain sites where unilateral nanoinjections of 5TG elicited food intake (Ritter, Dinh, and Zhang 2000). In contrast, none of these glucoregulatory responses were triggered when 5TG was injected into hypothalamic sites, even when higher doses were injected. Positive responses to hindbrain 5TG were just as robust as those evoked by systemic 2DG or insulin-induced hypoglycemia. A provocative outcome of the cannula mapping experiments discussed previously was that many of the sites positive for elicitation of glucoregulatory responses overlap CA subgroups that are preferentially activated by glucoprivation, as indicated by increased Fos-immunoreactivity (Ritter, Llewellyn-Smith, and Dinh 1998). These include the majority of neurons in A1 and C1, excepting the most rostral, retrofacial segment of C1 (or C1r). In comparison, a smaller proportion of the total CA population in A2 and C2 were activated by 2DG.

9.5.3   HINDBRAIN CA NEURONS ARE REQUIRED FOR ELICITING KEY
PROTECTIVE RESPONSES TO BRAIN GLUCOSE DEFICIT

The availability of a highly selective retrogradely transported immunotoxin, anti-DBH-saporin (DSAP), made it possible to rigorously test the hypothesis that hindbrain E/NE neurons mediate and are required for responses to glucoprivation. Unlike 6-hydroxydopamine or electrolytic lesion of CA projections used previously, DSAP produced deficits that are highly selective for NE and E neurons anatomically, neurochemically, and behaviorally. It does not lesion dopamine neurons (Picklo et al. 1994, 1995, Wiley and Kline 2000, Wrenn et al. 1996). DSAP consists of a monoclonal antibody against the uniquely expressed NE/E biosynthetic enzyme, DBH,

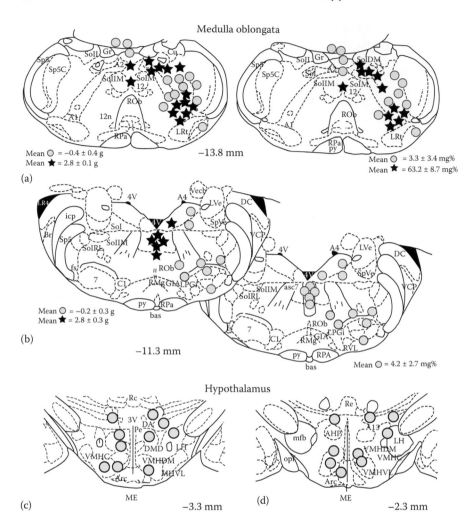

FIGURE 9.2 Cannula sites tested for feeding and blood glucose responses induced by unilateral injection of 5TG (24 μg in 200 nl). Positive sites (stars) and negative sites (circles) are shown. In (a) (caudal medulla) and (b) (rostral medulla), left and right maps show the two responses for each rat: feeding on the left and blood glucose on the right at the same rostrocaudal levels. In (c) and (d), maps are shown for two rostrocaudal hypothalamic levels: all hypothalamic cannula sites were negative for both feeding and blood glucose. Levels caudal to bregma (mm) are shown. Blood glucose was measured in the absence of food. Sites positive and negative for these 5TG-induced responses were very similar in distribution to sites positive for 5TG-induced corticosterone and glucagon secretion mapped in a separate study (Andrew et al. 2007). (From Ritter, S., Dinh, T.T., Zhang, Y., *Brain. Res.*, 856, 37–47, 2000.)

conjugated to the ribosomal toxin, saporin (SAP). As a ribosomal toxin, toxicity requires SAP internalization by cells. Due to the DBH antibody in the conjugate, DSAP selectively binds with and is internalized by DBH-containing synaptic vesicles and is retrogradely transported to the CA neuron cell body, where SAP disrupts protein synthesis, causing cell death. Although uptake of DSAP in CA terminal areas, with subsequent toxin transport to the cell bodies, is extraordinarily useful, DSAP internalization is not restricted to terminals of CA neurons but also occurs when injected into the vicinity of the CA cell bodies (Madden et al. 1999, Rinaman 2003, Schreihofer and Guyenet 2000).

Injection of DSAP into spinal and hypothalamic terminal sites produced different patterns of selective CA neuron degeneration and impaired distinct CRRs. Intraspinal DSAP injection retrogradely lesioned E/NE neurons known to innervate preganglionic sympathetic neurons and eliminated the adrenal medullary response to glucoprivation. Glucoprivic feeding was not impaired and rostrally projecting E/NE neurons in the hindbrain were not damaged. In contrast, injecting DSAP into the paraventricular nucleus of the hypothalamus (PVH) destroyed E/NE neurons with known projections to the hypothalamus and eliminated feeding (Ritter, Bugarith, and Dinh 2001), corticosterone secretion (Ritter et al. 2003), suppression of estrous cycles (I'Anson et al. 2003), and modulation of growth hormone secretion (Emanuel and Ritter 2010) in response to glucoprivation. In contrast to spinal DSAP, PVH DSAP injections did not impair the adrenal medullary hyperglycemic response.

Importantly, DSAP lesions did not appear to alter the ability of the feeding, neuroendocrine, and adrenal medullary systems to function normally under standard nonglucodeprived laboratory conditions, as shown in Figure 9.3. In animals with DSAP lesions, glucoprivic feeding was impaired without obvious impairment of feeding responses to nonglucoprivic stimuli such as the feeding responses to overnight food deprivation, mercaptoacetate (a fatty acid antagonist that stimulates feeding), the diurnal pattern of food intake, or the ability of rats to maintain their body weight (Ritter, Bugarith, and Dinh 2001). Although glucoprivation-induced corticosterone secretion was significantly impaired by PVH DSAP, DSAP did not damage CRH neurons themselves, nor did DSAP treatment disrupt the circadian pattern of corticosterone secretion or the corticosterone response to swim stress, both of which remained intact (Ritter et al. 2003). Rats in which DSAP was injected into the PVH did not exhibit suppression of estrous in response to glucoprivation, but the normal estrous cycles of the DSAP-treated rats were not impaired in the absence of glucoprivation (I'Anson et al. 2003). Neither PVH nor intraspinal DSAP impaired the ability of rats to maintain normal glucose levels during ad libitum access to food (Ritter, Bugarith, and Dinh 2001). This suggests that the glucoregulatory circuits mediating these responses to glucoprivation are distinct from circuits mediating the same responses to nonglucoprivic stimuli.

9.5.4   WHICH CA NEURONS MEDIATE GLUCOREGULATORY RESPONSES?

Despite their considerable functional heterogeneity (Guyenet et al. 2013) and complex neuroanatomical organization, progress has been made in determining the functional specificity of different CA subgroups. For example, groups C1 and C3

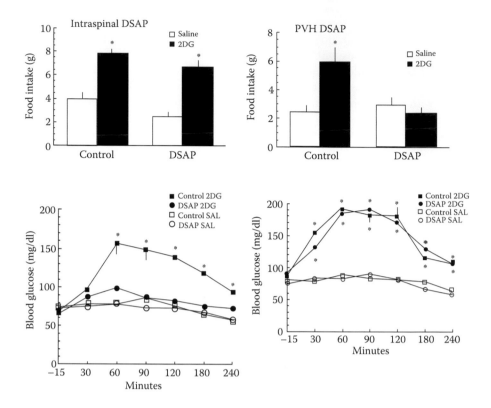

FIGURE 9.3 Food intake and blood glucose responses to systemic injection of saline (Control) or 2DG in rats previously injected with DSAP or SAP into the spinal cord (left panels) or into the PVN (right panels). Intraspinal injection of DSAP impaired the blood glucose response, but not the feeding response, to 2DG. PVH DSAP injections impaired the feeding response, but not the glucose response, to 2DG. (From Ritter, S., Bugarith, K., Dinh, T.T., *J. Comp. Neurol.*, 432, 197–216, 2001.)

each contain at least two distinct populations of neurons—those that innervate the spinal cord and those that innervate the hypothalamus. Spinally projecting neurons in C1 are sympathetic and adrenal medullary premotor neurons, some of which are involved in control of blood pressure (C1r), and others, in adrenal medullary secretion (Morrison and Cao 2000, Morrison, Milner, and Reis 1988).

Several lines of evidence indicate that the glucoprivic feeding response is heavily dependent on a subgroup of CA neurons located primarily within C1m and A1/C1 and coexpressing NPY and DBH (Li and Ritter 2004, Li, Wang, and Ritter 2006). Expression of mRNA for both DBH and NPY is increased in A1/Ca following glucoprivation (Li and Ritter 2004, Li, Wang, and Ritter 2006). Moreover, localized silencing of *Npy* and *Dbh* simultaneously, but not separately, significantly and reversibly reduces glucoprivic feeding (by 61%), as shown in Figure 9.4, without altering feeding elicited by the fatty acid antagonist, β-mercaptoacetate, or by overnight food deprivation (Li et al. 2009). These results suggest that CAs and NPY as cotransmitters act conjointly to control glucoprivic feeding in response to glucoprivation.

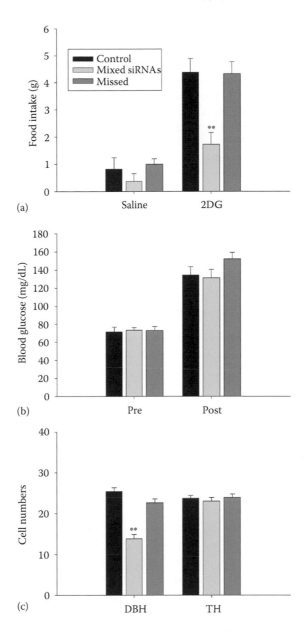

FIGURE 9.4 Effects of combined Npy and Dbh siRNAs ("mixed") injected into A1/C1 or dorsally to miss this area ("missed") on food intake (a) and blood glucose (b) responses to 2DG and control treatments. (c) Cell counts for DBH- and TH-ir cells show that expression of DBH, but not upstream TH, was reduced by siRNA. (From Li, A.J., Wang, Q., Dinh, T.T., Ritter, S., *J. Neurosci.*, 9, 280–287, 2009.)

The importance of A1/C1 neurons for stimulation of feeding has been confirmed using designer receptors exclusively activated by designer drug (DREADD) technology to selectively activate these neurons. hM3D(Gq), a "designer" receptor for the "designer drug" clozapine-*N*-oxide (CNO), was selectively expressed in A1/C1 CA neurons by injection of AAV-DIO-hM3D(Gq)-mCherry into the A1/C1 area of Th-Cre+ rats (Li et al. 2015b). Using this procedure, over 85% of mCherry-labeled neurons were double labeled for DBH, 92% of mCherry-labeled neurons were also TH-positive, and 90% of TH/mCherry cells expressed c-Fos after CNO treatment, which selectively activates only neurons transfected to express hM3D(Gq). Selective activation of A1/C1 neurons by a peripheral injection of CNO increased food intake. Rats consumed approximately 4 g of chow in the 4-hour test after CNO, compared to just 0.8 g after control injections. The magnitude of this response to CNO activation was equivalent to responses induced by systemic 2DG. These same rats, tested in the absence of food, did not exhibit increased blood glucose responses to CNO injections, supporting the hypothesis that the latter control is mediated by neurons distinct from those controlling food intake.

9.5.5 POTENTIAL INVOLVEMENT OF THE DORSOMEDIAL MEDULLA IN CRRs

In the NTS, expression of c-Fos in response to glucoprivation is present in A2, C2, and C3 (Ritter, Llewellyn-Smith, and Dinh 1998). However, very few A2 neurons in the medial and commissural subnuclei of the NTS express c-Fos in response to glucoprivation. Non-CA neurons throughout the NTS are also activated. Although it is tempting to conclude, based on work done to date, that the CA neurons in the dorsal vagal complex are less critical for CRR elicitation than those located in the ventrolateral medulla (VLM), it has been reported that electrolytic and aspiration lesions of the area postrema and underlying NTS (Bird, Cardone, and Contreras 1983, Contreras, Fox, and Drugovich 1982, Ritter and Taylor 1990) severely impair or abolish glucoprivic feeding, although not all studies have obtained this result (Hyde and Miselis 1983). Moreover, PVH DSAP lesions that eliminate glucoprivic feeding and corticosterone secretion not only eliminate most CA neurons in A1, A1/C1, and C1m but also destroy a significant percentage of the CA neurons in the dorsal vagal complex (Ritter, Bugarith, and Dinh 2001, Ritter et al. 2003), indicating that the contribution of the dorsal medulla to glucoregulation cannot be ruled out.

A plausible hypothesis is that the role of the dorsomedial medulla in glucose CRR may differ from that of the ventromedial medulla, as suggested by its anatomical connections. It is known that A2 neurons are heavily influenced by input from the vagus nerve. Electrophysiological experiments in hindbrain slices have shown that approximately half of the A2 neurons are activated by the gastrointestinal satiety peptide, cholecystokinin, via activation of presynaptic vagal afferent fibers (Appleyard et al. 2007). Data such as these suggest that A2 neurons are involved in integration of inputs that influence normal appetite and daily food intake (Contreras, Kosten, and Bird 1984), but perhaps not in glucoprivic feeding. Alternatively, the CA neurons involved may be inhibited during glucoprivation, and if so, their role may be to suppress competing effects of satiety or malaise on stimulation of feeding in response to glucoprivation.

9.6 INTERACTION OF CA NEURONS
WITH FOREBRAIN NEURONS

9.6.1 NPY/AGRP NEURONS AS DOWNSTREAM
COMEDIATORS OF GLUCOSE CRR CIRCUITRY

In contrast to the finding that localized A1/C1 silencing of both *Npy* and *Dbh* was required for impairment of glucoprivic feeding, Sindelar et al. (2004) have reported that global NPY knockout mice, with apparently intact CA neurons, have deficient feeding responses to glucoprivation but have normal neuroendocrine responses. This result further confirms the importance of NPY neurons for glucoprivic feeding and suggests that NPY neurons in the hypothalamic arcuate nucleus, which are downstream of those in A1/C1, in addition to those in A1/C1 itself, are critical for the feeding response. Alternatively, the effectiveness of the global knockout may be due to the more complete loss of *Npy* in the hindbrain CA neurons than could be achieved using localized gene silencing, overriding the necessity for a contribution from CA neurons.

In this regard, another SAP conjugate, NPY-SAP, has been useful in evaluating the importance of arcuate NPY/AGRP neurons in glucoprivic feeding (Bugarith et al. 2005). This conjugate binds to NPY receptors and presumably enters the cell by agonist-driven receptor internalization. Unlike DSAP, but like most other peptide-SAP conjugates, NPY-SAP is not retrogradely transported and therefore lesions only NPY receptive neurons at the injection site. When injected into the basomedial hypothalamus, NPY-SAP, but not blank-SAP (B-SAP) control, destroyed NPY-receptor-expressing neurons in the ARC, including NPY/AGRP and proopiomelanocortin (POMC)/ cocaine- and amphetamine-regulated transcript (CART) neurons. There was a virtually complete loss of NPY, AGRP, and CART mRNA expression in the NPY-SAP rats. In addition, NPY-Y1 receptor immunoreactivity in the ARC was profoundly reduced in the NPY-SAP-injected rats. Dopamine β-hydroxylase and NPY terminals (presumably from the hindbrain) remained abundant in the NPY-SAP injected area, despite the loss of hypothalamic NPY cell bodies. Hindbrain NPY/CA neurons with terminals at the injection site were not destroyed by NPY-SAP, confirming that this conjugate is not retrogradely transported to cell bodies of these neurons. Hypothalamic injection of NPY-SAP eliminated both weight loss and suppression of food intake induced by central leptin injection, as well as eliminated the stimulation of feeding by central ghrelin injection (Bugarith et al. 2005). Leptin and ghrelin are thought to produce their primary effects on feeding by actions on POMC/CART and NPY/AGRP neurons within the arcuate nucleus (Cone et al. 2001, Cowley et al. 2001, Elias et al. 1999, Elias et al. 1998a, 1998b, Elmquist 1998). Both deficits are therefore consistent with loss of arcuate NPY/AGRP and POMC/CART neurons. However, NPY-SAP did not impair the glucoprivic feeding and hyperglycemic or corticosterone responses. In short, DSAP injections that destroy hindbrain CA/NPY neurons impair glucoprivic feeding, despite the fact that arcuate NPY neurons remain intact. Arcuate NPY-SAP injections that destroy NPY/AGRP neurons, leaving the hindbrain CA/NPY neurons intact, do not impair glucoprivic feeding. A reasonable conclusion from these findings is that hindbrain, not arcuate, NPY neurons are required for glucoprivic feeding but that both populations are important contributors. This conclusion is consistent with the fact that supracollicular decerebration does not abolish glucoprivation-induced increase in food intake (Flynn and Grill 1983).

Although hypothalamic NPY/AgRP neurons are not required for glucoprivic feeding, they may be recruited by hindbrain CA neurons to facilitate glucoprivic responses, as suggested by Fraley et al. (Fraley, Dinh, and Ritter 2002, Fraley and Ritter 2003), who showed that hypothalamic *Npy* and *Agrp* expressions are increased in response to systemic glucoprivation and that PVH DSAP eliminates this increase. Another interesting aspect of this work is that the basal expression levels of these same genes are increased in DSAP rats, perhaps as a compensatory response to loss of hindbrain NPY/CA input.

9.6.2 Orexin and CA Neurons as Comediators of Glucose CRRs

Recent evidence suggests that orexinergic neurons contribute importantly to glucoregulation. Orexin is known to stimulate food intake when injected into the brain. Injections of orexin-A into the hypothalamus (Sakurai 2007, Yamanaka et al. 1999), lateral and fourth ventricles (Li et al. 2015a, 2015b, Yamanaka et al. 1999, Zhao et al. 2015, Zheng, Patterson, and Berthoud 2005), and the A1/C1 region of the ventrolateral medulla are all effective in stimulating feeding. Moreover, in vitro electrophysiological studies have determined that some orexin neurons are glucosensing and respond directly to extracellular glucose concentrations; that is, for some orexin neurons, glucose itself acts as a signaling agent, distinct from its role as a metabolic substrate, since some orexin neurons are inhibited by high glucose, as well as by elevated levels of nonmetabolic glucose analogues, such as 2DG (Burdakov and Gonzalez 2009, Burdakov and Lesage 2010, Gonzalez, Reimann, and Burdakov 2009). However, in vivo systemic 2DG also activates a large number of orexin neurons, presumably in response to glucoprivation. A role for orexin neurons as participants in control of glucose homeostasis would complement their role in coordinating states of arousal and activity and is an area of current research interest.

Of special interest for the present review is the interaction of orexin and CA neurons. Sites of orexin innervation in the brain and spinal cord are similar to those of the hindbrain CA neurons (Date et al. 1999, Nambu et al. 1999, Peyron et al. 1998). In addition, the C1 cell group contains E neurons that project to orexinergic areas of the hypothalamus (Bochorishvili et al. 2014, Card et al. 2006, Guyenet et al. 2013). Hypothalamically projecting C1 neurons identified by expression of the E biosynthetic enzyme, PNMT, forms synaptic connections with orexin cell bodies and dendrites, as shown by neuron-selective viral tracing, immunohistochemistry, and electron microscopy (Bochorishvili et al. 2014). In fact, the same study showed that a majority of PNMT-ir terminals in the hypothalamic area in which orexin neurons are concentrated originate from the C1 cell group and the majority form asymmetric (excitatory) synapses on orexin neurons. Thus, CA neurons are anatomically situated to communicate directly with orexin neurons and, based on studies of c-Fos expression, appear able to activate them.

Similarly, orexin neurons innervate sites containing CA neurons. Indeed, pivotal glucoregulatory CA cell populations and orexin neurons may be reciprocally innervated. Orexin fibers and receptors are expressed in close proximity to CA neurons in both the VLM and the NTS. In addition, injection of orexin into either the LV or 4V increases Fos expression in CA neurons.

Given the broad range of physiological functions associated with both orexin and CA neurons, two pertinent questions are (1) which of the sites they innervate control food intake and (2) are the responses elicited at these sites related to glucose counter-regulation? CA terminals are particularly dense within the perifornical lateral hypo-thalamus (PeFLH), and this area is an exceptionally sensitive site for stimulation of feeding by NPY (Stanley et al. 1993, Stanley and Thomas 1993), which is coex-pressed by nearly all C1 neurons with projections to the hypothalamus (Everitt et al. 1984, Sawchenko et al. 1985). Therefore, it is likely that some of the orexin neurons innervated by CA/NPY coexpressing neurons are involved in control of food intake.

As noted, LV and 4V injections of orexin A stimulate feeding. However, Zheng, Patterson, and Berthoud (2005), using a number of feeding paradigms, reported that injection of orexin-A into the NTS itself, an area concentrating rostrally projecting CA neurons and expressing orexin terminals and orexin receptors (A and B), did not increase food intake, although ventricular injections were effective. This puzzling dissociation of NTS and 4V effects requires further investigation. Nevertheless, orexin terminals are present in the A1/C1 area, and injection of orexin into that site stimulates feeding. Furthermore, injection of DSAP into the hypothalamus to lesion A1/C1 neurons eliminated the feeding response to both LV and 4V orexin administration (Figure 9.5), reduced 2DG-induced Fos expression in orexin neu-rons, and eliminated feeding induced by systemic 2DG, indicating that CA neurons are required for orexin-induced feeding. Perifornical lateral hypothalamic DSAP injections produced results that were similar to those reported previously after PVH DSAP injections, and not surprisingly, results of retrograde tracing experiments indicate that many CA neurons appear to project collaterally to innervate both PVH and PeFLH. An important role for CA neuron projections to orexin neurons has been

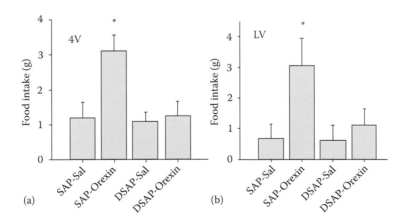

FIGURE 9.5   Food intake in response to 4V orexin and saline control in PVH DSAP- and SAP-injected rats in a 4-h test following 4V (a) or LV (b) injection of orexin-A (0.5 nmol in 3 μl) or saline control. (From Li, A.J., Wang, W., Davis, H., Wang, R., Ritter, S., *Am. J. Physiol. Regul. Integr. Comp. Physiol.* 309, R358–R567, 2015.)

supported by results of DREADD experiments in which hM3D(Gq) was selectively expressed in A1/C1 neurons of *Th*-Cre+ rats (Li et al. 2015b). The results showed that systemic CNO injections increased food intake and c-Fos expression in PVH neurons and in orexin neurons in the PeFLH, indicating that input from A1/C1 neurons mediates this activation. Neither LV, 4V, or A1/C1 injections of orexin in control rats nor A1/C1 injection of CNO altered blood glucose concentrations.

Taken together, these results suggest that CA-induced activation of orexin neurons may contribute to glucoprivic feeding. Due to their known roles in controlling arousal (Ohno and Sakurai 2008, Sakurai 2007), it is reasonable to speculate that they might contribute to glucoprivic feeding by increasing behavioral activation necessary for appetitive responses to glucose deficit. It also is conceivable that orexin neurons, which are reported as having unique glucoreceptive properties (Burdakov and Gonzalez 2009, Gonzalez, Reimann, and Burdakov 2009), provide input to engage CA neurons in glucoregulatory activity in the absence of glucoprivic crisis, for example, *in anticipation of* increased physical activity. In any case, there currently is not sufficient evidence to conclude whether or not orexin neurons are required for appetitive responses to glucose deficit.

9.6.3 FEEDING ELICITED BY VARIOUS GLUCOSE-SENSING MECHANISMS REQUIRES CA NEURONS

A number of cellular glucose-sensing mechanisms capable of stimulating food intake have been identified in brain tissue. 2DG and 5TG are glucose analogues that inhibit glucose utilization in all cells. In addition to insulin-induced hypoglycemia, these are the most extensively used experimental tools for elicitation of CRRs, and their effects have been discussed extensively in this review. 2DG is an antimetabolic glucose analogue that inhibits glycolysis via its phosphorylated product, 2DG-6-phosphate, which competitively inhibits phosphohexose isomerase (Brown 1962, Parniak and Kalant 1985). 5TG most potently inhibits phosphoglucomutase and G6P dehydrogenase, but it also inhibits hexokinases, including GK (Chen and Whistler 1975). Although the mechanisms responsible for blockade of glucose utilization by 2DG and 5TG have been delineated by biochemical studies, the specific mechanisms through which these agents trigger CRRs are not fully understood.

Many studies examining glucose-sensing mechanisms in the brain have now shown that AMPK, which is phosphorylated (activated) in response to increased ADP/ATP ratio, is a cellular fuel sensor that also contributes to control of food intake, suggesting that it may also contribute to control of CRRs. For example, in brain sites involved in control of food intake, AMPK phosphorylation is increased by food deprivation and decreased by feeding (Hayes et al. 2009). Intraparenchymal NTS injections of Compound C, an AMPK inhibitor, reduce food intake and body weight (Hayes et al. 2009). Results have also been reported showing that intracerebroventricular administration of the AMPK inhibitor, Compound C, reduced feeding, glucagon, and corticosterone responses to systemic hypoglycemia and, in addition, that hypoglycemia induced AMPK activity in medial hypothalamic nuclei (Han et al. 2005).

AMPK phosphorylation is also increased by systemic glucoprivation in tissue sampled from the A1/C1 area, but not in an adjacent non-CA site in the ventromedial medulla and not significantly in A2 (Li, Wang, and Ritter 2011). Furthermore, phosphorylation of AMPK is not increased by glucoprivation in the A1/C1 area in rats in which the CA neurons had been eliminated by PVH injection of DSAP, suggesting localization of the AMPK to the CA neurons. Fourth ventricular injection of the AMPK activator, AICAR, increased food intake during the first 60 min of a 4-h test. Fourth ventricle injection of Compound C, which boosts cellular metabolism, attenuated 2DG-induced feeding during the first 2 hours of a 4-hour test (Li, Wang, and Ritter 2011). Therefore, AMPK may participate in glucose sensing that activates CA neurons and elicits CRRs. However, it is interesting that neither stimulation nor inhibition of AMPK altered blood glucose concentrations in these experiments, again suggesting that the blood glucose response and the feeding response are mediated by distinctly different biochemical mechanisms.

In additional experiments, antagonists of two proposed glucose-sensing mechanisms were injected into the LV and 4V (Li et al. 2014). Glucosamine was used to inhibit GK (Iynedjian 2009), phloridzin was used to inhibit SGLT (Ehrenkranz et al. 2005), and 5TG was used to inhibit glucose metabolism by inhibition of glycolysis (Chen and Whistler 1975). The ability of these agents to stimulate feeding and blood glucose in DSAP-treated and unconjugated SAP control rats was examined. As shown previously by other investigators, glucosamine (Zhou et al. 2011), phloridzin (Flynn and Grill 1985, Glick and Mayer 1968, Tsujii and Bray 1990) and 5TG (Ritter, Slusser, and Stone 1981) all evoked increased feeding when injected into either LV or 4V of controls. However, these responses were absent in rats that had received PVH DSAP injections (Figure 9.6), indicating that feeding induced by glucosamine and phloridzin requires hindbrain CA neurons (Li et al. 2014).

Of the agents tested in the experiments discussed previously (AMPK, glucosamine, phloridzin, and 5TG), only 5TG elicited a blood glucose response (Li et al. 2014). GK and phloridzin were ineffective, even though they were injected into the same rats and into same sites at which 5TG was effective in robustly elevating blood

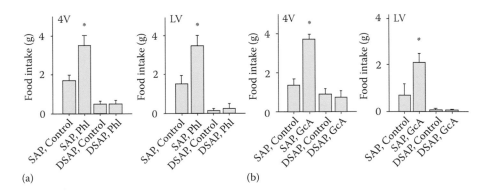

FIGURE 9.6 Food intake in response to 4V or LV injection of 0.6 mg glucosamine (a), 112.5 μg phloridzin (b), and saline control in PVH DSAP- and SAP-injected rats. Both drugs were administered in a 3 μl volume. Food intake was measured in a 4-h test. (From Li, A.J., Wang, Q., Dinh, T.T., Powers, B.R., Ritter, S., *Am. J. Physiol. Regul. Integr. Comp. Physiol.*, 306, R257–R264, 2014.)

glucose. The blood glucose response to 5TG was not impaired by PVH DSAP, even though the feeding response was abolished. As described previously, injections of DSAP at this hypothalamic site do not retrogradely lesion spinally projecting CA neurons that are critical for the adrenal medullary hyperglycemic response (Ritter, Bugarith, and Dinh 2001, Ritter et al. 2003). Together, these results suggest that AMPK, GK, and SGLT do not contribute to the activation of hindbrain CA neurons that mediate the hyperglycemic response to glucose deficit but may contribute to glucoprivic feeding. Whether they are expressed by CA neurons or are present in cells converging on them remains to be determined.

9.7 CHALLENGES FOR FUTURE RESEARCH

From this brief overview of glucose counterregulation, it is clear that significant progress is being made in this area but that major questions remain unanswered. Significant progress has been made in identifying potential mechanisms for cellular glucose-sensing, in characterizing the nature of stimuli that activate these mechanisms, and in defining the neuroanatomical localization of cell types that express them. The manner in which these sensing mechanisms interact at the cellular level also appears to be a rich area for future investigation. We can look forward to progress in determining the specific roles that these mechanisms play, locally and regionally, in maintaining glucose homeostasis.

Progress has also been made in identifying a pivotal central neural system comprised of hindbrain CA neurons and their projections that are required for elicitation of glucoregulatory responses to acute and profound glucose deficit. Progress has also been made in identifying a variety of glucose-sensing mechanisms that may contribute to the activation of this system and is beginning to identify functional interactions with forebrain NPY/AGRP and orexin neurons that refine and possibly expand their role in averting hypoglycemic conditions during predicted or ongoing changes in glucose requirements. Additional progress is anticipated in determining the mechanisms by which CA neurons are activated, specifically in determining whether these neurons are capable of responding directly to glucose, whether they depend upon converging inputs from other neurons, astrocytes, or tanycytes. A key requirement for progress in these areas is determination of which specific neurons, among the functionally diverse population of CA neurons, mediate CRRs.

Finally, progress has been made in the development of technical procedures that allow assessment of brain function under different pathological conditions in human and animal populations. Further research that will translate fundamental discoveries regarding brain glucose sensing to clinically beneficial treatments for complications of diabetes, obesity, and other conditions associated with impairment of glucose homeostasis, such as stroke, heart attack, and head injuries, is needed. However, our current appreciation of the variety of glucose-sensing mechanisms and the diversity of neural and nonneural systems involved in CRR caution that translational discoveries will be achieved only when we more fully appreciate the specific cellular mechanisms and brain circuits involved in the glucoregulatory responses extant during specific conditions.

LITERATURE CITED

Adachi, A., M. Kobashi, and M. Funahashi. 1995. Glucose-responsive neurons in the brainstem. *Obesity Res* 3 Suppl 5:735S–40S.

Adachi, A., N. Shimizu, Y. Oomura, and M. Kobashi. 1984. Convergence of hepatoportal glucose-sensitive afferent signals to glucose-sensitive units within the nucleus of the solitary tract. *Neurosci Let* 46:215–8.

Andrew, S. F., T. T. Dinh, and S. Ritter. 2007. Localized glucoprivation of hindbrain sites elicits corticosterone and glucagon secretion. *Am J Physiol Regul Interg Comp Physiol* 292:R1792–8.

Aou, S., Y. Oomura, L. Lenard, H. Nishino, A. Inokuchi, T. Minami, and H. Misaki. 1984. Behavioral significance of monkey hypothalamic glucose-sensitive neurons. *Brain Res* 302:69–74.

Appleyard, S. M., D. Marks, K. Kobayashi, H. Okano, M. J. Low, and M. C. Andresen. 2007. Visceral afferents directly activate catecholamine neurons in the solitary tract nucleus. *J Neurosci* 27:13292–302.

Ashford, M. L., P. R. Boden, and J. M. Treherne. 1990a. Glucose-induced excitation of hypothalamic neurones is mediated by ATP-sensitive K+ channels. *Pflugers Arch Eur J Physiol* 415:479–83.

Ashford, M. L., P. R. Boden, and J. M. Treherne. 1990b. Tolbutamide excites rat glucoreceptive ventromedial hypothalamic neurones by indirect inhibition of ATP-K+ channels. *Br J Pharmacol* 101:531–40.

Balfour, R. H., A. M. Hansen, and S. Trapp. 2006. Neuronal responses to transient hypoglycaemia in the dorsal vagal complex of the rat brainstem. *J Physiol* 570:469–84.

Bird, E., C. C. Cardone, and R. J. Contreras. 1983. Area postrema lesions disrupt food intake induced by cerebroventricular infusions of 5-thioglucose in the rat. *Brain Res* 270:193–6.

Bochorishvili, G., T. Nguyen, M. B. Coates, K. E. Viar, R. L. Stornetta, and P. G. Guyenet. 2014. The orexinergic neurons receive synaptic input from C1 cells in rats. *J Comp Neurol* 522:3834–46.

Bohland, M., A. V. Matveyenko, M. Saberi, A. M. Khan, A. G. Watts, and C. M. Donovan. 2014. Activation of hindbrain neurons is mediated by portal-mesenteric vein glucosensors during slow-onset hypoglycemia. *Diabetes* 63:2866–75.

Borg, W. P., R. S. Sherwin, M. J. During, M. A. Borg, and G. I. Shulman. 1995. Local ventromedial hypothalamus glucopenia triggers counterregulatory hormone release. *Diabetes* 44:180–4.

Bray, G. A. 1994. "Appetite control in adults." In *Appetite and Body Weight Regulation: Sugar, Fat, and Macronutrient Substitutes*, edited by J. D. Fernstrom and G. D. Miller, 17–31. Boca Raton, FL: CRC Press, Inc.

Briski, K. P., B. A. Ibrahim, and P. Tamrakar. 2014. Energy metabolism and hindbrain AMPK: Regulation by estradiol. *Horm Mol Biol Clin Investig* 17:129–36.

Brown, J. 1962. Effects of 2-deoxyglucose on carbohydrate metabolism: Review of the literature and studies in the rat. *Metabolism* 11:1098–112.

Bugarith, K., T. T. Dinh, A. J. Li, R. C. Speth, and S. Ritter. 2005. Basomedial hypothalamic injections of neuropeptide Y conjugated to saporin selectively disrupt hypothalamic controls of food intake. *Endocrinology* 146:1179–91.

Burcelin, R., and B. Thorens. 2001. Evidence that extrapancreatic GLUT2-dependent glucose sensors control glucagon secretion. *Diabetes* 50:1282–9.

Burdakov, D., and J. A. Gonzalez. 2009. Physiological functions of glucose-inhibited neurones. *Acta Physiol* 195:71–8.

Burdakov, D., and F. Lesage. 2010. Glucose-induced inhibition: How many ionic mechanisms? *Acta Physiol* 198:295–301.

Cannon, W. B., M. A. McIver, and S. W. Bliss. 1924. Studies on the conditions of activity in endocrine glands. *Am J Physiol* 69:46–66.

Card, J. P., J. C. Sved, B. Craig, M. Raizada, J. Vazquez, and A. F. Sved. 2006. Efferent projections of rat rostroventrolateral medulla C1 catecholamine neurons: Implications for the central control of cardiovascular regulation. *J Comp Neurol* 499:840–59.

Cersosimo, E., C. Triplitt, L. J. Mandarino, and R. A. DeFronzo. 2000. "'Pathogenesis of Type 2 Diabetes Mellitus.'" In *Endotext*, edited by L. J. De Groot, P. Beck-Peccoz, G. Chrousos, K. Dungan, A. Grossman, J. M. Hershman, C. Koch, R. McLachlan, M. New, R. Rebar, F. Singer, A. Vinik, and M. O. Weickert. South Dartmouth, MA, http://www.endotext.org.

Chen, M., and R. L. Whistler. 1975. Action of 5-thio-D-glucose and its 1-phosphate with hexokinase and phosphoglucomutase. *Arch Biochem Biophys* 169:392–6.

Cherian, A. K., and K. P. Briski. 2012. A2 noradrenergic nerve cell metabolic transducer and nutrient transporter adaptation to hypoglycemia: Impact of estrogen. *J Neurosci Res* 90:1347–58.

Clark, D., and L. Sokoloff. 1999. "Cerebral energy metabolism *in vivo*." In *Basic Neurochemistry: Molecular, Cellular, and Medical Aspects*. Sixth ed., edited by G. Siegel and B. Agranoff, 637–670. Philadelphia, PA: Lippincott Williams and Wilkins.

Cone, R. D., M. A. Cowley, A. A. Butler, W. Fan, D. L. Marks, and M. J. Low. 2001. The arcuate nucleus as a conduit for diverse signals relevant to energy homeostasis. *Int J Obes Relat Metab Disord* 25 Suppl 5:S63–7.

Contreras, R. J., E. Fox, and M. L. Drugovich. 1982. Area postrema lesions produce feeding deficits in the rat: Effects of preoperative dieting and 2-deoxy-D-glucose. *Physiol Behav* 29:875–84.

Contreras, R. J., T. Kosten, and E. Bird. 1984. Area postrema: Part of the autonomic circuitry of caloric homeostasis. *Fed Proc* 43:2966–8.

Cowley, M. A., J. L. Smart, M. Rubinstein, M. G. Cerdan, S. Diano, T. L. Horvath, R. D. Cone, and M. J. Low. 2001. Leptin activates anorexigenic POMC neurons through a neural network in the arcuate nucleus. *Nature* 411:480–4.

Cryer, P. E. 1997. Hierarchy of physiological responses to hypoglycemia: Relevance to clinical hypoglycemia in type I (insulin dependent) diabetes mellitus. *Horm Metab Res* 29:92–6.

Cryer, P. E. 1999. Symptoms of hypoglycemia, thresholds for their occurrence, and hypoglycemia unawareness. *Endocrinol Metab Clin North Am* 28:495–500, v–vi.

Cryer, P. E. 2001. Hypoglycemia-associated autonomic failure in diabetes. *Am J Physiol Endocrinol Metab* 281:E1115–21.

Dagogo-Jack, S. E., S. Craft, and P. E. Cryer. 1993. Hypoglycemia-associated autonomic failure in insulin-dependent diabetes mellitus. Recent antecedent hypoglycemia reduces autonomic responses to, symptoms of, and defense against subsequent hypoglycemia. *J Clin Invest* 91:819–28.

Dallaporta, M., J. Perrin, and J. C. Orsini. 2000. Involvement of adenosine triphosphate-sensitive K+ channels in glucose-sensing in the rat solitary tract nucleus. *Neurosci Lett* 278:77–80.

Date, Y., Y. Ueta, H. Yamashita, H. Yamaguchi, S. Matsukura, K. Kangawa, T. Sakurai, M. Yanagisawa, and M. Nakazato. 1999. Orexins, orexigenic hypothalamic peptides, interact with autonomic, neuroendocrine and neuroregulatory systems. *Proc Natl Acad Sci USA* 96:748–53.

Diez-Sampedro, A., B. A. Hirayama, C. Osswald, V. Gorboulev, K. Baumgarten, C. Volk, E. M. Wright, and H. Koepsell. 2003. A glucose sensor hiding in a family of transporters. *Proc Natl Acad Sci USA* 100:11753–8.

DiRocco, R. J., and H. J. Grill. 1979. The forebrain is not essential for sympathoadrenal hyperglycemic response to glucoprivation. *Science* 204:1112–4.

Donovan, C. M., and A. G. Watts. 2014. Peripheral and central glucose sensing in hypoglycemic detection. *Physiology* 29:314–24.

Dunn-Meynell, A. A., N. E. Rawson, and B. E. Levin. 1998. Distribution and phenotype of neurons containing the ATP-sensitive K+ channel in rat brain. *Brain Res* 814:41–54.

Dunn-Meynell, A. A., V. H. Routh, L. Kang, L. Gaspers, and B. E. Levin. 2002. Glucokinase is the likely mediator of glucosensing in both glucose-excited and glucose-inhibited central neurons. *Diabetes* 51:2056–65.

Ehrenkranz, J. R., N. G. Lewis, C. R. Kahn, and J. Roth. 2005. Phlorizin: A review. *Diab Metab Res Rev* 21:31–8.

Elias, C. F., C. Aschkenasi, C. Lee, J. Kelly, R. S. Ahima, C. Bjorbaek, J. S. Flier, C. B. Saper, and J. K. Elmquist. 1999. Leptin differentially regulates NPY and POMC neurons projecting to the lateral hypothalamic area. *Neuron* 23:775–86.

Elias, C. F., C. Lee, J. Kelly, C. Aschkenasi, R. S. Ahima, P. R. Couceyro, M. J. Kuhar, C. B. Saper, and J. K. Elmquist. 1998a. Leptin activates hypothalamic CART neurons projecting to the spinal cord. *Neuron* 21:1375–85.

Elias, C. F., C. B. Saper, E. Maratos-Flier, N. A. Tritos, C. Lee, J. Kelly, J. B. Tatro, G. E. Hoffman, M. M. Ollmann, G. S. Barsh, T. Sakurai, M. Yanagisawa, and J. K. Elmquist. 1998b. Chemically defined projections linking the mediobasal hypothalamus and the lateral hypothalamic area. *J Comp Neurol* 402:442–59.

Elmquist, J. K., R. S. Ahima, C. F. Elias, J S. Flier, and C. B. Saper. 1998. Leptin activates distinct projections from the dorsomedial and ventromedial hypothalamic nuclei. *Proc Natl Acad Sci U S A* 95:741–6.

Emanuel, A. J., and S. Ritter. 2010. Hindbrain catecholamine neurons modulate the growth hormone but not the feeding response to ghrelin. *Endocrinology* 151:3237–46.

Everitt, B. J., T. Hokfelt, L. Terenius, K. Tatemoto, V. Mutt, and M. Goldstein. 1984. Differential co-existence of neuropeptide Y (NPY)-like immunoreactivity with catecholamines in the central nervous system of the rat. *Neuroscience* 11:443–62.

Flynn, F. W., and H. J. Grill. 1983. Insulin elicits ingestion in decerebrate rats. *Science* 221:188–90.

Flynn, F. W., and H. J. Grill. 1985. Fourth ventricular phlorizin dissociates feeding from hyperglycemia in rats. *Brain Res* 341:331–6.

Fraley, G. S., and S. Ritter. 2003. Immunolesion of norepinephrine and epinephrine afferents to medial hypothalamus alters basal and 2DG-induced NPY and AGRP mRNA expression in the arcuate nucleus. *Endocrinology* 144:75–83.

Fraley, G. S., T. T. Dinh, and S. Ritter. 2002. Immunotoxic catecholamine lesions attenuate 2DG-induced increase of AGRP mRNA. *Peptides* 23:1093–9.

Fujita, S., and C. M. Donovan. 2005. Celiac-superior mesenteric ganglionectomy, but not vagotomy, suppresses the sympathoadrenal response to insulin-induced hypoglycemia. *Diabetes* 54:3258–64.

Fujita, S., M. Bohland, G. Sanchez-Watts, A. G. Watts, and C. M. Donovan. 2007. Hypoglycemic detection at the portal vein is mediated by capsaicin-sensitive primary sensory neurons. *Am J Physiol Endocrinol Metab* 293:E96–101.

Glick, Z., and J. Mayer. 1968. Hyperphagia caused by cerebral ventricular infusion of phloridzin. *Nature* 219:1374.

Gonzalez, J. A., F. Reimann, and D. Burdakov. 2009. Dissociation between sensing and metabolism of glucose in sugar sensing neurones. *J Physiol* 587:41–8.

Grabauskas, G., I. Song, S. Zhou, and C. Owyang. 2010. Electrophysiological identification of glucose-sensing neurons in rat nodose ganglia. *J Physiol* 588:617–32.

Grabauskas, G., S. Y. Zhou, Y. Lu, I. Song, and C. Owyang. 2013. Essential elements for glucosensing by gastric vagal afferents: Immunocytochemistry and electrophysiology studies in the rat. *Endocrinology* 154:296–307.

Guyenet, P. G., R. L. Stornetta, G. Bochorishvili, S. D. Depuy, P. G. Burke, and S. B. Abbott. 2013. C1 neurons: The body's EMTs. *Am J Physiol Regul Integr Comp Physiol* 305:R187–204.

Han, S. M., C. Namkoong, P. G. Jang, I. S. Park, S. W. Hong, H. Katakami, S. Chun, S. W. Kim, J. Y. Park, K. U. Lee, and M. S. Kim. 2005. Hypothalamic AMP-activated protein kinase mediates counter-regulatory responses to hypoglycaemia in rats. *Diabetologia* 48:2170–8.

Havel, P. J., S. J. Parry, J. S. Stern, J. O. Akpan, R. L. Gingerich, G. J. Taborsky, Jr., and D. L. Curry. 1994. Redundant parasympathetic and sympathoadrenal mediation of increased glucagon secretion during insulin-induced hypoglycemia in conscious rats. *Metabolism* 43:860–6.

Hayes, M. R., K. P. Skibicka, K. K. Bence, and H. J. Grill. 2009. Dorsal hindbrain 5′-adenosine monophosphate-activated protein kinase as an intracellular mediator of energy balance. *Endocrinology* 150:2175–82.

Hermann, G. E., E. Viard, and R. C. Rogers. 2014. Hindbrain glucoprivation effects on gastric vagal reflex circuits and gastric motility in the rat are suppressed by the astrocyte inhibitor fluorocitrate. *J Neurosci* 34:10488–96.

Hevener, A. L., R. N. Bergman, and C. M. Donovan. 2000. Portal vein afferents are critical for the sympathoadrenal response to hypoglycemia. *Diabetes* 49:8–12.

Hyde, T. M., and R. R. Miselis. 1983. Effects of area postrema/caudal medial nucleus of solitary tract lesions on food intake and body weight. *Am J Physiol* 244:R577–87.

I'Anson, H., C. A. Starer, and K. R. Bonnema. 2003. Glucoprivic regulation of estrous cycles in the rat. *Horm Behav* 43:388–93.

I'Anson, H., L. A. Sundling, S. M. Roland, and S. Ritter. 2003. Immunotoxic destruction of distinct catecholaminergic neuron populations disrupts the reproductive response to glucoprivation in female rats. *Endocrinology* 144:4325–31.

Iynedjian, P. B. 2009. Molecular physiology of mammalian glucokinase. *Cell Mol Life Sci* 66:27–42.

Jackson, P. A., S. Cardin, C. S. Coffey, D. W. Neal, E. J. Allen, A. R. Penaloza, W. L. Snead, and A. D. Cherrington. 2000. Effect of hepatic denervation on the counterregulatory response to insulin-induced hypoglycemia in the dog. *Am J Physiol Endocrinol Metab* 279:E1249–57.

Jackson, P. A., M. J. Pagliassotti, M. Shiota, D. W. Neal, S. Cardin, and A. D. Cherrington. 1997. Effects of vagal blockade on the counterregulatory response to insulin-induced hypoglycemia in the dog. *Am J Physiol* 273:E1178–88.

Jokiaho, A. J., C. M. Donovan, and A. G. Watts. 2014. The rate of fall of blood glucose determines the necessity of forebrain-projecting catecholaminergic neurons for male rat sympathoadrenal responses. *Diabetes* 63:2854–65.

Kahn, B. B., T. Alquier, D. Carling, and D. G. Hardie. 2005. AMP-activated protein kinase: Ancient energy gauge provides clues to modern understanding of metabolism. *Cell Metab* 1:15–25.

Kang, L., A. A. Dunn-Meynell, V. H. Routh, L. D. Gaspers, Y. Nagata, T. Nishimura, J. Eiki, B. B. Zhang, and B. E. Levin. 2006. Glucokinase is a critical regulator of ventromedial hypothalamic neuronal glucosensing. *Diabetes* 55:412–20.

Kang, L., V. H. Routh, E. V. Kuzhikandathil, L. D. Gaspers, and B. E. Levin. 2004. Physiological and molecular characteristics of rat hypothalamic ventromedial nucleus glucosensing neurons. *Diabetes* 53:549–59.

Levin, B. E., V. H. Routh, L. Kang, N. M. Sanders, and A. A. Dunn-Meynell. 2004. Neuronal glucosensing: What do we know after 50 years? *Diabetes* 53:2521–8.

Li, A. J., and S. Ritter. 2004. Glucoprivation increases expression of neuropeptide Y mRNA in hindbrain neurons that innervate the hypothalamus. *Eur J Neurosci* 19:2147–54.

Li, A. J., Q. Wang, H. Davis, R. Wang, and S. Ritter. 2015a. Orexin-A enhances feeding in male rats by activating hindbrain catecholamine neurons. *Am J Physiol Regul Integr Comp Physiol* 309:R358–67.

Li, A. J., Q. Wang, T. T. Dinh, B. R. Powers, and S. Ritter. 2014. Stimulation of feeding by three different glucose-sensing mechanisms requires hindbrain catecholamine neurons. *Am J Physiol Regul Integr Comp Physiol* 306:R257–64.

Li, A. J., Q. Wang, T. T. Dinh, and S. Ritter. 2009. Simultaneous silencing of Npy and Dbh expression in hindbrain A1/C1 catecholamine cells suppresses glucoprivic feeding. *J Neurosci* 9:280–7.

Li, A. J., Q. Wang, M. M. Elsarelli, R. L. Brown, and S. Ritter. 2015b. Hindbrain catecholamine neurons activate orexin neurons during systemic glucoprivation in male rats. *Endocrinology* 156:2807–20.

Li, A. J., Q. Wang, and S. Ritter. 2006. Differential responsiveness of dopamine-beta-hydroxylase gene expression to glucoprivation in different catecholamine cell groups. *Endocrinology* 147:3428–34.

Li, A. J., Q. Wang, and S. Ritter. 2011. Participation of hindbrain AMP-activated protein kinase in glucoprivic feeding. *Diabetes* 60:436–42.

Lynch, R. M., L. S. Tompkins, H. L. Brooks, A. A. Dunn-Meynell, and B. E. Levin. 2000. Localization of glucokinase gene expression in the rat brain. *Diabetes* 49:693–700.

Madden, C. J., S. Ito, L. Rinaman, R. G. Wiley, and A. F. Sved. 1999. Lesions of the C1 catecholaminergic neurons of the ventrolateral medulla in rats using anti-DbetaH-saporin. *Am J Physiol* 277:R1063–75.

Maekawa, F., Y. Toyoda, N. Torii, I. Miwa, R. C. Thompson, D. L. Foster, S. Tsukahara, H. Tsukamura, and K. Maeda. 2000. Localization of glucokinase-like immunoreactivity in the rat lower brain stem: For possible location of brain glucose-sensing mechanisms. *Endocrinology* 141:375–84.

Marty, N., M. Dallaporta, M. Foretz, M. Emery, D. Tarussio, I. Bady, C. Binnert, F. Beermann, and B. Thorens. 2005. Regulation of glucagon secretion by glucose transporter type 2 (glut2) and astrocyte-dependent glucose sensors. *J Clin Invest* 115:3545–53.

Matveyenko, A. V., M. Bohland, M. Saberi, and C. M. Donovan. 2007. Portal vein hypoglycemia is essential for full induction of hypoglycemia-associated autonomic failure with slow-onset hypoglycemia. *Am J Physiol Endocrinol Metab* 293:E857–64.

Medeiros, N., L. Dai, and A. V. Ferguson. 2012. Glucose-responsive neurons in the subfornical organ of the rat—A novel site for direct CNS monitoring of circulating glucose. *Neurosci* 201:157–65.

Miki, T., B. Liss, K. Minami, T. Shiuchi, A. Saraya, Y. Kashima, M. Horiuchi, F. Ashcroft, Y. Minokoshi, J. Roeper, and S. Seino. 2001. ATP-sensitive K+ channels in the hypothalamus are essential for the maintenance of glucose homeostasis. *Nat Neurosci* 4:507–12.

Miselis, R. R., and A. N. Epstein. 1975. Feeding induced by intracerebroventricular 2-deoxy-D-glucose in the rat. *Am J Physiol* 229:1438–47.

Mizuno, Y., and Y. Oomura. 1984. Glucose responding neurons in the nucleus tractus solitarius of the rat: In vitro study. *Brain Res* 307:109–16.

Moriyama, R., H. Tsukamura, M. Kinoshita, H. Okazaki, Y. Kato, and K. Maeda. 2004. In vitro increase in intracellular calcium concentrations induced by low or high extracellular glucose levels in ependymocytes and serotonergic neurons of the rat lower brainstem. *Endocrinology* 145:2507–15.

Morrison, S. F., and W. H. Cao. 2000. Different adrenal sympathetic preganglionic neurons regulate epinephrine and norepinephrine secretion. *Am J Physiol Regul Integr Comp Physiol* 279:R1763–75.

Morrison, S. F., T. A. Milner, and D. J. Reis. 1988. Reticulospinal vasomotor neurons of the rat rostral ventrolateral medulla: Relationship to sympathetic nerve activity and the C1 adrenergic cell group. *J Neurosci* 8:1286–301.

Mueckler, M., and B. Thorens. 2013. The SLC2 (GLUT) family of membrane transporters. *Mol Asp Med* 34:121–38.

Nagatani, S., D. C. Bucholtz, K. Murahashi, M. A. Estacio, H. Tsukamura, D. L. Foster, and K. I. Maeda. 1996. Reduction of glucose availability suppresses pulsatile luteinizing hormone release in female and male rats. *Endocrinology* 137:1166–70.

Nakano, Y., Y. Oomura, L. Lenard, H. Nishino, S. Aou, T. Yamamoto, and K. Aoyagi. 1986. Feeding-related activity of glucose- and morphine-sensitive neurons in the monkey amygdala. *Brain Res* 399:167–72.

Nambu, T., T. Sakurai, K. Mizukami, Y. Hosoya, M. Yanagisawa, and K. Goto. 1999. Distribution of orexin neurons in the adult rat brain. *Brain Res* 827:243–60.

O'Malley, D., F. Reimann, A. K. Simpson, and F. M. Gribble. 2006. Sodium-coupled glucose cotransporters contribute to hypothalamic glucose sensing. *Diabetes* 55:3381–6.

Ohno, K., and T. Sakurai. 2008. Orexin neuronal circuitry: Role in the regulation of sleep and wakefulness. *Front Neuroendocrinol* 29:70–87.

Oomura, Y., T. Ono, H. Ooyama, and M. J. Wayner. 1969. Glucose and osmosensitive neurones of the rat hypothalamus. *Nature* 222:282–4.

Parniak, M., and N. Kalant. 1985. Incorporation of glucose into glycogen in primary cultures of rat hepatocytes. *Can J Biochem Cell Biol = Rev Can Biochim Biol Cell* 63:333–40.

Paxinos, G., and C. Watson. 1997. *The Rat Brain in Stereotaxic Coordinates*. Fourth ed. San Diego, CA: Academic Press.

Peyron, C., D. K. Tighe, A. N. van den Pol, L. de Lecea, H. C. Heller, J. G. Sutcliffe, and T. S. Kilduff. 1998. Neurons containing hypocretin (orexin) project to multiple neuronal systems. *J Neurosci* 18:9996–10015.

Picklo, M. J., R. G. Wiley, D. A. Lappi, and D. Robertson. 1994. Noradrenergic lesioning with an anti-dopamine beta-hydroxylase immunotoxin. *Brain Res* 666:195–200.

Picklo, M. J., R. G. Wiley, S. Lonce, D. A. Lappi, and D. Robertson. 1995. Anti-dopamine beta-hydroxylase immunotoxin-induced sympathectomy in adult rats. *J Pharmacol Exp Ther* 275:1003–10.

Rinaman, L. 2003. Hindbrain noradrenergic lesions attenuate anorexia and alter central cFos expression in rats after gastric viscerosensory stimulation. *J Neurosci* 23: 10084–92.

Ritter, S., and J. S. Taylor. 1990. Vagal sensory neurons are required for lipoprivic but not glucoprivic feeding in rats. *Am J Physiol* 258:R1395–401.

Ritter, S., K. Bugarith, and T. T. Dinh. 2001. Immunotoxic destruction of distinct catecholamine subgroups produces selective impairment of glucoregulatory responses and neuronal activation. *J Comp Neurol* 432:197–216.

Ritter, S., T. T. Dinh, and A. J. Li. 2006. Hindbrain catecholamine neurons control multiple glucoregulatory responses. *Physiol Behav* 89:490–500.

Ritter, S., T. T. Dinh, and Y. Zhang. 2000. Localization of hindbrain glucoreceptive sites controlling food intake and blood glucose. *Brain Res* 856:37–47.

Ritter, S., A. J. Li, Q. Wang, and T. T. Dinh. 2011. Minireview: The value of looking backward: The essential role of the hindbrain in counterregulatory responses to glucose deficit. *Endocrinology* 152:4019–32.

Ritter, S., I. Llewellyn-Smith, and T. T. Dinh. 1998. Subgroups of hindbrain catecholamine neurons are selectively activated by 2-deoxy-D-glucose induced metabolic challenge. *Brain Res* 805:41–54.

Ritter, R. C., P. G. Slusser, and S. Stone. 1981. Glucoreceptors controlling feeding and blood glucose: Location in the hindbrain. *Science* 213:451–2.

Ritter, S., A. G. Watts, T. T. Dinh, G. Sanchez-Watts, and C. Pedrow. 2003. Immunotoxin lesion of hypothalamically projecting norepinephrine and epinephrine neurons differentially affects circadian and stressor-stimulated corticosterone secretion. *Endocrinology* 144:1357–67.

Roland, A. V., and S. M. Moenter. 2011. Glucosensing by GnRH neurons: Inhibition by androgens and involvement of AMP-activated protein kinase. *Mol Endocrinol* 25:847–58.

Saberi, M., M. Bohland, and C. M. Donovan. 2008. The locus for hypoglycemic detection shifts with the rate of fall in glycemia: The role of portal-superior mesenteric vein glucose sensing. *Diabetes* 57:1380–6.

Sakurai, T. 2007. The neural circuit of orexin (hypocretin): Maintaining sleep and wakefulness. *Nat Rev Neurosci* 8:171–81.

Sawchenko, P. E., L. W. Swanson, R. Grzanna, P. R. Howe, S. R. Bloom, and J. M. Polak. 1985. Colocalization of neuropeptide Y immunoreactivity in brainstem catecholaminergic neurons that project to the paraventricular nucleus of the hypothalamus. *J Comp Neurol* 241:138–53.

Schreihofer, A. M., and P. G. Guyenet. 2000. Sympathetic reflexes after depletion of bulbospinal catecholaminergic neurons with anti-DbetaH-saporin. *Am J Physiol Regul Integr Comp Physiol* 279:R729–42.

Silver, I. A., and M. Erecinska. 1994. Extracellular glucose concentration in mammalian brain: Continuous monitoring of changes during increased neuronal activity and upon limitation in oxygen supply in normo-, hypo-, and hyperglycemic animals. *J Neurosci* 14:5068–76.

Sindelar, D. K., L. Ste Marie, G. I. Miura, R. D. Palmiter, J. E. McMinn, G. J. Morton, and M. W. Schwartz. 2004. Neuropeptide Y is required for hyperphagic feeding in response to neuroglucopenia. *Endocrinology* 145:3363–8.

Smith, G. P., and A. N. Epstein. 1969. Increased feeding in response to decreased glucose utilization in the rat and monkey. *Am J Physiol* 217:1083–7.

Song, Z., B. E. Levin, J. J. McArdle, N. Bakhos, and V. H. Routh. 2001. Convergence of pre- and postsynaptic influences on glucosensing neurons in the ventromedial hypothalamic nucleus. *Diabetes* 50:2673–81.

Stanley, B. G., and W. J. Thomas. 1993. Feeding responses to perifornical hypothalamic injection of neuropeptide Y in relation to circadian rhythms of eating behavior. *Peptides* 14:475–81.

Stanley, B. G., W. Magdalin, A. Seirafi, W. J. Thomas, and S. F. Leibowitz. 1993. The perifornical area: The major focus of (a) patchily distributed hypothalamic neuropeptide Y-sensitive feeding system(s). *Brain Res* 604:304–17.

Tamrakar, P., B. A. Ibrahim, A. D. Gujar, and K. P. Briski. 2015. Estrogen regulates energy metabolic pathway and upstream adenosine 5′-monophosphate-activated protein kinase and phosphatase enzyme expression in dorsal vagal complex metabolosensory neurons during glucostasis and hypoglycemia. *J Neurosci Res* 93:321–32.

Thorens, B. 1996. Glucose transporters in the regulation of intestinal, renal, and liver glucose fluxes. *Am J Physiol* 270:G541–53.

Thorens, B., and M. Mueckler. 2010. Glucose transporters in the 21st century. *Am J Physiol Endocrinol Metab* 298:E141–5.

Troy, A. E., S. S. Simmonds, S. D. Stocker, and K. N. Browning. 2016. High fat diet attenuates glucose-dependent facilitation of 5-HT3-mediated responses in rat gastric vagal afferents. *J Physiol* 594:99–114.

Tsujii, S., and G. A. Bray. 1990. Effects of glucose, 2-deoxyglucose, phlorizin, and insulin on food intake of lean and fatty rats. *Am J Physiol* 258:E476–81.

Wild, S., G. Roglic, A. Green, R. Sicree, and H. King. 2004. Global prevalence of diabetes: Estimates for the year 2000 and projections for 2030. *Diabetes Care* 27:1047–53.

Wiley, R. G., and I. R. Kline. 2000. Neuronal lesioning with axonally transported toxins. *J Neurosci Meth* 103:73–82.

Wrenn, C. C., M. J. Picklo, D. A. Lappi, D. Robertson, and R. G. Wiley. 1996. Central noradrenergic lesioning using anti-DBH-saporin: Anatomical findings. *Brain Res* 740:175–84.

Yamanaka, A., T. Sakurai, T. Katsumoto, M. Yanagisawa, and K. Goto. 1999. Chronic intracerebroventricular administration of orexin-A to rats increases food intake in daytime, but has no effect on body weight. *Brain Res* 849:248–52.

Yu, A. S., B. A. Hirayama, G. Timbol, J. Liu, E. Basarah, V. Kepe, N. Satyamurthy, S. C. Huang, E. M. Wright, and J. R. Barrio. 2010. Functional expression of SGLTs in rat brain. *Am J Physiol Cell Physiol* 299:C1277–84.

Yu, A. S., B. A. Hirayama, G. Timbol, J. Liu, A. Diez-Sampedro, V. Kepe, N. Satyamurthy, S. C. Huang, E. M. Wright, and J. R. Barrio. 2013. Regional distribution of SGLT activity in rat brain in vivo. *Am J Physiol Cell Physiol* 304:C240–7.

Zhao, H., J. H. Peters, M. Zhu, S. J. Page, R. C. Ritter, and S. M. Appleyard. 2015. Frequency-dependent facilitation of synaptic throughput via postsynaptic NMDA receptors in the nucleus of the solitary tract. *J Physiol* 593:111–25.

Zheng, H., L. M. Patterson, and H. R. Berthoud. 2005. Orexin-A projections to the caudal medulla and orexin-induced c-Fos expression, food intake, and autonomic function. *J Comp Neurol* 485:127–42.

Zhou, L., C. Y. Yueh, D. D. Lam, J. Shaw, M. Osundiji, A. S. Garfield, M. Evans, and L. K. Heisler. 2011. Glucokinase inhibitor glucosamine stimulates feeding and activates hypothalamic neuropeptide Y and orexin neurons. *Behav Brain Res* 222:274–8.

10 Hindbrain Astrocyte Glucodetectors and Counterregulation

Richard C. Rogers, David H. McDougal, and Gerlinda E. Hermann

CONTENTS

10.1 INTRODUCTION

Astrocytes have classically been associated with maintenance of neurons. However, since the late 1990s, there has been a dramatic shift in the recognition of the role of astrocytes in central nervous system (CNS) function from passive supporter to active participant (Araque et al. 1999, Bushong et al. 2002, Halassa et al. 2007, Halassa and Haydon 2010, Perea, Navarrete, and Araque 2009, Vance, Rogers, and Hermann 2015). The degree to which astrocytes are involved in regulating central nervous system-wide synaptic function is controversial (Agulhon, Fiacco, and McCarthy 2010, Smith 2010). However, the hindbrain astrocyte has emerged as a powerful component in homeostatic regulation (Agulhon et al. 2013, Funk 2010, Gourine and Kasparov 2011, Gourine et al. 2010, Hermann et al. 2009, Lin et al. 2013, McDougal, Hermann, and Rogers 2013, Vance, Rogers, and Hermann 2015).

There are several reports of astrocyte involvement in the regulation of hindbrain synaptic activity (Accorsi-Mendonca, Bonagamba, and Machado 2012, Vance, Rogers, and Hermann 2015), neural inputs regulating astrocyte function (McDougal, Hermann, and Rogers 2011, Porter and McCarthy 1996), and astrocyte involvement as detectors of physiological parameters critical to the maintenance of homeostasis (Funk 2010, Gourine and Kasparov 2011, Accorsi-Mendonca, Bonagamba, and Machado 2012). This chapter reviews recent data that support a special function of astrocytes in the detection of hypoglycemic emergencies and initiation of the rapid, life-saving homeostatic adjustments to hypoglycemia together referred to as "counterregulation."

10.2   COUNTERREGULATORY RESPONSE TO GLUCOSE DEFICIT

Severe glucose deficits caused by acute food deprivation or medication errors can be life-threatening, physiological emergencies. Dangerous reductions in circulating glucose levels are resisted by a series of unique autonomic and behavioral mechanisms organized primarily by circuitry in the hindbrain. These "counterregulatory responses" (CRRs; reviewed extensively; Marty, Dallaporta, and Thorens 2007, Watts and Donovan 2010, Ritter et al. 2011) specifically detect low CNS glucose levels and engage several defensive reactions to restore glucose homeostasis. Physiological and behavioral CRRs include release of glucagon and epinephrine (to trigger glycogenolysis), release of corticosteroids (to shift dependence of nonneural tissues away from glucose toward fatty acids), initiation of glucoprivic feeding (to restore metabolic fuel), and a dramatic increase in gastrointestinal motility in anticipation of the arrival of food (to aid rapid digestion). These physiological responses are typically coupled with sensations of sweating, shaking, weakness, fatigue, headache, and hunger, collectively serving as hypoglycemia "awareness" for the individual.

The accurate and timely initiation of CRR is literally a matter of life and death to diabetics. An insulin-dependent diabetic may experience a couple of medication-induced hypoglycemic episodes per week. The CRR mechanism is desensitized by successive bouts of hypoglycemia in both clinical populations as well as in normal subjects (Cryer, Davis, and Shamoon 2003). The resultant hypoglycemia unawareness and hypoglycemia-associated autonomic failure (HAAF) can be lethal. It is not uncommon that a diabetic may suffer one such event annually that is serious enough to require the intervention by another for his or her survival. Approximately 1 in 20 diabetic dies as a consequence of iatrogenic hypoglycemia and the failure of CRR (Cryer, Davis, and Shamoon 2003).

The mechanisms connecting the physiological detection of CNS cytoglucopenia with the efferent neural systems that drive the various aspects of CRR are an active area of research. Until recently, it was assumed that the glucodetection mechanism was, like the integrative circuitry coordinating CRR, neuronal. However, compelling evidence has emerged suggesting that CRR critically depends on astrocytes as the principal chemosensors (Marty et al. 2005, McDougal, Hermann, and Rogers 2013).

10.3 CRR IN HISTORICAL PERSPECTIVE

Claude Bernard introduced the concept of autonomic control over glucose production in the mid-nineteenth century. Bernard conducted detailed experimental analyses of the origin and synthesis of glucose appearing in the circulation of carbohydrate-starved subjects. At the time, it was believed that only plants were capable of de novo synthesis of glucose, so Bernard was held to a very high standard of proof. His careful, stepwise demonstration that the liver is capable of the synthesis, storage, and release of glucose became the essential foundation of his concept of the physiological defense of the "milieu interieur." Part of this work included studies on the source of the physiological stimulus for the release of hepatic glucose. Bernard's vagal nerve section and stimulation studies produced equivocal results. In his subsequent studies, he stimulated the entry zone for the "pneumo-gastric nerve" (contemporary name for the vagus) on the floor of the fourth ventricle. His only available method for "site-specific" CNS stimulation involved applying pressure with a needle to the region containing the nucleus of the solitary tract (NST). This maneuver elicited a robust increase in glucose release from the liver, a "piqure diabetes." Bernard later attributed the effect to descending sympathetic activation of hepatic glucose release (Bernard 1848, 1849, 1877). WB Cannon used Bernard's seminal work to advance the concept of homeostatic regulation of circulating glucose. Specifically, Cannon identified the link between glucose deficit and the sympathetic activation of adrenal epinephrine and glucocorticoid release essential to hepatic glycogenolysis and gluconeogenesis (Cannon, McIver, and Bliss 1924).

Considerable attention has been directed toward hypothalamic glucoregulatory and feeding control mechanisms, yet, an unbroken chain of observations from Bernard to the present day clearly associate the hindbrain with the hyperglycemia portion of CRR. Chandler Brooks (working first in the Cannon and Bard laboratories at Harvard and then independently at Princeton in 1931) showed that hypothalamic stimulation can produce an elevation in blood glucose. However, using the decerebrate cat preparation, he also demonstrated that the critical circuitry necessary for electrical stimulation-driven hyperglycemia is the caudal medulla (Brooks 1931). Nearly 50 years later, DiRocco and Grill (1979) used the chronic, awake, decerebrate rat to verify that the critical glucodetection and integration machinery necessary to evoke an increase in blood glucose in response to cytoglucopenia is located in the hindbrain. The evidence is now clear that glucopenia-induced feeding behavior, adrenal hormone release, hepatic glucose production, and increases in gastric motility are all dependent on the intact hindbrain. In particular, it is clear that the hindbrain is essential for the detection of the glucopenic state and the translation of that data into physiological action (Marty, Dallaporta, and Thorens 2007, Ritter et al. 2011, Watts and Donovan 2010).

10.4 CONTEMPORARY VIEW OF CRR MECHANISMS

This CRR mechanism is dependent on two populations of catecholamine (CA) neurons in the hindbrain: the A2/C2 grouping in the NST and the A1/C1 group in the basolateral medulla (BLM) (Ritter et al. 2011, Watts and Donovan 2010). Localized glucoprivation (i.e., targeted microinjection of 2-deoxyglucose or 5-thioglucose) or site/phenotype-specific saporin lesions suggest that these neuron groups are necessary to glucoprivic feeding, as well as adrenal epinephrine and corticosterone secretion. That is, specific destruction of hindbrain CA neurons results in an inability to evoke CRR (Li et al. 2014). Thus, these CA neurons are a final common path for elicitation of these responses. Local glucoprivation of hindbrain CA regions drive sympathetically mediated glucagon secretion (Andrew, Dinh, and Ritter 2007). However, since a significant amount of pancreatic alpha cell activation is under local glycemic, paracrine, endocrine, and enteric control, removal of hindbrain CA circuits does not completely eliminate systemic hypoglycemia-mediated glucagon release (Ritter et al. 2011). While there is some evidence for segregating different CRR functions (i.e., glucoprivic feeding, corticosterone, glucagon, epinephrine secretion for the A1/C1 versus A2/C2 areas), there is also evidence for overlap in neurocircuitry involved in CRR function (Ritter et al. 2011, Watts and Donovan 2010). One exception may involve neurons in the dorsal vagal complex (DVC), which control glucoprivation-mediated increases in gastric motility. That is, this reflex control is mediated entirely by the DVC without any involvement of the BLM (Hermann, Nasse, and Rogers 2005). Nevertheless, at least some of the critical NST neurons regulating vago-vagal control of gastric function are also noradrenergic (Hermann, Nasse, and Rogers 2005, Rogers, Travagli, and Hermann 2003) not unlike other CRR circuits. Hindbrain CA neurons form highly divergent pathways that are in position to directly influence autonomic outflows controlling relevant hormone secretion, gastric motility, and feeding control (Hudson and Ritter 2004, Li et al. 2009, 2013, Rinaman 2011, Ritter et al. 2011). These hindbrain CA neurons form the integrative core of the CRRs.

The CRR response elicited by hindbrain CA neurons is produced by a unique, "protected" circuitry that can function to mobilize glucose and drive feeding behavior in an emergency without significant modulation of, or by, other homeostatic systems. The advantage of such a system in the management of a physiological emergency is that it retains its sensitivity to the defended parameter under practically all other physiological circumstances (Donovan and Watts 2014, Ritter et al. 2011). This exclusivity of CRR circuitry can help identify CRR versus non-CRR metabolic and feeding control elements. For example, CRR circuit elements are probably not affected by leptin or α-melanocyte-stimulating hormone (α-MSH) inputs, while non-CRR regulatory feeding and metabolic control elements are biased in their response to glucoprivic stimuli in the presence of signals corresponding to repletion state (Donovan and Watts 2014, Mimee and Ferguson 2015, Ritter et al. 2011, Watts and Donovan 2010).

The specific cellular mechanisms connecting low glucose detection with any local neurons, even the CA neurons in the hindbrain, are not clear. A small percentage of hindbrain CA neurons may autonomously behave like glucosensors and may express the components of hypothetical glucodetectors (e.g., K_{ATP} channels, glucokinase, AMP kinase, etc.; Marty, Dallaporta, and Thorens 2007, Ritter et al. 2011, Watts and Donovan 2010). However, it has not been clearly established whether any of these CA neurons are themselves sensitive to glucoprivation and are involved in CRR (Ritter et al. 2011). It is recognized that afferents to and cells within the dorsal medulla can sense glucose. However, the specific involvement of these processes in CRR (as opposed to circuits involved in the broader integrated control of metabolism; Ritter et al. 2011), is not understood (Marty, Dallaporta, and Thorens 2007, Ritter et al. 2011, Watts and Donovan 2010). Regardless of the details, until recently, it was assumed that the hindbrain cells responsible for sensing glucose availability in CRR were neurons. However, a couple of provocative papers (Klip and Hawkins 2005, Marty et al. 2005, Marty, Dallaporta, and Thorens 2007) have shown that astrocytes may be the primary detectors of low glucose conditions.

10.5 CLASSIC AND CONTEMPORARY VIEWS OF ASTROCYTE FUNCTION IN THE CNS

Classically, the astrocyte has been thought to play a subservient role to the neuron in the control of CNS function. In this view, the astrocyte maintains the extracellular nutrient, metabolite, and ionic environment for the neuron, while also working to dispose of and recycle released neurotransmitters and their breakdown products. Additionally, the astrocyte provides mechanical support, literally the "glue" that holds the nervous system together. This view is essentially the same as that proposed by Cajal (1995) in his "Histologie du système nerveux de l'homme & des vertébrés" of 1909. While the astrocyte is certainly responsible for these basic functions, the reputation of the glial cell as an active participant in CNS signaling and control has undergone a recent and dramatic rejuvenation (Haydon and Carmignoto 2006, Volterra and Meldolesi 2005).

The foundation for the glial–neuron interaction controversy was laid over 100 years ago by two of the most famous antagonists in neuroscience: Camillio Golgi and Santiago Ramon y Cajal. Golgi developed his silver chromate "black reaction" stains in 1872 to specifically investigate glial morphology. Based on his observations, Golgi correctly concluded that astrocytes are connected in a syncytial fashion but made the error of extending this argument to include neuronal interconnections (Mazzarello 2010). Cajal modified Golgi's procedure and used improved optical techniques to conclude correctly that neurons maintain synaptic relationships but concluded, incorrectly, that glial cells were unlikely to be involved in processes other than insulation of neurons. The fallout from Cajal winning the neuronal argument in Stockholm with the Nobel Prize in 1906 probably set glial–neural physiology back 100 years. The relatively recent discovery that glial–neural interactions could modify synaptic strength or initiate changes in neuronal excitability (Halassa and Haydon 2010, Pasti et al. 1997, Perea, Navarrete, and Araque 2009) were revolutionary, requiring a modern reexamination of the role of astrocytes in CNS function.

Astrocytes are the most abundant cells within the CNS. A single astrocyte may contact tens to hundreds of thousands of synapses and, along with presynaptic terminals and postsynaptic neurons, will form what has been termed the "tripartite synapse" (Araque et al. 1999, Bushong et al. 2002, Halassa et al. 2007, Halassa and Haydon 2010, Perea, Navarrete, and Araque 2009) in which presynaptic terminals and synaptic efficacy as well as the postsynaptic responsiveness to afferent input and neuronal excitability are regulated by astrocytes. Astrocytes, themselves, are subject to afferent synaptic input from neurons, completing the contemporary view of neural–glial interaction (McDougal, Hermann, and Rogers 2011).

This revised view of the significance of the astrocyte includes the observation that astrocytes are subject to modulation by neurotransmitters released from neuronal pre-synaptic terminals as well as gliotransmitters released by other astrocytes (Haydon and Carmignoto 2006, McDougal, Hermann, and Rogers 2011). Additionally, hormones, circulating factors such as thrombin, changes in endogenous physiological signals like O_2/CO_2, pH, and changes (especially reductions) in glucose concentration or metabolic availability can all increase astrocytic calcium levels. This increase in astrocytic calcium is coupled to a release of gliotransmitters in processes similar to neurotransmission (Araque, Carmignoto, and Haydon 2001, Halassa et al. 2007, Halassa and Haydon 2010, Perea, Navarrete, and Araque 2009). Currently recognized gliotransmitters include glutamate, adenosine triphosphate (ATP), adenosine, and D-serine, among others (Angulo et al. 2004, Bezzi et al. 1998, Coco et al. 2003, Fellin and Carmignoto 2004, Parpura and Haydon 2000, Martineau et al. 2013).

The astrocytic release of adenosine, in response to glucoprivation, may be especially relevant to the connection between low glucose detection and the activation of downstream CRR mechanisms. There is good evidence that adenosine is released rapidly within the CNS, in general (Dunwiddie and Masino 2001), and from astrocytes, in particular (Ciccarelli et al. 1999). This adenosine release is a consequence of the consumption of cellular ATP and the build-up of the dephosphorylated product. There are at least two mechanisms by which astrocytes subjected to hypoglycemia could increase the adenosine concentration in the vicinity of neurons. First, adenosine can be released directly from astrocytes through reversible equilibrating nucleoside transporters in the cell membrane (Meghji, Tuttle, and Rubio 1989), a release that is not coupled to cytoplasmic calcium. Second, ATP (released by calcium-dependent gliotransmission) is readily converted to adenosine via the action of ectonucleotidases (Halassa, Fellin, and Haydon 2009). While a number of downstream effects of CNS hypoglycemia are blocked by antagonists to the A1 adenosine receptor (Minor et al. 2001, Turner, Blackburn, and Rivkees 2004), a specific connection between astrocyte low glucose detection, adenosine release, and activation of downstream CRR mechanisms is still speculative.

10.5.1 GLUCOSE DETECTION MECHANISMS AND ASTROCYTE SENSITIVITY TO LOW GLUCOSE

Glucose detection and coupling to mechanisms regulating cellular excitability have been elegantly described for the pancreatic beta cell and for some neurons presumed to be involved in physiological and nutrient homeostasis. The critical element of this mechanism is a specialized transmembrane glucose transporter, GLUT2 (Klip and Hawkins 2005, Marty et al. 2005). GLUT2 is a reversible carrier in that it will transport glucose down a concentration gradient in either direction across the cell membrane. Further, GLUT2 operates at a high relative volume, but with a low affinity compared to other hexose transporters; e.g., Kds for transport in the 5–10 millimolar range for GLUT2 versus the high micromolar range for the high-affinity but low-volume GLUT1. Most important, however, is that the combination of the high volume of transport and low affinity characteristics makes the GLUT2 transporter the critical discriminator of physiological glucose concentrations (Klip and Hawkins 2005). The physiological consequences of these parameters are that glucose concentrations are rapidly equalized between the extracellular and intracellular compartments for cells that possess a significant number of GLUT2 transporters. Increases in extracellular glucose concentrations are rapidly translated into elevated intracellular glucose. Newly available utilizable glucose is metabolized through glycolysis to produce lactate and ATP. The intracellular ATP concentration, in this instance, mirrors the supply of intracellular glucose. This information is converted to proportional changes in excitation through the action of ATP on a specialized potassium ion channel, K_{ATP}. In glucodetecting cells, this tonically open potassium conductance helps hold the resting membrane in a hyperpolarized state. ATP inactivates this conductance, causing localized membrane depolarization. In beta cells, this depolarization triggers the opening of voltage-gated calcium channels and calcium-induced calcium release (CICR). CICR is a process by which calcium entering the cytoplasm binds to ryanodine channels in the endoplasmic reticulum (ER), discharging large amounts of calcium into the cytoplasm. The resulting wave of cytoplasmic calcium, in turn, drives insulin secretion in proportion to the concentration of intracellular glucose (Islam 2010). In glucose-sensitive neurons, the process is similar with the distinction that localized membrane depolarization couples to the voltage-dependent sodium conductance, which generates action potentials in proportion to the amount of utilizable glucose (Ashcroft 1988). Since the GLUT2 transporter is bidirectional, any reduction in extracellular glucose would be rapidly reflected in a reduction in intracellular glucose available for the synthesis of ATP, hence a reduction in beta cell insulin secretion and a reduction in neuronal glucosensor excitability (Klip and Hawkins 2005).

The importance of GLUT2 to physiological glucose detection makes it a convenient marker for the identification of putative glucose-sensing cells. This logic propelled the work of Marty et al. in a search for the cells necessary for the detection of low glucose and the initiation of the CRR (Marty et al. 2005, Marty, Dallaporta, and Thorens 2007). A complex transgenic scheme was required to show that CNS astrocytes, probably localized to the hindbrain, are essential components of the CRR glucodetection mechanism. A global knockout of GLUT2 is not survivable given the dependence of normal beta cell insulin secretion on GLUT2, as discussed earlier. To solve this problem, GLUT2 knockouts were paired with a transgenic modification of beta cells such that these insulin secreting cells now expressed the GLUT1 transporter. This manipulation produced the global GLUT2 deletion while leaving beta cells sufficiently sensitive to glucose to allow normal basal insulin secretion. However, GLUT2 deletion eliminated the initiation of CNS hypoglycemia-triggered CRR. Surprisingly, rescue expression of GLUT2 in *neurons* had no effect to reverse the elimination of CRR. Even more surprising was the observation that reexpression of GLUT2 in CNS astrocytes rescued CRR. The conclusion of this ground-breaking study is that astrocytes are key elements in the direct sensing of declines in glucose (Klip and Hawkins 2005), a view supported by recent investigations from our laboratory (McDougal, Hermann, and Rogers 2013) as well as suspected by earlier studies (Young, Baker, and Montes 2000).

While this chapter focuses on the role of hindbrain astrocytes in CRR, the authors would be remiss for not mentioning evidence that astrocytes in other brain regions may also contribute to glucoregulatory phenomena. Injection of glucose into the central carotid artery provokes a transient yet significant elevation of insulin secretion. Several loci in the forebrain (in addition to the hindbrain) can contribute to this effect. In particular, glucose probably has direct effects on hypothalamic structures such as the arcuate nucleus (ARC), the paraventricular nucleus (PVN), and the ventromedial nucleus (VMH) to regulate glycemia, metabolism, and feeding behavior (Guillod-Maximin et al. 2004, Levin, Dunn-Meynell, and Routh 1999, Penicaud et al. 2006, Watts and Donovan 2010). Immunostaining for cFOS reveals that the ARC, in particular, is highly activated by carotid glucose. Double immunostain studies also show that astrocytes in the ARC (but not PVN or VMH) are significantly activated by the challenge. Selective suppression of astrocyte signaling and metabolism with methionine sulfoxamine blocks both the glucose activation of ARC cFOS as well as the spike in insulin (Guillod-Maximin et al. 2004). These data strongly suggest that astrocytes in structures outside the hindbrain can detect glucose transients (both high and low) and command changes in glucostatic mechanisms.

10.5.2 Physiological Evidence for Astrocyte Involvement in Homeostatic Processes

Our laboratory arrived at the concept of astrocytic regulation of CRR mechanisms through a circuitous route. One of our principal interests is in determining mechanistic explanations for autonomic failure to control gastric function in chronic disease or following traumatic injury (Hermann et al. 2009, Vance, Rogers, and Hermann 2015). For example, head injuries, burns, and severe bleeding trauma have all been known to cause severe suppression of gastric motility, resulting in a high degree of gastric feeding intolerance and predisposition toward nausea and emesis. While the effects of head injuries on autonomic dysregulation might reasonably be blamed on increased intracranial pressure, this connection has been difficult to defend (Garrick et al. 1988, Larson et al. 1984). Furthermore, intracranial pressure changes cannot be responsible for the autonomic failures produced by burns or corporeal injury. Therefore, some other "product" of injury must be responsible for changes in CNS–autonomic control. We turned to thrombin, a product of traumatic injury, as a potential link between injury and autonomic dysfunction. Thrombin is a potent serine proteinase that triggers the initiation of fibrinogenesis in blood clotting. Additionally, this proteinase can act on an unusual class of G-protein-coupled receptors: proteinase-activated receptors (PARs). PAR type I is widely expressed in the brain. Thrombin, generated as a consequence of head injury or peripheral trauma, can access these central receptors via the circulation (Traynelis and Trejo 2007). Early studies suggested that the DVC of the hindbrain contained a high density of PARs (Weinstein et al. 1995). This dorsal hindbrain region regulates vago-vagal control of the stomach as well as other complex autonomic responses such as CRR.

Originally, we hypothesized that traumatic injury and thrombin production were linked to the suppression of gastric motility via PAR receptors on neurons on the NST. Gastric-NST neurons are excited by vagal afferents from the stomach. These neurons, in turn, inhibit adjacent vagal motor neurons in the dorsal motor nucleus (DMN). Inhibition of gastric-DMN neurons withdraws a source of tonic parasympathetic excitation to the stomach, the result being a dramatic relaxation of the stomach and a suppression of motility. This vago-vagal reflex normally regulates gastric tone and motility based on the degree to which the stomach is filled (i.e., monitored by NST neurons). Activation of these gastric-NST neurons by other means (e.g., PAR receptors) would produce the same gastric effects (relaxation or gastric stasis) (Rogers and Hermann 2012).

We were surprised to find that all PAR1 receptors in the DVC were located on *astrocytes*, rather than on neurons (Hermann et al. 2009). Activation of PARs on astrocytes in the NST produced a dramatic increase in cytoplasmic calcium signal in NST astrocytes that was translated, with a delay, into activation of neurons in the NST. Subsequent work showed that PAR activation of NST astrocytes produces a calcium-mediated gliotransmission of glutamate onto neuronal NST NMDA receptors (Vance, Rogers, and Hermann 2015). We were certainly aware of the fact that CRR control circuitry shared this region of the hindbrain and were also aware that one of the earliest physiological hallmarks of CRR involves a dramatic increase in gastric motility.

While CRR is typically associated with autonomically mediated increases in glucose release from the liver and increases in feeding behavior to make up for metabolic fuel deficits, it has been recognized for more than 100 years that hypoglycemia and acute food deprivation also increase gastric motility (Bulatao and Carlson 1924, Cannon and Washburn 1912). The increase in gastric motility in anticipation of glucoprivic feeding speeds digestion and metabolism and is an obligatory feature of CRR glucose homeostasis. Therefore, we extended our original hypothesis concerning the role of astrocytes in the hindbrain to include the regulation of gastric-vago-vagal reflex control during low glucose availability. Thus, we reasoned that some astrocytes in the DVC might be sensitive to reductions in the local concentration of glucose, and if so, would act to increase gastric motility.

Fluorocitrate (FC) is an astrocyte-selective metabolic antagonist that blocks astrocyte metabotropic signaling while leaving neuronal function intact (Bonansco et al. 2011, Hassel et al. 1992). If astrocytes in the DVC are sensitive to low glucose availability, and, if they are involved in triggering a vagally mediated increase in gastric motility, then locally applied (fourth ventricular; 4V) FC should block the increase in motility seen following localized hindbrain cytoglucopenia induced by 4V 2-deoxy-glucose (2DG; competitive antagonist of glycolysis). 4V-FC should also reduce gastric motility responses to systematic hypoglycemia produced by subcutaneous insulin. As Figure 10.1 shows, FC applied to 4V blocks the increase in gastric motility produced by either central or peripheral cytoglucopenia. Additionally, in vivo single unit recordings (Figure 10.2) of physiologically identified neurons in the DVC show that hypoglycemic conditions ("4V 2DG") alter the sensitivity of both NST and DMN neurons responding to slight gastric distension. While FC, alone, has no effect on the sensitivity of either NST or DMN neurons responding to gastric distension, it is clear that interfering with astrocytic function via the pretreatment of FC prior to hypoglycemic conditions ("4V FC + 2DG") blocks the sensitization of both NST and DMN neurons to afferent information. Lastly, preliminary evidence suggests that 4V-FC blocks the increase in blood glucose evoked by 2DG (Figure 10.3). These data

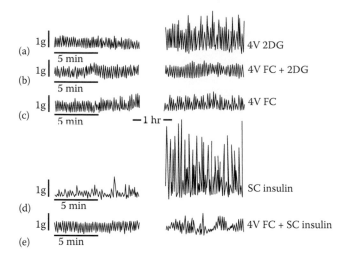

FIGURE 10.1 Glucoprivic stimuli evoke increases in gastric motility that can be blocked by fourth ventricular application of fluorocitrate (FC) in the anesthetized rat. Plots on the left are gastric strain gauge recordings taken before any experimental manipulation. Plots on the right represent strain gauge recordings an hour after the application of a stimulus. (a) 2DG applied to the floor of the fourth ventricle (4V 2DG) causes a significant increase in gastric motility. (b) Fluorocitrate, an astrocyte-specific metabolic antagonist, applied to the fourth ventricle before 2DG (4V FC + 2DG) blocks the 2DG effect. (c) FC applied to the fourth ventricle (4V FC) alone has no effect on basal gastric motility pattern. (d) Subcutaneous insulin produces a dramatic increase in gastric motility (SC Insulin). (e) Fourth ventricular FC largely blocks the effects of insulin to increase gastric motility (4V FC + SC insulin). These data suggest that astrocytes in the hindbrain detect glucoprivic conditions and can activate vagal pro-motility circuits. (Modified from Hermann, G.E., Viard, E., Rogers R.C., *J. Neurosci.*, 34, 10488–10496, 2014.)

and the results obtained by Marty et al. (Marty et al. 2005, Marty, Dallaporta, and Thorens 2007) argue persuasively in favor of hindbrain astrocyte involvement in counterregulatory control of glucose production. Note, however, that the CRR is itself a complex collection of responses. Thus, while astrocyte involvement in the CNS cytoglucopenia-triggered increase in gastric motility (Hermann, Viard, and Rogers 2014) and glucagon mediated increase in plasma glucose (Marty et al. 2005) is highly likely, it is not clear if astrocytes are directly involved in triggering the feeding, epinephrine, or corticosterone dependent aspects of CRR.

10.5.3 Physiological Evidence for Low-Glucose-Sensitive Astrocytes in the Hindbrain

While compelling, the data discussed so far concerning astrocyte low glucose detection were collected using indirect methods. Direct physiological study of astrocyte "activation" is difficult since these cells are not electrically excitable cells and produce no obvious electrical signatures of activation as do neuronal or beta cell glucosensors.

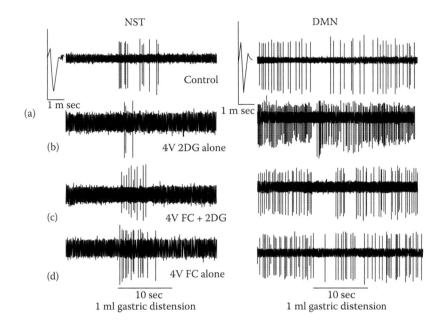

FIGURE 10.2 Effects of 4V 2DG glucoprivation and fluorocitrate (FC) on single identified gastric reflex control neurons in the hindbrain. Left panel: single-unit NST neuron responses to gastric balloon distension (1 ml). Note that 2DG reduces the excitation of the NST neuron responding to vagal afferent distension information (b). While the astrocytic metabolic blocker (fluorocitrate; FC) alone has no effect on NST neuron responsiveness (d). FC blunts the 2DG effect (c). Right panels: These DMN neurons are reflexly inhibited by NST neurons, as can be readily observed from their response to the same gastric distension signal. 2DG greatly accelerates basal DMN firing and obstructs the firing rate inhibition normally caused by gastric distension. Again, FC has no effect of and by itself on DMN firing; however, the 2DG effect on DMN responsiveness is blocked by FC. Insets in (a) (both left and right panels): multiple extracellular action potentials of the neuron being monitored are superimposed on an expanded time scale to show the unitary nature of the recordings. Compression of the spike train records for the purpose of evaluating 10-sec intervals causes an apparent distortion of spike shape and amplitude. All spike train records analyzed for this study were confirmed to be from single units. These results suggest that NST-astrocytes detect glucopenia and, via gliotransmission, inhibit NST-neurons that receive inputs from the gut. NST neurons inhibit DMN neurons that excite the stomach; the end result is that glial effects to reduce NST excitability ultimately increases gastric motility. (Modified from Hermann, G.E., Viard, E., Rogers R.C., *J. Neurosci.*, 34, 10488–10496, 2014.)

So, unlike neurons, they cannot be studied with direct electrophysiological methods (Araque et al. 1999). Astrocyte signaling is based on calcium flux (Araque, Carmignoto, and Haydon 2001, Vance, Rogers, and Hermann 2015). Calcium signals can be generated by membrane channel activities, but as in other cell types, transmembrane calcium flux is usually coupled to mass calcium release from storage in the ER via CICR through ER ryanodine channels. However, mass release of calcium from ER storage can also occur through a completely separate but parallel inositol

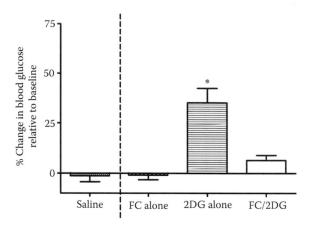

FIGURE 10.3 Hindbrain glucoprivation (fourth ventricular 2DG alone; 3 mg) in Inactin anesthetized rats increased blood glucose levels an average of 35% above baseline levels. While 4V application of the metabolic blocker of astrocytes, fluorocitrate (FC; 5 nanomoles), alone has no effect on basal blood glucose levels, pretreatment with FC prevented 2DG stimulation to increase blood glucose relative to baseline. These data suggest that hindbrain astrocytes are critical detectors of glucoprivation and triggers of CRR. (From Rogers, R. et al., Astrocytes in the hindbrain trigger counterregulation, abstract presented at annual meeting of Society for Study of Ingestive Behavior, Denver, CO, http://www.ssib.org/web/past_programs /SSIB_2015_Abstracts.pdf, 2015.)

tris-phosphate (IP3) channel. This mechanism for ER calcium release is activated by G-protein receptors coupled to phospholipase C (PLC). When activated by Gq-type receptors (such as the PAR receptor), PLC cleaves the membrane phospholipid PIP2 into diacyl glycerol and IP3. The "wave" of cytoplasmic calcium released from the ER due to membrane receptor signaling initiates a cascade of signal transduction events, most notably vesicle secretion from beta cells and gliotransmission from astrocytes (Satin 2000, Zorec et al. 2012). The ER calcium-ATPase pumps are largely responsible for the restoration of cytoplasmic calcium to low levels after signaling events. Reestablishing the transmembrane and ER to cytoplasm concentration gradients is necessary for renewed calcium signaling. Modulation of the calcium ATPase pump and changes in the rate of removal of cytoplasmic calcium could alter the dynamics of the calcium signal as well (Nett, Oloff, and McCarthy 2002).

Astrocyte calcium signaling can be observed directly, in real time, only under physiological conditions with the aid of exogenously applied calcium-sensitive fluorescent intracellular dyes (or genetic constructs such as GCaMP; a genetically encoded calcium indicator fused with green fluorescent protein) in combination with laser confocal in vitro and ex vivo tissue slice recording methods. Our laboratory originally used these methods to determine that PAR signaling in the hindbrain operated through gliotransmission to neurons in the NST (Hermann et al. 2009). Using similar confocal live cell imaging methods, we have recently produced unambiguous evidence that astrocytes in the NST produce cytoplasmic calcium signals proportional to a reduction in glucose concentration or the intracellular store of utilizable

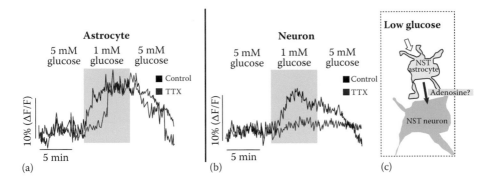

FIGURE 10.4 Astrocytic glucodetection is independent of neuronal glucodetection. Mixed fields of NST-astrocytes and neurons were exposed to 1 mM glucose concentrations with and without the presence of TTX (blocker of neuron action potential) in the perfusion bath. (a) Response of NST-astrocytes to a low-glucose challenge is shown by black trace; the presence of 1 μM TTX did not effectively alter the astrocytic response (red trace). In contrast, (b) the response of NST-neurons to low-glucose challenge was nearly abolished in the presence of bath TTX (black trace = control condition; red trace = TTX condition). (c) These data suggest that NST neuronal responses to low glucose are driven by gliotransmitter inputs from astrocytes. The literature suggests that adenosine could be the candidate gliotransmitter. (Modified from McDougal, D.H., Hermann, G.E., Rogers, R.C., *Front. Neurosci.*, 7, 249, 2013.)

glucose (McDougal, Hermann, and Rogers 2013). In these studies, astrocytes and neurons in the NST were labeled with CalciumGreen 1-AM, an intracellular calcium reporter dye. Astrocytes were discriminated from neurons with the aid of an astrocyte-specific vital stain, SR101. Reductions of bath glucose concentrations from "normal" level (5 mM; 90 mg%) to hypoglycemic levels (1 mM; 18 mg%) produced a robust increase in calcium signal in astrocytes that returned to basal levels in the presence of normal glucose Krebs solution. This effect was also seen with 2DG (in 5 mM glucose), thus demonstrating that astrocyte calcium signaling is related to changes in utilizable intracellular glucose (Figure 10.4).

NST neurons also produced an increase in cytoplasmic calcium, but after a significant delay relative to astrocytic activation (Figure 10.5). Further, pharmacologic inactivation of neuronal excitability and synaptic transmission with TTX eliminated increases in calcium signal in *neurons*, but not in *astrocytes* (Figure 10.5). These results correspond well with those of Marty et al. (2005) and suggest that astrocytes in the NST are intrinsically responsive to reductions in metabolizable glucose.

10.5.4 ASTROCYTE GLUCOSE DETECTION; DIFFERENCES FROM "CLASSIC" MODELS

The mechanism by which a reduction in glucose availability signals an increase in cytoplasmic calcium in the NST-astrocyte remains a matter for speculation. While astrocytic expression of GLUT2 appears necessary for proper glucose counterregulation (Marty et al. 2005), the "classic" transduction mechanisms coupled to GLUT2 in beta cells and neurons produce changes in calcium that run in the opposite direction to that observed for astrocytes (Figure 10.6). For example, pancreatic beta

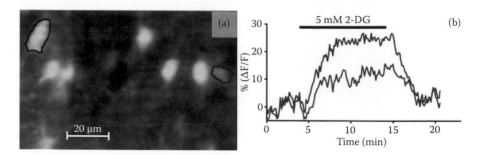

FIGURE 10.5 Low glucose and glucoprivic challenges and effects on NST astrocytes and neurons. (a) Live cell calcium imaging from the rat NST slice preparation. Astrocytes and neurons are preloaded with Calcium Green (an intracellular dye whose fluorescence is proportional to calcium concentration). Astrocytes are stained red with a selective astrocyte vital stain, SR101. Therefore, astrocytes are double labeled and appear yellow (example is circled in red); neurons only take up the Calcium Green (example circled in blue). (b) Plots of the change in calcium signal produced by perfusing the slice with 5 mM 2DG (blocker of glucose utilization). Responses to 2DG block of cellular glucose utilization of an astrocyte (red line = cell circled in red in panel [a]) and a neuron (blue line = cell circled in blue in panel [a]). Astrocytes respond with larger amplitude, larger integrated response (area under the curve), and more rapidly than neurons. (Modified from McDougal, D.H., Hermann, G.E., Rogers, R.C., *Front. Neurosci.*, 7, 249, 2013.)

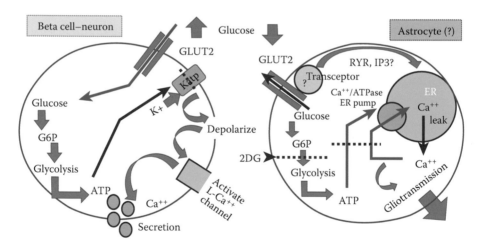

FIGURE 10.6 Fundamental differences in how the "classic model" (i.e., beta cell) of glucodetection must differ from the astrocyte mechanism: (1) activating levels of glucose are opposite. That is, glucopenia activates astrocytes, while elevated glucose activates beta cells and glucose-sensitive neurons. (2) The mechanism of glucose activation of beta cells is well known; ATP generated by glycolysis inhibits a dominant K+ conductance, causing depolarization. Depolarization opens voltage-gated cation channels triggering action potential generation and/or secretion. (3) Mechanisms for activating calcium entry/release after low glucose exposure are not known but may involve ATP "starvation" induced shutdown of ER calcium storage followed by calcium leakage from the ER. The role of "transceptors" attached to GLUT2, possibly mediating ER calcium release (via inhibition or activation) are common in yeast and may exist in vertebrates, but this is not yet clear.

cells respond with an increase in intracellular calcium levels in response to increasing extracellular glucose. As discussed earlier, glucose is transported through the GLUT2 transporter and metabolized via glycolysis and the tricarboxylic acid cycle to CO_2, producing ATP. Increased cellular ATP energy charge acts to phosphorylate and inactivate K_{ATP} channels, leading to depolarization, activation of voltage gated calcium channels, and ending in excitation-secretion coupling in the beta cell (Holsbeeks et al. 2004, Levin et al. 2004, Schuit et al. 2001).

However, not unlike our observations, others have reported that glucose restriction in cultured astrocytes causes an increase in astrocytic cytoplasmic calcium signals. Similar to our present studies, this increase in cytoplasmic calcium is reversed with the restoration of normal levels of glucose in the perfusion bath. Astrocytes are highly dependent on glycolysis for ATP production; removal of glucose or blocking glucose utilization may rapidly starve astrocytes of glucose for ATP production. With impaired glycolysis and subsequent low ATP following low extracellular glucose availability, the calcium-ATPase pump in the ER of astrocytes fails and ER calcium is released to the cytoplasm (Arnold 2005, Kahlert and Reiser 2000). These results are consistent with our observations in the slice preparation. However, it is not clear if this mechanism is actually responsible for the cytoplasmic calcium signal seen by our laboratory in in situ NST-astrocytes. One reason for doubt is that the response time for astrocytes in our NST slice preparation (McDougal, Hermann, and Rogers 2013) is about fivefold faster than that reported for cultured hippocampal astrocytes (Arnold 2005, Kahlert and Reiser 2000).

Rapid signaling of glucose status in intact hindbrain astrocytes may involve the action of a GLUT2-glucose "transceptor" (that may not be present in hippocampal or cultured astrocytes). GLUT2 is the only mammalian glucose transporter that may act as a "transceptor," i.e., a protein that functions as both a transporter and receptor (Figure 10.6). A GLUT2-based transceptor could detect changes in extracellular glucose concentration and then rapidly initiate a calcium-based transduction event. This system would function somewhat like a ligand-gated cation channel or a membrane G-protein-based receptor linked to ER calcium release. Transgenic mice generated to knock down a GLUT2-intracellular loop domain yielded animals that demonstrated an inability to detect glucose but left the GLUT2-dependent glucose transport unaffected (Stolarczyk et al. 2010, 2007). While the possibility of the GLUT2 "transceptor" is intriguing, any mechanism connecting GLUT2 transceptor-like activation with downstream changes in calcium remains uninvestigated.

10.6 GLIAL ADAPTATION IN HAAF

Astrocytes appear to be important detectors and triggers for the initiation of hypoglycemic CRR. It makes sense then, to consider the astrocyte as a potential target for the disruption of CRR by repeated, usually iatrogenic bouts of hypoglycemia that produce HAAF (i.e., the conscious and physiological inability to detect and correct the hypoglycemic state). It has long been known that astrocyte-neural substrate-product interactions are the fundamental elements of overall cerebral metabolism. Recent evidence suggests that these interactions may be altered by exposure to recurrent hypoglycemia, especially in individuals with HAAF.

As early as the 1960–70s, experimental evidence suggested that cerebral metabo-lism could be divided into two separate metabolic compartments, one that relied primarily on glycolysis for energy production and another that relied on mitochon-drial oxidative phosphorylation to supply energy (Berl et al. 1962, Garfinkel 1970, Lajtha, Berl, and Waelsch 1959, van den Berg and Garfinkel 1971). The Krebs cycle in the glycolytic compartment was overwhelmingly "synthetic," meaning it was used to synthesize amino acids, primarily glutamine, rather than to generate energy. It was subsequently determined this compartmentalization was a function of the dis-tinct metabolic signatures of glia and neurons, with the glycolytic compartment and synthetic Krebs cycle lodged within the glial cell (Cruz and Cerdan 1999, Fonnum, Johnsen, and Hassel 1997, Hertz et al. 1999).

Although distinct, there is a high degree of metabolic interdependence between glia and neurons. It is generally accepted that under conditions of high fuel demand, neurons rely on the metabolism of glial-derived lactate to supplement their energy needs (Magistretti et al. 1999, Pellerin et al. 2007). The glial and neural Krebs cycles are also linked via the transfer of intermediates and related metabolites. Glial-derived glutamine is transported to adjacent neurons, where it is converted into glu-tamate, while neurons supply GABA to glia, which is used to generate Krebs cycle intermediates (Cruz and Cerdan 1999, Hertz et al. 1999, van den Berg and Garfinkel 1971). This interdependence makes measurement of specific alterations in glial or neuronal metabolism challenging.

However, one mechanism for overcoming these analytical challenges is through the use of substrates, which are exclusively metabolized by glial cells, such as acetate (Deelchand et al. 2009, Muir, Berl, and Clarke 1986, Waniewski and Martin 1998). Similar to other monocarboxylate substates such as lactate and ketone bodies, acetate is transported into cells via monocarboxylate transporters (MCTs), where it enters the Krebs cycle following conversion into acetyl-coenzyme A (CoA). In contrast to glial cells, neurons do not express the MCT isoforms necessary for transport of acetate (Deelchand et al. 2009, Muir, Berl, and Clarke 1986, Waniewski and Martin 1998). This allows acetate to be used for direct measurement of glial metabolism, specifically alteration in the flux through the glial Krebs cycle. More specifically, the labeling of specific acetate carbon(s) molecules permits the measurement of acetate metabolism by tracking the time course of the label's incorporation into downstream metabolites, mainly glutamine (Cruz and Cerdan 1999, Lebon et al. 2002).

Historically, astrocyte-specific carbon flux analysis involved radioisotopic labeling techniques, which confined the technique to the animal model. More recently, advances in ^{13}C magnetic resonance spectroscopy (MRS) have permit-ted the measurement of cell-specific metabolic fluxes in human subjects. MRS is a companion technique to magnetic resonance imaging, which is used to nonin-vasively assess metabolism in a variety of tissues. When endogenous compounds (such as glucose, lactate, and acetate) are labeled with ^{13}C, a naturally occurring stable isotope of carbon, the ^{13}C MRS spectra measured can be used to determine the concentrations of their metabolic by-products. When used in conjunction with intravenous infusion of ^{13}C acetate, MRS can be implemented for the targeted measurement of human glial metabolism in both the normal and diseased state, e.g., HAAF.

Interestingly, ^{13}C MRS studies investigating alterations in cerebral metabolism have demonstrated that HAAF exposure to hypoglycemia is generally associated specifically with perturbations in glial metabolism, as opposed to changes in global cerebral glucose metabolism. More specifically, exposure to acute hypoglycemia does not alter metabolic fluxes associated with neuronal glucose metabolism, the kinetics of cerebral glucose transport, or the cerebral metabolic rate of glucose consumption (van de Ven et al. 2011, 2012). Furthermore, individuals with long-standing type 1 diabetes (T1DM; a population that is likely to experience frequent bouts of iatrogenic hypoglycemia) show little indication of alterations in neuronal glucose metabolism relative to nondiabetic subjects (Brooks et al. 1986, Grill et al. 1990, Segel et al. 2001, van de Ven et al. 2012). Therefore, the cerebral oxidative metabolism of glucose, which is largely confined to neurons, appears to be largely unaffected by both acute and chronic exposure to hypoglycemia.

In contrast, changes in astrocyte metabolism are observed in response to acute hypoglycemia in individuals with T1DM (Mason et al. 2006), as well as in diabetic patients with HAAF under hypoglycemic conditions (Gulanski et al. 2013). Furthermore, these changes in astrocyte metabolism are significantly correlated with reductions in the CRR magnitude of the autonomic response to severe hypoglycemia (Gulanski et al. 2013). These observations are supported by similar changes in astrocyte metabolism which have been reported in an animal model of HAAF (Jiang et al. 2009). In addition, T1DM patients display an increase in brain lactate concentrations (lactate is monocarboxylic acid similar to acetate) during hypoglycemia relative to nondiabetic patients (De Feyter et al. 2013). Similar changes in astrocyte metabolism, as measured by metabolic flux of ^{13}C acetate, have also been observed in an animal model of HAAF (Jiang et al. 2009). Taken together, these findings suggest that astrocyte metabolism is preferentially altered by exposure to hypoglycemia. These changes may represent metabolic adaptations aimed at increasing the utilization of nonglucose substrates, such as lactate, to meet energy demands during periods of low glucose availability, i.e., hypoglycemia.

10.7   CONCLUSION

It is very likely that these astrocytic metabolic adaptations to repeated bouts of hypoglycemia are reflected in a subsequent lack of sensitivity to reductions in glucose. In adapting to the utilization of fuels other than glucose, the astrocyte detection of glucose or the ability to produce physiologically relevant gliotransmission communications with critical CRR-generating neurons in the hindbrain may be suppressed. Understanding the detailed mechanisms connecting glial metabolism with gliotransmission will be instrumental to formulating therapies to overcome HAAF.

LITERATURE CITED

Accorsi-Mendonca, D., L. G. H. Bonagamba, and B. H. Machado. 2012. ATP released by glia increases the excitatory neurotransmission onto NTS neurons related to the peripheral chemoreflex. *Soc Neurosci*:824.09.

Agulhon, C., K. M. Boyt, A. X. Xie, F. Friocourt, B. L. Roth, and K. D. McCarthy. 2013. Modulation of the autonomic nervous system and behaviour by acute glial cell Gq protein-coupled receptor activation in vivo. *J Physiol* 591:5599–609.

Agulhon, C., T. A. Fiacco, and K. D. McCarthy. 2010. Hippocampal short- and long-term plasticity are not modulated by astrocyte Ca2+ signaling. *Science* 327:1250–4.

Andrew, S. F., T. T. Dinh, and S. Ritter. 2007. Localized glucoprivation of hindbrain sites elicits corticosterone and glucagon secretion. *Am J Physiol Regul Integr Comp Physiol* 292:R1792–8.

Angulo, M. C., A. S. Kozlov, S. Charpak, and E. Audinat. 2004. Glutamate released from glial cells synchronizes neuronal activity in the hippocampus. *J Neurosci* 24:6920–7.

Araque, A., G. Carmignoto, and P. G. Haydon. 2001. Dynamic signaling between astrocytes and neurons. *Annu Rev Physiol* 63:795–813.

Araque, A., V. Parpura, R. P. Sanzgiri, and P. G. Haydon. 1999. Tripartite synapses: Glia, the unacknowledged partner. *Trends Neurosci* 22:208–15.

Arnold, S. 2005. Estrogen suppresses the impact of glucose deprivation on astrocytic calcium levels and signaling independently of the nuclear estrogen receptor. *Neurobiol Dis* 20:82–92.

Ashcroft, F. M. 1988. Adenosine 5′-triphosphate-sensitive potassium channels. *Annu Rev Neurosci* 11:97–118.

Berl, S., G. Takagaki, D. D. Clarke, and H. Waelsch. 1962. Metabolic compartments in vivo. Ammonia and glutamic acid metabolism in brain and liver. *J Biol Chem* 237:2562–9.

Bernard, C. 1848. De l'origine de sucre dans l'économie animale. *Arch Gén de Méd.* 4e:303–19. http://www.claude-bernard.co.uk/page2.htm.

Bernard, C. 1849. Magendie annonce à l'Académie des Sciences que Bernard a achevé une augmentation de glucose dans le sang par une blessure d'un certain point du cerveau. *C R Hebd Acad Sci T* 28:393–4. http://www.claude-bernard.co.uk/page2.htm.

Bernard, C. 1877. *Leçons sur le diabète et la glycogenèse animale.* Paris, Baillière: 576. Cours du Collège de France, rec: Mathias Duval. http://www.claude-bernard.co.uk/page2.htm.

Bezzi, P., G. Carmignoto, L. Pasti, S. Vesce, D. Rossi, B. L. Rizzini, T. Pozzan, and A. Volterra. 1998. Prostaglandins stimulate calcium-dependent glutamate release in astrocytes. *Nature* 391:281–5.

Bonansco, C., A. Couve, G. Perea, C. A. Ferradas, M. Roncagliolo, and M. Fuenzalida. 2011. Glutamate released spontaneously from astrocytes sets the threshold for synaptic plasticity. *Eur J Neurosci* 33:1483–92.

Brooks, C. M. 1931. A delimitation of the central nervous mechanism involved in reflex hyperglycemia. *Am J Physiol* 99:64–76.

Brooks, D. J., J. S. Gibbs, P. Sharp, S. Herold, D. R. Turton, S. K. Luthra, E. M. Kohner, S. R. Bloom, and T. Jones. 1986. Regional cerebral glucose transport in insulin-dependent diabetic patients studied using [11C]3-*O*-methyl-D-glucose and positron emission tomography. *J Cereb Blood Flow Metab* 6:240–4.

Bulatao, E., and A. J. Carlson. 1924. Contributions to the physiology of the stomach: Influence of experimental changes in blood sugar level on gastric hunger contractions *Am J Physiol* 69:107–15.

Bushong, E. A., M. E. Martone, Y. Z. Jones, and M. H. Ellisman. 2002. Protoplasmic astrocytes in CA1 stratum radiatum occupy separate anatomical domains. *J Neurosci* 22:183–92.

Cajal, S. R. 1995. *Histology of the nervous system.* Translated by N. Swanson and L. W. Swanson. 2 vols. Vol. 1. New York: Oxford University Press.

Cannon, W. B., and A. L. Washburn. 1912. An explanation of hunger. *Am J Physiol* 29:441–54.

Cannon, W. B., M. A. McIver, and S. W. Bliss. 1924. Studies on the conditions of activity in endocrine glands. *Am J Physiol* 69:46–66.

Ciccarelli, R., P. Di Iorio, P. Giuliani, I. D'Alimonte, P. Ballerini, F. Caciagli, and M. P. Rathbone. 1999. Rat cultured astrocytes release guanine-based purines in basal conditions and after hypoxia/hypoglycemia. *Glia* 25:93–8.

Coco, S., F. Calegari, E. Pravettoni, D. Pozzi, E. Taverna, P. Rosa, M. Matteoli, and C. Verderio. 2003. Storage and release of ATP from astrocytes in culture. *J Biol Chem* 278:1354–62.

Cruz, F., and S. Cerdan. 1999. Quantitative 13C NMR studies of metabolic compartmentation in the adult mammalian brain. *NMR Biomed* 12:451–62.

Cryer, P. E., S. N. Davis, and H. Shamoon. 2003. Hypoglycemia in diabetes. *Diabetes Care* 26:1902–12.

De Feyter, H. M., G. F. Mason, G. I. Shulman, D. L. Rothman, and K. F. Petersen. 2013. Increased brain lactate concentrations without increased lactate oxidation during hypoglycemia in type 1 diabetic individuals. *Diabetes* 62:3075–80.

Deelchand, D. K., A. A. Shestov, D. M. Koski, K. Ugurbil, and P. G. Henry. 2009. Acetate transport and utilization in the rat brain. *J Neurochem* 109 Suppl 1:46–54.

DiRocco, R. J., and H. J. Grill. 1979. The forebrain is not essential for sympathoadrenal hyperglycemic response to glucoprivation. *Science* 204:1112–4.

Donovan, C. M., and A. G. Watts. 2014. Peripheral and central glucose sensing in hypoglycemic detection. *Physiology (Bethesda)* 29:314–24.

Dunwiddie, T. V., and S. A. Masino. 2001. The role and regulation of adenosine in the central nervous system. *Annu Rev Neurosci* 24:31–55.

Fellin, T., and G. Carmignoto. 2004. Neurone-to-astrocyte signalling in the brain represents a distinct multifunctional unit. *J Physiol* 559:3–15.

Fonnum, F., A. Johnsen, and B. Hassel. 1997. Use of fluorocitrate and fluoroacetate in the study of brain metabolism. *Glia* 21:106–13.

Funk, G. D. 2010. The 'connexin' between astrocytes, ATP and central respiratory chemoreception. *J Physiol* 588:4335–7.

Garfinkel, D. 1970. A simulation study of brain compartments. I. Fuel sources, and GABA metabolism. *Brain Res* 23:387–406.

Garrick, T., S. Mulvihill, S. Buack, M. Maeda-Hagiwara, and Y. Tache. 1988. Intracerebroventricular pressure inhibits gastric antral and duodenal contractility but not acid secretion in conscious rabbits. *Gastroenterology* 95:26–31.

Gourine, A. V., and S. Kasparov. 2011. Astrocytes as brain interoceptors. *Exp Physiol* 96:411–6.

Gourine, A. V., V. Kasymov, N. Marina, F. Tang, M. F. Figueiredo, S. Lane, A. G. Teschemacher, K. M. Spyer, K. Deisseroth, and S. Kasparov. 2010. Astrocytes control breathing through pH-dependent release of ATP. *Science* 329:571–5.

Grill, V., M. Gutniak, O. Bjorkman, M. Lindqvist, S. Stone-Elander, R. J. Seitz, G. Blomqvist, P. Reichard, and L. Widen. 1990. Cerebral blood flow and substrate utilization in insulin-treated diabetic subjects. *Am J Physiol* 258:E813–20.

Guillod-Maximin, E., A. Lorsignol, T. Alquier, and L. Penicaud. 2004. Acute intracarotid glucose injection towards the brain induces specific c-fos activation in hypothalamic nuclei: Involvement of astrocytes in cerebral glucose-sensing in rats. *J Neuroendocrinol* 16:464–71.

Gulanski, B. I., H. M. De Feyter, K. A. Page, R. Belfort-DeAguiar, G. F. Mason, D. L. Rothman, and R. S. Sherwin. 2013. Increased brain transport and metabolism of acetate in hypoglycemia unawareness. *J Clin Endocrinol Metab* 98:3811–20.

Halassa, M. M., and P. G. Haydon. 2010. Integrated brain circuits: Astrocytic networks modulate neuronal activity and behavior. *Annu Rev Physiol* 72:335–55.

Halassa, M. M., T. Fellin, and P. G. Haydon. 2009. Tripartite synapses: Roles for astrocytic purines in the control of synaptic physiology and behavior. *Neuropharmacology* 57:343–6.

Halassa, M. M., T. Fellin, H. Takano, J. H. Dong, and P. G. Haydon. 2007. Synaptic islands defined by the territory of a single astrocyte. *J Neurosci* 27:6473–7.

Hassel, B., R. E. Paulsen, A. Johnsen, and F. Fonnum. 1992. Selective inhibition of glial cell metabolism in vivo by fluorocitrate. *Brain Res* 576:120–4.

Haydon, P. G., and G. Carmignoto. 2006. Astrocyte control of synaptic transmission and neurovascular coupling. *Physiol Rev* 86:1009–31.

Hermann, G. E., J. S. Nasse, and R. C. Rogers. 2005. Alpha-1 adrenergic input to solitary nucleus neurones: Calcium oscillations, excitation and gastric reflex control. *J Physiol* 562:553–68.

Hermann, G. E., M. J. Van Meter, J. C. Rood, and R. C. Rogers. 2009. Proteinase-activated receptors in the nucleus of the solitary tract: Evidence for glial-neural interactions in autonomic control of the stomach. *J Neurosci* 29:9292–300.

Hermann, G. E., E. Viard, and R. C. Rogers. 2014. Hindbrain glucoprivation effects on gastric vagal reflex circuits and gastric motility in the rat are suppressed by the astrocyte inhibitor fluorocitrate. *J Neurosci* 34:10488–96.

Hertz, L., R. Dringen, A. Schousboe, and S. R. Robinson. 1999. Astrocytes: Glutamate producers for neurons. *J Neurosci Res* 57:417–28.

Holsbeeks, I., O. Lagatie, A. Van Nuland, S. Van de Velde, and J. M. Thevelein. 2004. The eukaryotic plasma membrane as a nutrient-sensing device. *Trends Biochem Sci* 29:556–64.

Hudson, B., and S. Ritter. 2004. Hindbrain catecholamine neurons mediate consummatory responses to glucoprivation. *Physiol Behav* 82:241–50.

Islam, M. S. 2010. Calcium signaling in the islets. *Adv Exp Med Biol* 654:235–59.

Jiang, L., R. I. Herzog, G. F. Mason, R. A. de Graaf, D. L. Rothman, R. S. Sherwin, and K. L. Behar. 2009. Recurrent antecedent hypoglycemia alters neuronal oxidative metabolism in vivo. *Diabetes* 58:1266–74.

Kahlert, S., and G. Reiser. 2000. Requirement of glycolytic and mitochondrial energy supply for loading of Ca(2+) stores and InsP(3)-mediated Ca(2+) signaling in rat hippocampus astrocytes. *J Neurosci Res* 61:409–20.

Klip, A., and M. Hawkins. 2005. Desperately seeking sugar: Glial cells as hypoglycemia sensors. *J Clin Invest* 115:3403–5.

Lajtha, A., S. Berl, and H. Waelsch. 1959. Amino acid and protein metabolism of the brain. IV. The metabolism of glutamic acid. *J Neurochem* 3:322–32.

Larson, G. M., S. Koch, T. M. O'Dorisio, B. Osadchey, P. McGraw, and J. D. Richardson. 1984. Gastric response to severe head injury. *Am J Surg* 147:97–105.

Lebon, V., K. F. Petersen, G. W. Cline, J. Shen, G. F. Mason, S. Dufour, K. L. Behar, G. I. Shulman, and D. L. Rothman. 2002. Astroglial contribution to brain energy metabolism in humans revealed by 13C nuclear magnetic resonance spectroscopy: Elucidation of the dominant pathway for neurotransmitter glutamate repletion and measurement of astrocytic oxidative metabolism. *J Neurosci* 22:1523–31.

Levin, B. E., A. A. Dunn-Meynell, and V. H. Routh. 1999. Brain glucose sensing and body energy homeostasis: Role in obesity and diabetes. *Am J Physiol* 276:R1223–31.

Levin, B. E., V. H. Routh, L. Kang, N. M. Sanders, and A. A. Dunn-Meynell. 2004. Neuronal glucosensing: What do we know after 50 years? *Diabetes* 53:2521–8.

Li, A. J., Q. Wang, T. T. Dinh, B. R. Powers, and S. Ritter. 2014. Stimulation of feeding by three different glucose-sensing mechanisms requires hindbrain catecholamine neurons. *Am J Physiol Regul Integr Comp Physiol* 306:R257–64.

Li, A. J., Q. Wang, T. T. Dinh, and S. Ritter. 2009. Simultaneous silencing of Npy and Dbh expression in hindbrain A1/C1 catecholamine cells suppresses glucoprivic feeding. *J Neurosci* 29:280–7.

Li, A. J., Q. Wang, T. T. Dinh, M. F. Wiater, A. K. Eskelsen, and S. Ritter. 2013. Hindbrain catecholamine neurons control rapid switching of metabolic substrate use during glucoprivation in male rats. *Endocrinology* 154:4570–9.

Lin, L. H., S. A. Moore, S. Y. Jones, J. McGlashon, and W. T. Talman. 2013. Astrocytes in the rat nucleus tractus solitarii are critical for cardiovascular reflex control. *J Neurosci* 33:18608–17.

Magistretti, P. J., L. Pellerin, D. L. Rothman, and R. G. Shulman. 1999. Energy on demand. *Science* 283:496–7.

Martineau, M., T. Shi, J. Puyal, A. M. Knolhoff, J. Dulong, B. Gasnier, J. Klingauf, J. V. Sweedler, R. Jahn, and J. P. Mothet. 2013. Storage and uptake of D-serine into astrocytic synaptic-like vesicles specify gliotransmission. *J Neurosci* 33:3413–23.

Marty, N., M. Dallaporta, M. Foretz, M. Emery, D. Tarussio, I. Bady, C. Binnert, F. Beermann, and B. Thorens. 2005. Regulation of glucagon secretion by glucose transporter type 2 (glut2) and astrocyte-dependent glucose sensors. *J Clin Invest* 115:3545–53.

Marty, N., M. Dallaporta, and B. Thorens. 2007. Brain glucose sensing, counterregulation, and energy homeostasis. *Physiology (Bethesda)* 22:241–51.

Mason, G. F., K. F. Petersen, V. Lebon, D. L. Rothman, and G. I. Shulman. 2006. Increased brain monocarboxylic acid transport and utilization in type 1 diabetes. *Diabetes* 55: 929–34.

Mazzarello, P. 2010. *Golgi: Biography of the founder of modern neuroscience.* New York, New York: Oxford University Press.

McDougal, D. H., G. E. Hermann, and R. C. Rogers. 2011. Vagal afferent stimulation activates astrocytes in the nucleus of the solitary tract via AMPA receptors: Evidence of an atypical neural–glial interaction in the brainstem. *J Neurosci* 31:14037–45.

McDougal, D. H., G. E. Hermann, and R. C. Rogers. 2013. Astrocytes in the nucleus of the solitary tract are activated by low glucose or glucoprivation: Evidence for glial involvement in glucose homeostasis. *Front Neurosci* 7:249.

Meghji, P., J. B. Tuttle, and R. Rubio. 1989. Adenosine formation and release by embryonic chick neurons and glia in cell culture. *J Neurochem* 53:1852–60.

Mimee, A., and A. V. Ferguson. 2015. Glycemic state regulates melanocortin, but not nesfatin-1, responsiveness of glucose-sensing neurons in the nucleus of the solitary tract. *Am J Physiol Regul Integr Comp Physiol* 308:R690–9.

Minor, T. R., M. K. Rowe, R. F. Soames Job, and E. C. Ferguson. 2001. Escape deficits induced by inescapable shock and metabolic stress are reversed by adenosine receptor antagonists. *Behav Brain Res* 120:203–12.

Muir, D., S. Berl, and D. D. Clarke. 1986. Acetate and fluoroacetate as possible markers for glial metabolism in vivo. *Brain Res* 380:336–40.

Nett, W. J., S. H. Oloff, and K. D. McCarthy. 2002. Hippocampal astrocytes in situ exhibit calcium oscillations that occur independent of neuronal activity. *J Neurophysiol* 87:528–37.

Parpura, V., and P. G. Haydon. 2000. Physiological astrocytic calcium levels stimulate glutamate release to modulate adjacent neurons. *Proc Natl Acad Sci U S A* 97:8629–34.

Pasti, L., A. Volterra, T. Pozzan, and G. Carmignoto. 1997. Intracellular calcium oscillations in astrocytes: A highly plastic, bidirectional form of communication between neurons and astrocytes in situ. *J Neurosci* 17:7817–30.

Pellerin, L., A. K. Bouzier-Sore, A. Aubert, S. Serres, M. Merle, R. Costalat, and P. J. Magistretti. 2007. Activity-dependent regulation of energy metabolism by astrocytes: An update. *Glia* 55:1251–62.

Penicaud, L., C. Leloup, X. Fioramonti, A. Lorsignol, and A. Benani. 2006. Brain glucose sensing: A subtle mechanism. *Curr Opin Clin Nutr Metab Care* 9:458–62.

Perea, G., M. Navarrete, and A. Araque. 2009. Tripartite synapses: Astrocytes process and control synaptic information. *Trends Neurosci* 32:421–31.

Porter, J. T., and K. D. McCarthy. 1996. Hippocampal astrocytes in situ respond to glutamate released from synaptic terminals. *J Neurosci* 16:5073–81.

Rinaman, L. 2011. Hindbrain noradrenergic A2 neurons: Diverse roles in autonomic, endocrine, cognitive, and behavioral functions. *Am J Physiol Regul Integr Comp Physiol* 300:R222–35.

Ritter, S., A. J. Li, Q. Wang, and T. T. Dinh. 2011. Minireview: The value of looking backward: The essential role of the hindbrain in counterregulatory responses to glucose deficit. *Endocrinology* 152:4019–32.

Rogers, R. C., and G. E. Hermann. 2012. "Brainstem control of gastric function." In *Physiology of the gastrointestinal tract*, edited by L. R. Johnson, 861–92. London, Waltham, MA, San Diego, CA: Elsevier Academic Press.

Rogers, R. C., R. A. Travagli, and G. E. Hermann. 2003. Noradrenergic neurons in the rat solitary nucleus participate in the esophageal–gastric relaxation reflex. *Am J Physiol Regul Integr Comp Physiol* 285:R479–89.

Rogers, R., S. Ritter, D. McDougal, and G. Hermann. 2015. Astrocytes in the hindbrain trigger counterregulation. Abstract presented at annual meeting of Society for Study of Ingestive Behavior, Denver, CO. http://www.ssib.org/web/past_programs/SSIB_2015 _Abstracts.pdf.

Satin, L. S. 2000. Localized calcium influx in pancreatic beta-cells: Its significance for Ca2+- dependent insulin secretion from the islets of Langerhans. *Endocrine* 13:251–62.

Schuit, F. C., P. Huypens, H. Heimberg, and D. G. Pipeleers. 2001. Glucose sensing in pancreatic beta-cells: A model for the study of other glucose-regulated cells in gut, pancreas, and hypothalamus. *Diabetes* 50:1–11.

Segel, S. A., C. G. Fanelli, C. S. Dence, J. Markham, T. O. Videen, D. S. Paramore, W. J. Powers, and P. E. Cryer. 2001. Blood-to-brain glucose transport, cerebral glucose metabolism, and cerebral blood flow are not increased after hypoglycemia. *Diabetes* 50:1911–7.

Smith, K. 2010. Neuroscience: Settling the great glia debate. *Nature* 468:160–2.

Stolarczyk, E., C. Guissard, A. Michau, P. C. Even, A. Grosfeld, P. Serradas, A. Lorsignol, L. Penicaud, E. Brot-Laroche, A. Leturque, and M. Le Gall. 2010. Detection of extracellular glucose by GLUT2 contributes to hypothalamic control of food intake. *Am J Physiol Endocrinol Metab* 298:E1078–87.

Stolarczyk, E., M. Le Gall, P. Even, A. Houllier, P. Serradas, E. Brot-Laroche, and A. Leturque. 2007. Loss of sugar detection by GLUT2 affects glucose homeostasis in mice. *PLoS One* 2:e1288.

Traynelis, S. F., and J. Trejo. 2007. Protease-activated receptor signaling: New roles and regulatory mechanisms. *Curr Opin Hematol* 14:230–5.

Turner, C. P., M. R. Blackburn, and S. A. Rivkees. 2004. A1 adenosine receptors mediate hypoglycemia-induced neuronal injury. *J Mol Endocrinol* 32:129–44.

van de Ven, K. C., B. E. de Galan, M. van der Graaf, A. A. Shestov, P. G. Henry, C. J. Tack, and A. Heerschap. 2011. Effect of acute hypoglycemia on human cerebral glucose metabolism measured by (1)(3)C magnetic resonance spectroscopy. *Diabetes* 60:1467–73.

van de Ven, K. C., M. van der Graaf, C. J. Tack, A. Heerschap, and B. E. de Galan. 2012. Steady-state brain glucose concentrations during hypoglycemia in healthy humans and patients with type 1 diabetes. *Diabetes* 61:1974–7.

van den Berg, C. J., and D. Garfinkel. 1971. A stimulation study of brain compartments. Metabolism of glutamate and related substances in mouse brain. *Biochem J* 123:211–8.

Vance, K. M., R. C. Rogers, and G. E. Hermann. 2015. PAR1-activated astrocytes in the nucleus of the solitary tract stimulate adjacent neurons via NMDA receptors. *J Neurosci* 35:776–85.

Volterra, A., and J. Meldolesi. 2005. Astrocytes, from brain glue to communication elements: The revolution continues. *Nat Rev Neurosci* 6:626–40.

Waniewski, R. A., and D. L. Martin. 1998. Preferential utilization of acetate by astrocytes is attributable to transport. *J Neurosci* 18:5225–33.

Watts, A. G., and C. M. Donovan. 2010. Sweet talk in the brain: Glucosensing, neural networks, and hypoglycemic counterregulation. *Front Neuroendocrinol* 31:32–43.

Weinstein, J. R., S. J. Gold, D. D. Cunningham, and C. M. Gall. 1995. Cellular localization of thrombin receptor mRNA in rat brain: Expression by mesencephalic dopaminergic neurons and codistribution with prothrombin mRNA. *J Neurosci* 15:2906–19.

Young, J. K., J. H. Baker, and M. I. Montes. 2000. The brain response to 2-deoxy glucose is blocked by a glial drug. *Pharmacol Biochem Behav* 67:233–9.

Zorec, R., A. Araque, G. Carmignoto, P. G. Haydon, A. Verkhratsky, and V. Parpura. 2012. Astroglial excitability and gliotransmission: An appraisal of Ca2+ as a signalling route. *ASN Neuro* 4.

11 Vagal Afferent Signaling and the Integration of Direct and Indirect Controls of Food Intake

Robert C. Ritter, Carlos A. Campos,
Jason Nasse, and James H. Peters

CONTENTS

11.1 INTEGRATION OF SENSORY INFORMATION—THE FOUNDATION FOR CONTROL OF FOOD INTAKE

In terms of individual survival, feeding arguably is the most important behavior in which animals engage, because all physiological functions, including other behaviors, depend on the energy and nutrients obtained only through food intake. Consequently, control of feeding behavior is of high priority for the brain, the organ of behavior. Indeed, it is tempting to argue that selective pressures driving the evolution of ganglia or brains near the oral opening of the digestive system included efficient detection, pursuit, capture, and ingestion of food. Moreover, the anatomical concentration of sensory inputs in ganglia or brain facilitates network interactions between modalities that represent distinct qualities of food, such as chemical composition (taste) and bulk or mass (gut stretch). The integration of afferent information from disparate peripheral sources is the foundation for control of food intake. For a concise review of nervous system and behavioral evolution see Dethier and Stellar (1964).

11.1.1 DIRECT AND INDIRECT CONTROLS OF FOOD INTAKE

Smith (1996) has proposed separating controls of food intake into two distinct categories based on the sources of afferent information from which they derive. Controls derived from preabsorptive stimulation by food itself are "direct controls" of food intake. Taste, gastrointestinal (GI) distension, or gut hormones released in response to food in the digestive tract are examples of direct controls, because they are directly activated by food itself. Controls that do not originate from food-mediated preabsorptive stimuli are "indirect" controls. Hormones, like insulin, leptin or estrogen, circulating metabolites, like glucose or ketoacids, as well as cognitively dependent influences, like advertising, exemplify indirect controls of food intake, because they are derivatives of energy storage, reproductive state, metabolic condition, or cognition, but are not generated from stimulation by food itself. Direct controls are activated transiently by food that is being eaten and, therefore, provide the sensory basis for satiation, the process that leads to meal termination. In contrast to the transient and episodic activation of direct controls of food intake, indirect controls appear to exert effects on feeding in a more tonic fashion, and are engaged over multiple meals. Nevertheless, most indirect controls of food intake are manifested by alterations of meal size, rather than meal frequency, suggesting that indirect controls of food intake might work by modulating the strength or salience of direct, within-meal controls. Modulation of one afferent input by another is a mechanism of integration, i.e., to make integral as one whole, resulting in a unified sensory experience to which an animal responds by altering meal size and total food intake.

11.1.2 INTEGRATING SENSORY SIGNALS TO CONTROL MEAL SIZE—LESSONS FROM FLIES

The adaptive value of direct controls of food intake is exemplified by the observation that nearly all animals possess them, including invertebrates. Studies in blowflies by Vincent Dethier and his colleagues provide an informative example of the importance of direct controls of food intake and of the integration of distinct sensory stimuli in the interest of adaptive ingestive behavior (Dethier and Gelperin 1967). Flies have chemoreceptors in the tarsal hairs on their legs as well as on mouthparts, the labella. Feeding behavior involves walking about until a nutrient is detected by the tarsal receptors (for a review of chemoreception in flies, see Dethier 1976). Detection of nutrient by the tarsal chemoreceptors activates afferents that arrive in the "brain" and trigger reflex lowering of the proboscis into the nutrient. When the proboscis contacts the nutrient, the labellar chemoreceptors and their associated afferents are activated, triggering ingestion. As the fly consumes its meal, stretch receptors in its crop are activated, sending volleys of spikes to the "brain" via the recurrent nerve. The recurrent nerve afferent activity is integrated with labellar and tarsal chemoreceptor inputs, ultimately resulting in withdrawal of the proboscis and termination of the meal. The integration of tarsal, labellar, and crop sensory information is important to fly survival. When the recurrent nerve was cut, flies consumed much more than they could carry aloft (Figure 11.1). In fact, some flies with severed recurrent nerves consumed so much that their abdomens ruptured.

The studies of Dethier and colleagues revealed that the size of a fly's meal is determined by integrating tarsal and labellar chemoreceptor signals with feedback from the crop (Dethier and Gelperin 1967). However, recent experiments in fruit flies have identified populations of neurons in the fly's head ganglion that control food intake in response to stored nutrients (Sassu et al. 2012, Docherty et al. 2015). It is not yet known just how stored nutrients effect changes in fly feeding behavior. It seems likely, however, that feedback signals from stores are integrated with signals from tarsal, labellar, and crop sensors to reduce meal size.

11.1.3 A VERY BRIEF HISTORY OF DIRECT INHIBITORY CONTROL OF FOOD INTAKE IN MAMMALS

Ivan Pavlov (1910) inferred GI control of food intake during his landmark investigations of digestive secretions during the early twentieth century. To facilitate his studies of gastric secretion, Pavlov developed a sham feeding procedure, in which ingested food was prevented from entering the stomach by allowing it to drain from

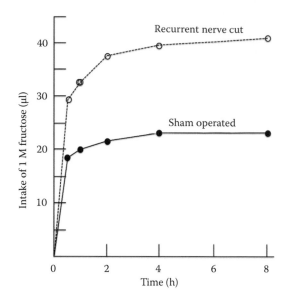

FIGURE 11.1 Increased food intake by blowfly following removal of inhibitory feedback from the digestive tract. (Data redrawn from Dethier, V.G., Gelperin, A., *J. Exp. Biol.*, 47, 191–200, 1967; fly images excerpted from Dethier, V.G., Bodenstein, D., *Z. Tierpsychol.*, 15, 120–140, 1958.)

an open esophageal fistula, enabling collections of secretions uncontaminated by food. Pavlov observed that dogs would continue to eat for hours when the esophageal fistula was open and inferred that rapid termination of eating during real feeding involved inhibitory signals from the GI tract (for an exposition of Pavlov's views on neural control of food intake, see the English translation of his 1910 lecture in Pavlov 1928 and G.P Smith's synopsis and analysis in Smith 1995). Morton Grossman and his collaborators presented direct experimental evidence of inhibitory feedback control of food intake in sham feeding dogs and rats in the late 1940s. They found that infusions of nutrients into the stomach during sham feeding reduced food intake, whereas parenteral infusions of nutrients did not (Janowitz and Grossman 1948, 1949, Janowitz, Hanson, and Grossman 1949). Subsequently, the sham feeding technique has been used by many investigators to establish the importance of gastric and intestinal signals in meal termination in rodents. These studies reveal that direct inhibitory signals that control meal size arise from mechanical stimulation of the stomach (Phillips and Powley 1996) and nutrient stimulation of the intestine (Yox, Stokesberry, and Ritter 1991, Yox and Ritter 1988).

Appreciation of mechanisms by which GI stimuli are transduced to control food intake took a major leap forward in the 1970s, when Smith and coworkers identified the gut peptide, cholecystokinin (CCK), as a putative inhibitory control of food intake that is released from the intestine in response to luminal nutrients (Gibbs, Young, and Smith 1973). Subsequent experiments by the Smith group and others revealed that CCK contributed to the process of satiation (Antin et al. 1975) and that it did so by activating primary afferent neurons in the vagus nerve (Ritter and Ladenheim 1985, Smith, Jerome, and Norgren 1985, South and Ritter 1988). In addition, a number of investigators demonstrated that CCK potentiated responses to other GI stimuli, such as gastric distension, to enhance vagal activation and reduce food intake (see, for example, Moran and McHugh 1988, Schwartz et al. 1991, van de Wall, Duffy, and Ritter 2005). The initial reports of CCK's effects on food intake were followed by several decades of progress during which participation of other GI peptides in the direct control of food intake was uncovered. Similar to CCK, the majority of these peptides appear to act, at least in part, by exciting vagal afferents (Abbott et al. 2005, Labouesse et al. 2012), thereby bolstering a working hypothesis that vagal afferents from the digestive tract are an important avenue by which the brain receives signals that mediate direct control of food intake.

Although, inhibition of food intake by GI signals is extensively documented, it would be incorrect to assume that all direct controls of food intake are inhibitory. For example, rodents, as well as other animals, form preferences for flavors that are associated with postoral nutrient stimuli, including carbohydrates, fats, and amino acid (for a review, see Sclafani and Ackroff 2012). Sclafani (2013) has coined the term *appetition* for the postoral processes that enhance food intake. The neural substrates that mediate appetition are poorly understood and appear to differ between macronutrient classes. For example, the abdominal vagus is necessary for conditioning flavor preferences with the amino acid glutamate (Uematsu et al. 2010), but is not required for conditioning preferences with carbohydrates (Sclafani and Lucas 1996). Similarly, mice in which the fatty acid receptors, GPR40 and GPR120, are knocked out do not form flavor preferences in response to GI long chain fatty acids (Sclafani, Zukerman, and Ackroff 2013), whereas mice in which sweet taste receptors are knocked out are unimpaired with regard to flavor preferences conditioned by GI carbohydrate infusion. While appetition has important effects on food intake, currently, little is known regarding mechanisms for integration of these conditioned effects with other controls of food intake.

11.1.4   Indirect Controls Decrease Food Intake by Reducing Meal Size

11.1.4.1   Control of Food Intake by Estrogen—An Example of Integrating Direct and Indirect Controls

As detailed earlier, indirect controls of food intake do not arise from preabsorptive digestive tract stimulation by food. Nevertheless, it appears that indirect controls of food intake, like direct controls, manifest themselves largely by varying the size of individual meals. For example, food intake of female rats varies with the phase of the estrus cycle, consumption being lower when estrogen levels are peaking and higher when the hormone is at its nadir (for a review of gonadal steroid effects on food intake, see Asarian and Geary 2006). Ovariectomy produces increased food intake, resulting from increased meal size, while estrogen replacement therapy decreases meal size and overall food intake (Asarian and Geary 2002). Observations like these led to the inference that estrogen might control food intake by enhancing direct GI signals, leading to more rapid satiation and reduced meal size. Estrogen receptors are expressed by neurons at multiple sites in the central and peripheral nervous systems, including by vagal primary afferents and neurons in the nucleus of the solitary tract (NTS). As such, estrogen receptor expression is appropriately situated to modulate sensory inputs responsible for GI controls of food intake. In fact, extensive work by Asarian and Geary indicates that estrogen does indeed enhance responsiveness to GI feedback signals, such as CCK (Geary et al. 1994, Asarian and Geary 1999, Geary 2001).

11.1.4.2 Leptin—Indirect Control of Food Intake by Body Fat Stores

Injection of leptin, a 16KD adipokine protein, which arguably is the most intensively investigated indirect control of food intake, potently reduces food intake, almost entirely by reducing meal size (Eckel et al. 1998, Kahler et al. 1998). Furthermore, reduced leptin signaling increases food intake by increasing meal size (Alingh Prins et al. 1986). Leptin is secreted mainly by adipocytes in white fat depots and appears to be the principal endocrine afferent for a negative feedback control of food intake by stored fat (for brief reviews of leptin and negative feedback control of adipose mass, see Harris 2013b, Friedman 2014). Average plasma leptin concentrations are proportional to white adipose mass (Maffei et al. 1995). Rats or humans that are leptin-deficient or leptin-insensitive are hyperphagic and become obese, while administration of recombinant leptin triggers reduction of food intake, increased energy expenditure and loss of body fat (reviewed in Dubern and Clement 2012, Vatier, Gautier, and Vigouroux 2012).

11.1.4.3 Leptin Controls Food Intake by Acting at Multiple Nervous System Sites

Investigation of brain sites where leptin acts to control food intake has focused intensively on the hypothalamus, specifically, the hypothalamic arcuate nucleus (ARC), which contains neurons that express high levels of leptin receptor transcript. Moreover, hypothalamic neurons expressing proopiomelanocortin (POMC) and cocaine-amphetamine-related transcript (CART) or neuropeptide Y and agouti-related protein are of particular importance for leptin's effects on food intake and body weight (Schwartz et al. 1996, 1997, Seeley et al. 1997). Nevertheless, leptin receptor is expressed in neuronal subpopulations throughout the brain (Scott et al. 2009), and localized leptin injections into several brain areas well away from the hypothalamus have been shown to alter feeding behavior. For example, leptin injection into the ventral tegmental area alters dopamine neuron activity and alters the response to palatable foods (Hommel et al. 2006). In the hippocampus, leptin facilitates neuroplasticity (reviewed in Irving and Harvey 2014) and modulates food-related learning (Kanoski et al. 2011). Therefore, it is evident that leptin, an indirect endocrine control of food intake, acts at multiple sites that affect multiple facets of a complex behavior—feeding behavior.

11.1.4.4 Integrating Leptin Signaling with GI Stimuli—Focus on the Vagus and Hindbrain

The actions of leptin at midbrain and forebrain sites are interesting and likely to be important for the control of food intake and perhaps, for control of other behaviors as well. Nonetheless, the fact remains that leptin controls food intake entirely by

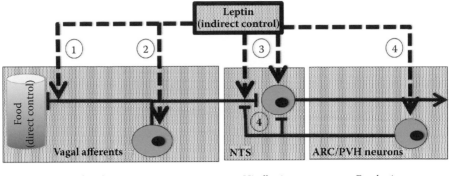

Peripheral nervous system   Hindbrain   Forebrain

FIGURE 11.2   Some putative sites (circled numerals) for integration of an indirect control of food intake, leptin, with direct controls of food intake mediated by vagal afferents innervating the GI tract. (1) Leptin acts directly on peripheral GI vagal afferent endings. (2) Leptin triggers transcriptionally mediated changes in GI vagal afferent function. (3) Leptin acts directly at receptors in central vagal afferent endings or NTS neurons that receive input from the GI tract. (4) Leptin activates forebrain neurons that release modulatory peptides to alter response of NTS vagal terminals or NTS neuron responses to GI signals.

reducing meal size, suggesting that it affects satiation, the process that leads to meal termination. As outlined earlier, direct controls triggered by food in the digestive tract appear to provide the primary signals for meal termination, and these signals reach the central nervous system via primary vagal afferents synapsing in the caudal hindbrain, specifically in the NTS. Therefore, the vagal afferent/NTS synapse constitutes the first opportunity for brain integration of direct GI controls of food intake and indirect controls such as leptin. This review will focus on mechanisms by which an indirect control of food intake, typified by leptin, exerts its effect by modulating signaling of primary vagal afferents and neurons in the NTS. Figure 11.2 illustrates several avenues by which leptin interacts with vagal afferent transmission and direct controls of food intake.

11.2   LEPTIN ACTS ON THE VAGUS TO MODULATE DIRECT CONTROLS OF FOOD INTAKE

Leptin receptor (lepRb) transcript and immunoreactivity have been detected in vagal afferent nerve cell bodies in the nodose ganglia of rats and humans (Burdyga et al. 2002). Moreover, using ratiometric calcium imaging of cultured rat nodose ganglion neurons, Peters, Ritter, and Simasko (2006) found that 42%–48% of vagal afferent neurons that innervate the stomach or duodenum were activated by leptin. Significantly, CCK also activated nearly all of these leptin responsive neurons (Figure 11.3). Subsequent voltage clamp studies further indicated that both CCK and leptin depolarize vagal afferent neurons and that leptin enhances CCK-evoked depolarization (Peters et al. 2004). Thus, vagal afferents express the required receptors to enable the interaction of an indirect control of food intake, leptin, with a direct

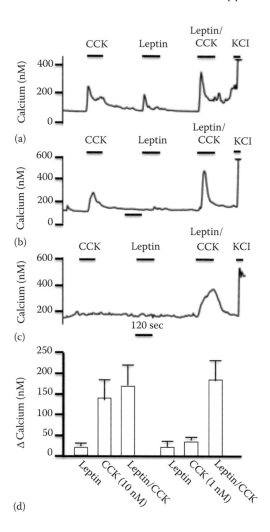

FIGURE 11.3 Intracellular calcium responses by cultured vagal afferent neurons in response to bath application of leptin and CCK applied alone or together. Panels A–C show typical responses. 55 mM KCl response indicates viable neuron at then completion of each experiment. Panel D summarizes averaged responses from individual neurons from nine cultures. Note the marked enhancement of CCK-evoked calcium response by leptin. (Data redrawn from Peters, J.H. et al., *Endocrinology*, 145, 3652–3657, 2004.)

control of food intake, CCK. Indeed, numerous behavioral and immunohistochemical observations are consistent with the hypothesis that leptin enhances responses to GI controls of food intake. For example, leptin enhances reduction of food intake and NTS Fos expression evoked by gastric preloads (Emond et al. 2001). Similarly, reductions of food intake and increases of NTS Fos expression, evoked by either CCK (Emond et al. 1999) or bombesin (Ladenheim, Emond, and Moran 2005), are also enhanced by leptin.

11.2.1   A ROLE FOR PERIPHERAL VAGAL AFFERENT LEPTIN RECEPTORS IN CONTROL OF FOOD INTAKE

The forgoing observations indicate that vagal afferent neuron excitability is enhanced by leptin but do not indicate whether central or peripheral expression of vagal leptin receptors contributes to enhanced vagal responsiveness and control of food intake. However, Wang et al. (1997) observed that bath application of leptin excited a subpopulation of teased vagal afferent fibers in an ex vivo rat stomach/duodenum preparation. They found that application of CCK enhanced the response to leptin. Therefore, it appears that leptin action on peripheral vagal endings, or the organs they innervate, triggers increased vagal afferent activity that might modulate responses to GI signals involved in control of food intake. Results from Peters et al. (2005) suggest that leptin action at peripheral vagal endings or their innervation targets indeed can alter food intake. Using near celiac arterial infusion in rats, they observed that leptin infused into the celiac arterial bed transiently reduced the size of a deprivation-induced meal, whereas the same or higher leptin doses, infused into the systemic venous circulation, were without effect. Furthermore, they demonstrated that intraceliac infusions of leptin and CCK, at doses that failed to alter food intake individually, significantly reduced meal size when coinfused by the near celiac arterial route (Figure 11.4). The branches of celiac artery perfuse the stomach and small intestine. Therefore, these data suggest that CCK and leptin cooperate to activate peripheral GI vagal afferent endings in vivo. In other words, direct and indirect controls of food intake can be integrated in the periphery prior to afferent signals reaching the brain.

11.2.2   TRANSCRIPTIONAL EFFECTS OF LEPTIN ON VAGAL AFFERENTS AND POTENTIAL FOR CONTROL OF FOOD INTAKE

In addition to acutely enhancing vagal afferent excitation by altering membrane conductance, leptin also engages transcriptional mechanisms that alter responses to CCK and other direct controls of food intake. Systemic leptin administration triggers phosphorylation of the signal transducer and activator of transcription 3 (STAT3) (Heldsinger et al. 2011) in the nodose ganglion and also induces nodose neuronal synthesis of another transcription factor early growth response protein 1 (EGR1) (de Lartigue et al. 2011). Leptin is reported to enhance CCK-induced nuclear translocation of EGR1 in nodose neurons (de Lartigue et al. 2010b). EGR1 translocation is associated with increased expression of CART peptide in a subpopulation of vagal afferents, and there is evidence that release of CART peptide, centrally or peripherally, modulates reduction of food intake by CCK (de Lartigue et al. 2010a). Hence, a second mode of leptin modulation of direct GI controls maybe through induction, increased synthesis, and release of neuromodulators by primary vagal afferent neurons themselves.

11.2.3   VAGAL LEPTIN RECEPTORS AND SPONTANEOUS FOOD INTAKE

Understanding of the contribution of vagal afferent leptin receptors in control of spontaneous food intake is in the early stages of investigation. Recently, however,

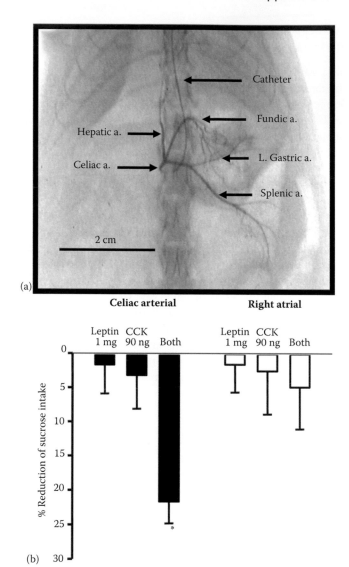

FIGURE 11.4 Reduction of meal size in response to coadministration of leptin and CCK via near-celiac arterial infusion, as compared to systemic venous infusion via the right atrial catheter. Panel a is a contrast radiograph illustrating the localized distribution of a radio-opaque contrast medium following its administration via the celiac arterial catheters. This route of infusion limits effective distribution of the infusate to areas innervated by abdominal vagal afferents. Panel b shows that coadministration of leptin and CCK, at doses that are ineffective when given individually, significantly reduces meal size via the celiac arterial infusion route, but not by the right atrial route. (Data from Peters, J.H. et al., *Am. J. Physiol. Regul. Integr. Comp. Physiol.*, 288, R879–R884, 2005.)

de Lartigue, Ronveaux, and Raybould (2014) selectively knocked down leptin receptor expression in a subpopulation of vagal afferent neurons in mice. As far as we know, these mice lack leptin receptors only in a subpopulation of primary sensory neurons that express Nav 1.8, a tetrodotoxin insensitive sodium channel that is present in 60%–70% of vagal afferents. Mice with the Nav 1.8-targeted knockdown of the leptin receptor exhibited mild hyperphagia that was entirely due to increased meal size. Moreover, the increased food intake was sufficient to account for a mild to moderate increase in adiposity. Assuming the behavioral effects of leptin receptor knockdown are due solely to reduced leptin signaling in primary afferents of the vagus, these results implicate leptin modulation of vagal function, and by inference modulation of direct controls of food intake, in the pathogenesis of obesity.

11.2.4 DIET—THE VAGUS AND ALTERED RESPONSE TO LEPTIN AND CCK

The observation that knock down of vagal afferent leptin receptors results in increased meal size complements extensive earlier results from Covasa and coworkers demonstrating that adaptation to high-fat diet, which results in development of obesity, attenuates the satiation effects of low doses of exogenous CCK (Covasa and Ritter 1998) or of intraintestinal fatty acid infusion (Covasa and Ritter 1999). Covasa, Grahn, and Ritter (2000a,b) also found that vagal activity, evoked by exogenous CCK or intestinal fatty acid, was attenuated in high-fat diet adapted rats, suggesting reduced vagal sensitivity or responsiveness to CCK. Subsequent work by others revealed that reduced CCK responsiveness in high-fat fed animals is associated with down-regulation of vagal afferent CCK receptor expression (Nefti et al. 2009). Recent results, however, also determined that attenuated CCK-induced reduction of food intake in high-fat fed and diet-induced obese rats is associated with vagal afferent leptin resistance (de Lartigue et al. 2012). Collectively, the foregoing observations indicate that significant integration of direct and indirect controls of food intake may be mediated, in part, by transcriptional changes in vagal afferents. Specifically, indirect controllers of food intake, like leptin, can alter responses to vagal stimulation by increasing expression and release of vagal afferent neuromodulatory substances, while direct controllers, like CCK, can regulate vagal afferent expression of leptin receptors thereby limiting modulation by this indirect controller. Potentially, imbalance between such opposing transcriptional changes could contribute to either positive or negative energy balance and result in weight gain or weight loss.

11.3 MECHANISMS FOR INTEGRATION OF DIRECT AND INDIRECT CONTROLS OF FEEDING IN THE HINDBRAIN

11.3.1 HINDBRAIN LEPTIN RECEPTORS AND CONTROL OF FOOD INTAKE AND BODY WEIGHT

Injection of leptin into the fourth ventricle or directly into the NTS of intact rats, at doses that, when systemically injected, do not alter food intake (Grill et al. 2002, Ruiter et al. 2010), reduces food intake, suggesting that the hindbrain is a site of leptin action. Consistent with this hypothesis, leptin receptor transcript is expressed in the NTS (Scott et al. 2009), and systemic leptin administration triggers STAT3 phosphorylation in NTS neurons (Maniscalco and Rinaman 2014). Moreover, many of the same NTS neurons that exhibit increased STAT3 phosphorylation after leptin injection are also excited by gastric distension (Huo et al. 2007). This observation and others support the hypothesis that leptin receptors on NTS neurons are positioned to control food intake by modulating GI signals, such as gastric distension.

Immunohistochemical studies and studies utilizing targeted transgenic expression of fluorescent proteins reveal that leptin-sensitive neurons constitute a relatively small proportion of NTS neurons, which include POMC-, CCK-, and pro-glucagon-expressing, GLP-1, neuronal phenotypes (Ellacott, Halatchev, and Cone 2006, Garfield et al. 2012). It is not clear, however, whether any or all of these NTS neuronal phenotypes contribute to control of food intake by leptin. In addition, some results suggest that there may be substantial interspecies differences in NTS neuronal leptin sensitivity. For example, in mice, leptin receptor transcript is expressed by NTS pro-glucagon neurons (Huo et al. 2008, Garfield et al. 2012) and leptin triggers phosphorylation of STAT3 in these neurons (Huo et al. 2008). Finally, bath-applied leptin triggers increased firing of identified proglucagon neurons in mouse hindbrain slice preparations (Hisadome et al. 2010). Surprisingly, however, proglucagon neurons in the rat NTS appear to be unresponsive to leptin (Huo et al. 2008), an observation that seems to fly in the face of earlier reports that intraventricular GLP-1 receptor antagonist injection attenuates reduction of food intake by systemic leptin administration (Goldstone et al. 1997).

Additional results that appear to contradict previous behavioral and immunohistochemical observations come from Williams and Smith (2006), who reported that leptin applied to rat or mouse hindbrain slices actually inhibits the activity of 58% of neurons in the NTS, including neurons that were excited by gastric distension. Intuitively, these results suggest that leptin receptors in the hindbrain might antagonize GI signals that reduce food intake or favor weight gain. In fact, a series of meticulous studies by Harris and coworkers supports the hypothesis that activation of hindbrain leptin receptors actually favors weight gain. Briefly, she and her collaborators found that decerebrate rats, in which the forebrain is disconnected from the hindbrain by transecting the brainstem at the level of the colliculi, did not lose weight, but rather gained fat when treated chronically with leptin (Harris, Bartness, and Grill 2007). Furthermore, if leptin was chronically infused into the hindbrain of intact rats, these rats also exhibited reduced energy expenditure and increased body fat gain. On the other hand, simultaneous infusion of leptin into both the third and the fourth ventricles produced marked reduction food intake and loss of body fat. Finally, complimentary work with mutated leptin protein infusions suggested that reduction of food intake and weight loss may depend on reciprocal neural projections between the hindbrain and the forebrain (Harris 2013a). Collectively, these results suggest that caution is indicated when interpreting results gathered in reduced or compromised preparations and highlight the importance of considering such findings in the context of neural circuits that might include forms of negative feedback signaling.

11.3.2 BRAIN PEPTIDES IN THE INTEGRATION OF DIRECT AND INDIRECT CONTROLS OF FOOD INTAKE

Electrophysiological recordings indicate that most neurons in the NTS receive direct synaptic input from primary vagal afferent endings. However, the vagus is not the only source of NTS afferents. The NTS also receives afferent input from other brain areas. These afferents arise from neurons in other hindbrain nuclei, such as the ventrolateral medullary catecholamine neurons and medullary raphe, the pontine lateral parabrachial nuclei, periaqueductal gray matter, the hypothalamus (paraventricular nucleus [PVN], lateral hypothalamus, ARC, and dorsomedial nucleus), amygdala, bed nucleus of the stria terminalis, insular, and medial prefrontal cortex. Therefore, anatomical lines of communication are in place for central modulation of sensory signals arriving from the GI tract at their very point of entry into the central nervous system. Moreover, the observations of Harris et al., briefly reviewed in the previous section, suggest that connections between the forebrain and the hindbrain play a critical role in leptin signaling in intact animals and are likely critical for integration of leptin signaling with mechanisms regulating the direct control of food intake by GI signals.

Several laboratories have reported results indicating that hypothalamic neurons control food intake via projections to the NTS. For example, observations by Blevins and colleagues suggest that NTS projections from oxytocin neurons in the hypothalamic PVN contribute to inhibitory control food intake (Blevins et al. 2003, Blevins, Schwartz, and Baskin 2004). The results of Bi and colleagues (Yang et al. 2009) are consistent with a working hypothesis that dorsomedial hypothalamic neuropeptide Y (NPY) projections to NTS participate in control of food intake. Finally, several reports indicate that leptin-responsive POMC neuronal inputs to the NTS control food intake, perhaps by modulating GI signals in the NTS (Zheng et al. 2005, 2010).

Leptin excites POMC neurons in the ARC of the hypothalamus (Cowley et al. 2001, 2003). Activation of POMC neurons is associated with inhibition of food intake and body fat loss, primarily through activation of type 4 melanocortin receptors (MC4R) (recently reviewed in Koch and Horvath 2014). Although most attention has focused on melanocortinergic projections within the hypothalamus, Zheng et al. (2010) have reported that hindbrain injection of a melanocortin 3/4 receptor antagonist attenuates reduction of food intake following leptin injection into the ARC. These results suggest that hypothalamic melanocortinergic projections to the hindbrain are responsible, at least in part, for reduction of food intake by leptin. Of further interest are reports indicating that hindbrain MC4R receptors participate in control of meal size (Zheng et al. 2005) and reduction of food intake by CCK (Fan et al. 2004, Sutton et al. 2005). Specifically, injection of a melanocortin receptor agonist into the hindbrain reduces food intake by reducing meal size, and reduction of food intake following intraperitoneal injection of CCK is attenuated by hindbrain injection of an MC3/4 receptor antagonist. The foregoing results strongly suggest that melanocortin receptors in the hindbrain modulate GI signals that control food intake. Until very recently, however, specific cellular mechanisms for modulation of direct GI control by hindbrain melanocortin receptors were not identified.

Examination of food intake and weight gain in transgenic mice suggests that both type 3 (MC3R) and type 4 (MC4R) melanocortin receptors participate in control of food intake and body weight (Butler and Cone 2002, Marks et al. 2006, Rowland et al. 2010). The bulk of experimental evidence, however, indicates that the MC4R is more prominent in the control of food intake. In this regard, expression of MC3R is rare or absent from neurons in the NTS (Roselli-Rehfuss et al. 1993, Kistler-Heer, Lauber, and Lichtensteiger 1998), while subpopulations of NTS neurons do express MC4R transcript (Mountjoy et al. 1994, Kishi et al. 2003). Similarly, MC4R mRNA is expressed by neurons in the nodose ganglia, but MC3R transcript is not detectable in nodose neurons (Wan et al. 2008, Gautron et al. 2010, 2012). Hence, it is likely that melanocortinergic modulation of GI signals in the hindbrain is mediated by MC4R activation.

11.3.3 GLUTAMATE AND VAGAL AFFERENT NEUROTRANSMISSION: IMPLICATIONS FOR INTEGRATION OF CONTROLS

A wealth of electrophysiological and anatomical data indicate that virtually all vagal afferents release glutamate from their endings in the NTS (Allchin et al. 1994, Andresen and Mendelowitz 1996, Lachamp, Crest, and Kessler 2006). During very brief stimulation, glutamatergic excitatory currents are mediated by AMPA-type glutamate receptors (Andresen and Mendelowitz 1996). However, Zhao et al. (2015) recently demonstrated that nearly 70% of total charge transfer during more sustained vagal afferent stimulation depends on N-methyl-D-aspartate-type glutamate receptors (NMDAR). Moreover, the throughput and fidelity of vagal afferent to NTS neuron transmission depend on the NMDAR current. Consistent with NMDAR participation in vagal glutamatergic transmission, injection of NMDAR antagonists into the NTS increases meal size by attenuating inhibitory GI feedback from ingested food (Burns and Ritter 1997, 1998). Moreover, NTS injection of NMDAR antagonists prevents reduction of food intake following intraperitoneal CCK injection (Guard et al. 2009, Wright et al. 2011). Thus, glutamatergic transmission and NMDAR activation play key roles in channeling direct signals from the GI tract to the CNS.

Because GI signals that control food intake are relayed to the brain via glutamatergic vagal afferents, modulation of glutamate release is an attractive avenue by which neuropeptides could influence those signals to control food intake. Therefore, it is intriguing that vagal afferents themselves express transcript coding for cognate receptors that bind a variety of central neuropeptides that alter food intake. A noncomprehensive list of peptide receptors expressed by vagal afferent neurons includes transcript coding for orexin1 receptors (Burdyga et al. 2003), oxytocin receptors (Welch et al. 2009), NPY receptors (Zhang et al. 1997), and MC4R (Wan et al. 2008). While some, if not all, of these receptor types are expressed by NTS neurons (Kopp et al. 2002, Gould and Zingg 2003, Stanic et al. 2006) as well as vagal afferents, electrophysiological studies indicate that many neuropeptide effects are mediated largely by altering glutamate release from presynaptic vagal afferent endings. For example, multiple groups have demonstrated that CCK acts on vagal afferent nerve endings in the NTS to increase both spontaneous and evoked vagal afferent release of glutamate (Appleyard et al. 2005, Baptista et al. 2005). Similarly, Peters et al. (2008) demonstrated that oxytocin acts presynaptically to enhance spontaneous and evoked release of glutamate from vagal afferents. Wan et al. (2008) have reported that activation of MC4R in the NTS increased spontaneous glutamate release from vagal afferent endings. Finally, our own preliminary results suggest that presynaptic MC4R activation also enhances the strength of vagal afferent neurotransmission by increasing the readily releasable pool of vagal afferent glutamate. Collectively, these patch clamp recording results suggest the intriguing hypothesis that peptides released within the brain could control food intake by modulating the synaptic strength of central vagal afferent endings in the NTS.

The concept that neuropeptides could control food intake by acting presynaptically to alter the function of vagal endings in the NTS is supported by a series of recent reports. First, results from our lab revealed that systemic CCK treatment increases phosphorylation of extracellular receptor kinases (ERK1/2) in vagal afferent endings, as well as in NTS neurons (Sutton, Patterson, and Berthoud 2004, Campos et al. 2012). Furthermore, we found that increased pERK1/2-catalyzed phosphorylation of the synaptic vesicle protein, synapsin 1 (Syn1), selectively at serines 62 and 67 (Campos et al. 2013). pERK1/2-mediated phosphorylation of synapsin 1 results in transiently increased trafficking of synaptic vesicles from a reserve pool to a readily releasable pool, thereby facilitating the increased release of glutamate and increasing synaptic strength (for review see Cesca et al. 2010). Increased synapsin phosphorylation following CCK injection persisted for just 15–20 minutes, about the same time period over which CCK acts to reduce meal size (Campos et al. 2013). Pharmacological inhibition of ERK1/2 phosphorylation prevented CCK-induced phosphorylation of synapsin and prevented reduction of food intake by CCK. Finally, when we inhibited dephosphorylation of serines 62 and 67, using a calcineurin inhibitor, pERK1/2-mediated phosphorylation of synapsin 1 was increased and prolonged, and so was the reduction of food intake by CCK (Campos et al. 2013) (Figure 11.5). These results are consistent with live cell imaging (Rogers and Hermann 2008) and electrophysiological data showing that CCK acts on vagal afferent CCK-A receptors to increase glutamate release (Appleyard et al. 2005, Baptista et al. 2005). The results suggest that CCK does more than simply activate vagal afferent fibers to reduce food intake. It also modulates the strength of vagal synaptic transmission by changing the dynamics of synaptic vesicle trafficking at vagal afferent endings. Endogenous CCK is secreted by the intestinal enteroendocrine cells (I cells) in response to nutrients in food, but CCK also is expressed by neurons in the NTS (Beinfeld and Palkovits 1982, Cortes et al. 1990). Currently, one can only speculate as to the source of endogenous CCK that contributes to control of food intake through action at central vagal afferent endings.

11.3.4   CENTRAL VAGAL AFFERENT ENDINGS AND MELANOCORTIN CONTROL OF FOOD INTAKE

The fact that reduction of food intake by CCK-A receptor activation involves modulation of vagal afferent transmission via synapsin phosphorylation raises the

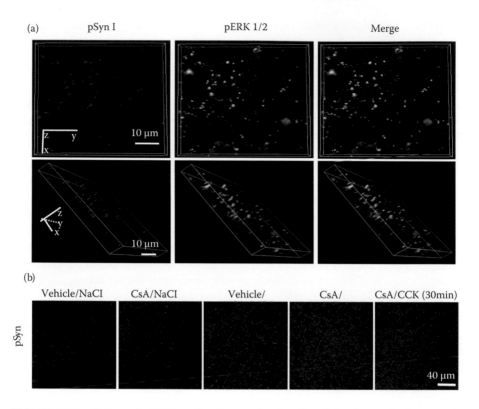

FIGURE 11.5 Enhanced pERK-mediated synapsin phosphorylation in vagal afferent endings and enhancement of CCK-induced reduction of food intake following inhibition of calcineurin by fourth ventricle cyclosporin A. (a) Three-dimensional images rendered from high-magnification (100×) optical sections (24 sections 0.5 μm apart for a total thickness of 12 μm) showing colocalization of pERK1/2 and pSyn in vagal afferent endings in the NTS. The top row is a view from the z-plane and the bottom row is a rotated view of the same rendering. Note the high degree of colocalization between pERK1/2 and its phosphorylation product pSyn1 (serines 62, 67). (b and c) Enhanced CCK-induced phosphorylation of synapsin 1 in the NTS following fourth ventricle injection of cyclosporine A (CsA). B, Representative images of hindbrain sections from rats injected intraperitoneally with CCK (2 g/kg) or saline depicting pSyn 1 (red) immunofluorescence 1 hour after fourth ventricle injection of CsA (12 μg) or vehicle.   (*Continued*)

possibility that activation of other peptide receptors expressed by vagal afferents also might modulate vagal synaptic function to control food intake. Vagal afferent MC4Rs are of special interest in this regard because of the key role played by this receptor in mediating leptin's effects on food intake and body weight. Injection of MC4R agonist into the fourth ventricle or directly into the NTS triggers a rapid reduction of food intake that persists for hours following injection (Grill et al. 1998, Campos, Shiina, and Ritter 2014, Campos and Ritter 2015). Reduction of

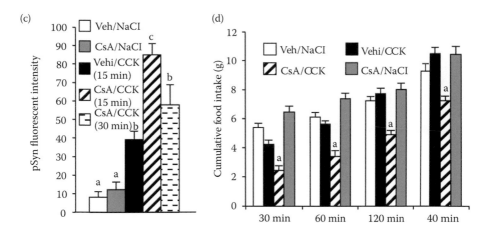

FIGURE 11.5 (CONTINUED) Enhanced pERK-mediated synapsin phosphorylation in vagal afferent endings and enhancement of CCK-induced reduction of food intake following inhibition of calcineurin by fourth ventricle cyclosporin A. (c) Quantification of pSyn immunofluorescence. Note that fourth ventricle pretreatment with CsA more than doubles the level of CCK-induced synapsin phosphorylation. In addition, CsA pretreatment extends the length of time that synapsin remains phosphorylated. (d) Fourth ventricle injection of calcineurin inhibitor CsA potentiates CCK-induced reduction of food intake by rats following a 16-hour fast. Graph shows cumulative intake at 30, 60, 120, and 240 minutes after IP injection of CCK (2 g/kg) or saline administration preceded by a fourth ventricle injection of CsA (12 μg) or vehicle 1 hour prior to the IP injections. (Data from Campos, C.A. et al. *Endocrinology*, 154, 2613–2625, 2013.)

food intake following hindbrain MC4R activation is entirely due to reduction of meal size, with little if any effect on meal frequency. Significantly, reduction of food intake following injection of MC4R agonist into the NTS does not require peripheral vagal fibers (Williams, Kaplan, and Grill 2000) but does depend on the presence of intact vagal afferent endings in the NTS (Campos, Shiina, and Ritter 2014). Sectioning the vagus below the diaphragm, or just distal to the nodose ganglion, results in degeneration of vagal afferent innervation to peripheral organs. However, vagal afferent neurons in the nodose ganglia and vagal afferent terminals in the NTS survive. Unilateral nodose ganglion removal, however, results in degeneration of the majority of vagal afferent endings ipsilateral to nodose removal, while vagal endings in the NTS contralateral to ganglion removal are not diminished. When melanotan-II (MTII), an MC3/4 receptor agonist, is injected into the NTS, contralateral to nodose removal, food intake is reduced, as it is in intact rats. However, if MTII is injected ipsilateral to nodose removal, where vagal afferent endings have degenerated, food intake is not significantly decreased by MTII (Figure 11.6). These results suggest that vagal afferent endings in the NTS are necessary participants in reduction of food intake by MC4R activation. The possibility that reduction of food intake by hindbrain MC4R activation depends on release of glutamate, perhaps from vagal afferent endings, is supported by the finding that

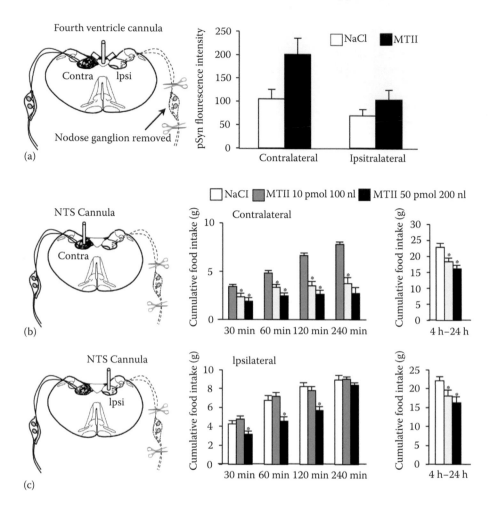

FIGURE 11.6 Attenuation of MTII-induced PKA catalyzed synapsin I phosphorylation (serine 9) and reduction of food intake in rats following destruction of central vagal afferent endings. (a) Schematics on the left side of the figure illustrate unilateral removal of a nodose ganglion and degeneration of central vagal afferent endings in the ipsilateral but not contralateral NTS of fourth-ventricle-cannulated rats. The graph summarizes attenuation of synapsin phosphorylation, 30 minutes after fourth ventricle MTII injection, ipsilateral, but not contralateral, to nodose ganglion removal (n = 4/treatment condition). (b) Schematic depicts placement of cannula in the NTS contralateral to nodose ganglion removal. Bar graphs show cumulative food intake following injection of saline or MTII into the contralateral NTS (n = 8). (c) Diagram shows placement of cannula into the NTS ipsilateral to nodose ganglion removal, where central vagal afferent endings were destroyed. Right, Cumulative food intake following injection of saline or MTII into the ipsilateral NTS (n = 8). Data are means SEM. *Values significantly different (p < 0.05) from saline control injection. Brackets are used to illustrate a significant difference in pSyn immunoreactivity between the contralateral and ipsilateral NTS. (Data from Campos, C.A., Shiina, H., Ritter, R.C., *J. Neurosci.*, 34, 12636–12645, 2014.)

hindbrain injection of an NMDAR antagonist prevents reduction of food intake by MTII injection (Campos and Ritter 2015). Importantly (see Section 11.3.5) reduction of food intake following hindbrain injection of MC4R agonist is attenuated by pretreatment, either with U0126, which inhibits ERK1/2 phosphorylation (Sutton et al. 2005), or by pretreatment with an inhibitor of cyclic adenosine monophosphate (cAMP)-dependent protein kinase (PKA) (Campos, Shiina, and Ritter 2014). Collectively, these observations are consistent with the hypothesis that activation of MC4R on vagal afferent endings reduces food intake, at least in part, by enhancing vagal release of glutamate, thereby reducing meal size. The results also suggest that the mechanisms for reduction of feeding by hindbrain MC4R activation involve both mitogen-activated protein kinase (MAPK) and PKA.

11.3.5 PKA-MEDIATED SYNAPSIN PHOSPHORYLATION AND MC4R MODULATION OF VAGAL FUNCTION

Anatomical and immunochemical evaluation of vagal afferent changes following MC4R activation provides additional support for the hypothesis that activation of vagal afferent MC4R reduces food intake by modulating vagal afferent synaptic function. Fourth ventricle injection of MTII triggers increased ERK1/2 phosphorylation in NTS neurons (Zheng et al. 2005, Campos and Ritter 2015). Surprisingly, however, it does not increase pERK1/2 in vagal afferent endings (Campos, Shiina, and Ritter 2014). Consistent with this observation, MTII does not trigger synapsin phosphorylation at serines 62 and 67 in vagal afferents (Campos, Shiina, and Ritter 2014). Hence, the reported role of pERK1/2 in reduction of food intake by hindbrain MTII appears to be confined to postsynaptic neurons. However, consistent with $G_{\alpha s}$ coupling of MC4R, we found that MTII triggers a marked increase of synapsin 1 phosphorylation, but this time at serine 9, a site selectively phosphorylated by PKA (Campos, Shiina, and Ritter 2014). MTII-induced synapsin 1 serine 9 phosphorylation was localized in vagal afferent endings, was diminished ipsilateral to unilateral nodose ganglion removal and was abolished by pretreatment with a PKA inhibitor. Finally, synapsin phosphorylation following hindbrain MTII persisted for at least 6 hours after injection, consistent with the long-lasting reduction of food intake and meal size following MTII injection (Figure 11.7). Similar to pERK-mediated synapsin phosphorylation, PKA-catalyzed phosphorylation of synapsin 1 at serine 9 increases the size of readily releasable glutamate and increases synaptic strength (Valente et al. 2012). Consistent with enhanced presynaptic glutamate release, MC4R activation increases the frequency of spontaneous excitatory postsynaptic currents (ePSCs) at vagal afferent NTS neuronal synapses (Wan et al. 2008). Taken together, the results of behavioral, pharmacological, and electrophysiological experiments support a model by which melanocortins acting at cognate MC4R control food intake, at least in part, by modulating glutamate release from vagal afferent endings in the NTS. A schematic of MC4R modulation of the vagal afferent/NTS neuron synapse is shown in Figure 11.8. The putative effect of increasing glutamate release would be to enhance the strength of food-related GI signals, leading to reduction of meal size.

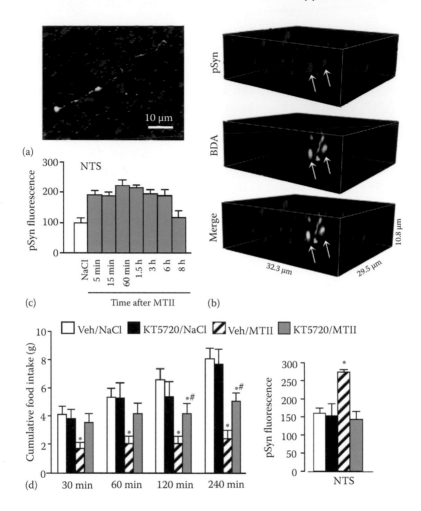

FIGURE 11.7 (a and b) Vagal afferent endings in the NTS were anterogradely labeled with biotintylated dextran (BDA) injected into the nodose ganglia. Following fourth ventricle MTII injection, sections were stained to reveal pSyn (serine 9) (red) and BDA (green). (a) A single z plane-merged image revealing colocalization of pSyn and BDA as yellow in vagal afferent endings ($n = 4$). (b) Three-dimensional images rendered from high-magnification (100×) optical sections showing colocalization (arrows) of MTII-induced pSyn and BDA-labeled vagal afferent endings. Red channel is pSyn, green is BDA, and merge shows colocalization in yellow. (c) Shows time course for elevation of pSyn (serine 9) in NTS following fourth ventricle injection of MTII. Note that pSyn is elevated for at least 6 hours following MTII. (d) Left panel: reduction of food intake by fourth ventricle MTII is attenuated by fourth ventricle pretreatment with KT5720, a PKA inhibitor. Right panel: KT5720 attenuates MTII-induced increase in NTS pSyn. (Data from Campos, C.A., Shiina, H., Ritter, R.C., *J. Neurosci.*, 34, 12636–12645, 2014.)

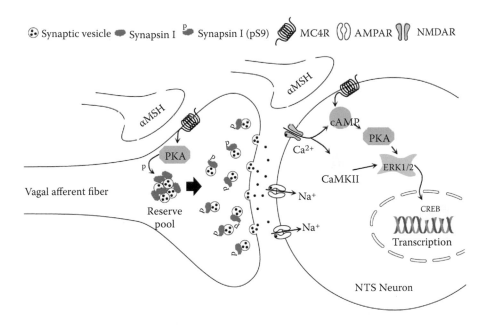

FIGURE 11.8 Postulated contributions of NTS presynaptic and postsynaptic MC4R activation in the control of food intake. PKA-catalyzed phosphorylation of synapsin I in central vagal afferent endings is downstream of presynaptic MC4R activation, which may contribute to reduction of food intake by increasing synaptic vesicle mobilization and thereby increasing glutamatergic neurotransmission from vagal afferent endings. In conjunction with presynaptic MC4R activation, postsynaptic MC4R activation of NTS neurons may modulate food intake by activating ERK and other signaling pathways that result in transcriptional changes. Note that activation of vagal afferent endings and subsequent activation of postsynaptic glutamate receptors could also contribute to activation of the ERK signaling cascade and changes in transcription. AMPAR, AMPA receptor; NMDAR, NMDA receptor; CaMKII, calcium/calmodulin-dependent protein kinase II; ERK1/2, extracellular signal-related kinases 1 and 2; CREB, cAMP response element-binding protein. (Diagram from Campos, C.A., Shiina, H., Ritter, R.C., *J. Neurosci.*, 34, 12636–12645, 2014.)

11.3.6 HINDBRAIN MC4R AND NMDAR PARTICIPATE IN REDUCTION OF FOOD INTAKE BY HYPOTHALAMIC LEPTIN

The potential role of endogenous melanocortins in control of food intake via activation of vagal afferent MC4R is intriguing but has only begun to be investigated. However, consistent with modulation of vagal afferent function, fibers immunoreactive for melanocyte-stimulating hormone (MSH), the endogenous MC4R agonist released by POMC neurons, make intimate contacts with vagal afferent endings in the NTS (Campos, Shiina, and Ritter 2014). Furthermore, injection of an MC4R antagonist into the NTS is reported to attenuate reduction of food intake following injection of leptin into the ARC (Zheng et al. 2010). Intriguingly, NTS injection of an NMDAR antagonist also attenuates reduction of food intake by ARC leptin injection (Campos, Shiina, and Ritter 2013), suggesting that glutamatergic neurotransmission in the NTS participates in reduction of food intake by leptin acting in the hypothalamus. Finally, ARC leptin injection triggers increased synapsin phosphorylation in vagal afferent endings in the NTS (Campos, Shiina, and Ritter 2013). Collectively, these findings support the hypothesis that presynaptic modulation of vagal function by endogenously released melanocortins is a mechanism by which indirect controls of food intake, such as leptin, may be integrated with direct inhibitory controls arising from food intake.

11.4 VAGAL AFFERENT MODULATION AND THE SENSORY EXPERIENCE OF SATIATION

By acting at the interface between primary vagal afferents and second order sensory neurons in the NTS, indirect controls of food intake, like leptin and brain neuropeptides released by leptin, may be able to modulate the sensory experience engendered by satiation. Modulation of sensation at the level of vagal afferent/NTS neurotransmission is fundamentally different from modulating the affective responses to food in the forebrain, where overall affective responses are assembled. However, probing the actual sensory experience that accompanies satiation in rodents is difficult. Nevertheless, Davidson and Carretta (1993), using a novel stimulus generalization design, have provided tantalizing experimental evidence that exogenous CCK engenders a sensory experience similar to satiation. More recently, the same group presented results suggesting that leptin, at a dose that has no effect by itself, enhanced the ability of exogenous CCK to produce a satiation-like sensory experience (Kanoski, Walls, and Davidson 2007). A more detailed understanding of cell and molecular mechanisms of vagal signaling at the vagal afferent/NTS synapse should provide cellular- and molecular-level understanding of the sensory experiences produced by integration of direct and indirect controls of food intake. Together with behavioral techniques for detecting and quantifying these experiences in non-human animals, this cellular/molecular understanding may prescribe selective tools with which to therapeutically modify the sensory experience of satiation and thereby control excessive food intake and weight gain.

LITERATURE CITED

Abbott, C. R., M. Monteiro, C. J. Small, A. Sajedi, K. L. Smith, J. R. Parkinson, M. A. Ghatei, and S. R. Bloom. 2005. The inhibitory effects of peripheral administration of peptide YY (3–36) and glucagon-like peptide-1 on food intake are attenuated by ablation of the vagal-brainstem-hypothalamic pathway. *Brain Res* 1044:127–31.

Alingh Prins, A., A. de Jong-Nagelsmit, J. Keijser, and J. H. Strubbe. 1986. Daily rhythms of feeding in the genetically obese and lean Zucker rats. *Physiol Behav* 38:423–6.

Allchin, R. E., T. F. Batten, P. N. McWilliam, and P. F. Vaughan. 1994. Electrical stimulation of the vagus increases extracellular glutamate recovered from the nucleus tractus solitarii of the cat by in vivo microdialysis. *Exp Physiol* 79:265–8.

Andresen, M. C., and D. Mendelowitz. 1996. Sensory afferent neurotransmission in caudal nucleus tractus solitarius—Common denominators. *Chem Senses* 21:387–95.

Antin, J., J. Gibbs, J. Holt, R. C. Young, and G. P. Smith. 1975. Cholecystokinin elicits the complete behavioral sequence of satiety in rats. *J Comp Physiol Psychol* 89:784–90.

Appleyard, S. M., T. W. Bailey, M. W. Doyle, Y. H. Jin, J. L. Smart, M. J. Low, and M. C. Andresen. 2005. Proopiomelanocortin neurons in nucleus tractus solitarius are activated by visceral afferents: Regulation by cholecystokinin and opioids. *J Neurosci* 25:35788–5.

Asarian, L., and N. Geary. 1999. Cyclic estradiol treatment phasically potentiates endogenous cholecystokinin's satiating action in ovariectomized rats. *Peptides* 20:445–50.

Asarian, L., and N. Geary. 2002. Cyclic estradiol treatment normalizes body weight and restores physiological patterns of spontaneous feeding and sexual receptivity in ovariectomized rats. *Horm Behav* 42:461–71.

Asarian, L., and N. Geary. 2006. Modulation of appetite by gonadal steroid hormones. *Philos Trans R Soc Lond B Biol Sci* 361:1251–63.

Baptista, V., Z. L. Zheng, F. H. Coleman, R. C. Rogers, and R. A. Travagli. 2005. Cholecystokinin octapeptide increases spontaneous glutamatergic synaptic transmission to neurons of the nucleus tractus solitarius centralis. *J Neurophysiol* 94:2763–71.

Beinfeld, M. C., and M. Palkovits. 1982. Distribution of cholecystokinin (CCK) in the rat lower brain stem nuclei. *Brain Res* 238:260–5.

Blevins, J. E., T. J. Eakin, J. A. Murphy, M. W. Schwartz, and D. G. Baskin. 2003. Oxytocin innervation of caudal brainstem nuclei activated by cholecystokinin. *Brain Res* 993:30–41.

Blevins, J. E., M. W. Schwartz, and D. G. Baskin. 2004. Evidence that paraventricular nucleus oxytocin neurons link hypothalamic leptin action to caudal brain stem nuclei controlling meal size. *Am J Physiol Regul Integr Comp Physiol* 287:R87–96.

Burdyga, G., S. Lal, D. Spiller, W. Jiang, D. Thompson, S. Attwood, S. Saeed, D. Grundy, A. Varro, R. Dimaline, and G. J. Dockray. 2003. Localization of orexin-1 receptors to vagal afferent neurons in the rat and humans. *Gastroenterology* 124:129–39.

Burdyga, G., D. Spiller, R. Morris, S. Lal, D. G. Thompson, S. Saeed, R. Dimaline, A. Varro, and G. J. Dockray. 2002. Expression of the leptin receptor in rat and human nodose ganglion neurones. *Neuroscience* 109:339–47.

Burns, G. A., and R. C. Ritter. 1997. The non-competitive NMDA antagonist MK-801 increases food intake in rats. *Pharmacol Biochem Behav* 56:145–9.

Burns, G. A., and R. C. Ritter. 1998. Visceral afferent participation in delayed satiation following NMDA receptor blockade. *Physiol Behav* 65:361–6.

Butler, A. A., and R. D. Cone. 2002. The melanocortin receptors: Lessons from knockout models. *Neuropeptides* 36:77–84.

Campos, C. A., and R. C. Ritter. 2015. NMDA-type glutamate receptors participate in reduction of food intake following hindbrain melanocortin receptor activation. *Am J Physiol Regul Integr Comp Physiol* 308:R1–9.

Campos, C. A., H. Shiina, and R. C. Ritter. 2013. *Hindbrain NMDA-receptors participate in reduction of food intake by hypothalamic leptin*. Society for the Study of Ingestive Behavior, New Orleans, LA, USA.

Campos, C. A., H. Shiina, and R. C. Ritter. 2014. Central vagal afferent endings mediate reduction of food intake by melanocortin-3/4 receptor agonist. *J Neurosci* 34:12636–45.

Campos, C. A., H. Shiina, M. Silvas, S. Page, and R. C. Ritter. 2013. Vagal afferent NMDA receptors modulate CCK-induced reduction of food intake through synapsin I phosphorylation in adult male rats. *Endocrinology* 154:2613–25.

Campos, C. A., J. S. Wright, K. Czaja, and R. C. Ritter. 2012. CCK-induced reduction of food intake and hindbrain MAPK signaling are mediated by NMDA receptor activation. *Endocrinology* 153:2633–46.

Cesca, F., P. Baldelli, F. Valtorta, and F. Benfenati. 2010. The synapsins: Key actors of synapse function and plasticity. *Prog Neurobiol* 91:313–48.

Cortes, R., U. Arvidsson, M. Schalling, S. Ceccatelli, and T. Hokfelt. 1990. In situ hybridization studies on mRNAs for cholecystokinin, calcitonin gene-related peptide and choline acetyltransferase in the lower brain stem, spinal cord and dorsal root ganglia of rat and guinea pig with special reference to motoneurons. *J Chem Neuroanat* 3:467–85.

Covasa, M., and R. C. Ritter. 1998. Rats maintained on high-fat diets exhibit reduced satiety in response to CCK and bombesin. *Peptides* 19:1407–15.

Covasa, M., and R. C. Ritter. 1999. Reduced sensitivity to the satiation effect of intestinal oleate in rats adapted to high-fat diet. *Am J Physiol* 277:R279–85.

Covasa, M., J. Grahn, and R. C. Ritter. 2000a. High fat maintenance diet attenuates hindbrain neuronal response to CCK. *Regul Pept* 86:83–8.

Covasa, M., J. Grahn, and R. C. Ritter. 2000b. Reduced hindbrain and enteric neuronal response to intestinal oleate in rats maintained on high-fat diet. *Auton Neurosci* 84:8–18.

Cowley, M. A., R. Cone, P. Enriori, I. Louiselle, S. M. Williams, and A. E. Evans. 2003. Electrophysiological actions of peripheral hormones on melanocortin neurons. *Ann N Y Acad Sci* 994:175–86.

Cowley, M. A., J. L. Smart, M. Rubinstein, M. G. Cerdan, S. Diano, T. L. Horvath, R. D. Cone, and M. J. Low. 2001. Leptin activates anorexigenic POMC neurons through a neural network in the arcuate nucleus. *Nature* 411:480–4.

Davidson, T. L., and J. C. Carretta. 1993. Cholecystokinin, but not bombesin, has interoceptive sensory consequences like 1-h food deprivation. *Physiol Behav* 53:737–45.

de Lartigue, G., C. Barbier de la Serre, E. Espero, J. Lee, and H. E. Raybould. 2011. Diet-induced obesity leads to the development of leptin resistance in vagal afferent neurons. *Am J Physiol Endocrinol Metab* 301:E187–95.

de Lartigue, G., C. Barbier de la Serre, E. Espero, J. Lee, and H. E. Raybould. 2012. Leptin resistance in vagal afferent neurons inhibits cholecystokinin signaling and satiation in diet induced obese rats. *PLoS One* 7:e32967.

de Lartigue, G., R. Dimaline, A. Varro, H. Raybould, C. B. De la Serre, and G. J. Dockray. 2010a. Cocaine- and amphetamine-regulated transcript mediates the actions of cholecystokinin on rat vagal afferent neurons. *Gastroenterology* 138:1479–90.

de Lartigue, G., G. Lur, R. Dimaline, A. Varro, H. Raybould, and G. J. Dockray. 2010b. EGR1 Is a target for cooperative interactions between cholecystokinin and leptin, and inhibition by ghrelin, in vagal afferent neurons. *Endocrinology* 151:3589–99.

de Lartigue, G., C. C. Ronveaux, and H. E. Raybould. 2014. Deletion of leptin signaling in vagal afferent neurons results in hyperphagia and obesity. *Mol Metab* 3:595–607.

Dethier, V. G. 1976. *The hungry fly: A physiological study of the behavior associated with feeding.* Cambridge, MA: Harvard University Press.

Dethier, V. G., and A. Gelperin. 1967. Hyperphagia in the blowfly. *J Exp Biol* 47:191–200.

Dethier, V. G., and E. Stellar. 1964. "Animal behavior: Its evolutionary and neurological basis." Edited by W. D. McElroy and C. P. Swanson. 2nd ed., *Foundations of modern biology series,* 1–118. Englewood Cliffs, NJ: Prentice-Hall Inc.

Docherty, J. E., J. E. Manno, J. E. McDermott, and J. R. DiAngelo. 2015. Mio acts in the Drosophila brain to control nutrient storage and feeding. *Gene* 568:190–5.

Dubern, B., and K. Clement. 2012. Leptin and leptin receptor-related monogenic obesity. *Biochimie* 94:2111–5.

Eckel, L. A., W. Langhans, A. Kahler, L. A. Campfield, F. J. Smith, and N. Geary. 1998. Chronic administration of OB protein decreases food intake by selectively reducing meal size in female rats. *Am J Physiol* 275:R186–93.

Ellacott, K. L., I. G. Halatchev, and R. D. Cone. 2006. Characterization of leptin-responsive neurons in the caudal brainstem. *Endocrinology* 147:3190–5.

Emond, M., E. E. Ladenheim, G. J. Schwartz, and T. H. Moran. 2001. Leptin amplifies the feeding inhibition and neural activation arising from a gastric nutrient preload. *Physiol Behav* 72:123–8.

Emond, M., G. J. Schwartz, E. E. Ladenheim, and T. H. Moran. 1999. Central leptin modulates behavioral and neural responsivity to CCK. *Am J Physiol* 276:R1545–9.

Fan, W., K. L. Ellacott, I. G. Halatchev, K. Takahashi, P. Yu, and R. D. Cone. 2004. Cholecystokinin-mediated suppression of feeding involves the brainstem melanocortin system. *Nat Neurosci* 7:335–6.

Friedman, J. 2014. 20 years of leptin: Leptin at 20: An overview. *J Endocrinol* 223:T1–8.

Garfield, A. S., C. Patterson, S. Skora, F. M. Gribble, F. Reimann, M. L. Evans, M. G. Myers, Jr., and L. K. Heisler. 2012. Neurochemical characterization of body weight-regulating leptin receptor neurons in the nucleus of the solitary tract. *Endocrinology* 153:4600–7.

Gautron, L., C. Lee, H. Funahashi, J. Friedman, S. Lee, and J. Elmquist. 2010. Melanocortin-4 receptor expression in a vago-vagal circuitry involved in postprandial functions. *J Comp Neurol* 518:6–24.

Gautron, L., C. E. Lee, S. Lee, and J. K. Elmquist. 2012. Melanocortin-4 receptor expression in different classes of spinal and vagal primary afferent neurons in the mouse. *J Comp Neurol* 520:3933–48.

Geary, N. 2001. Estradiol, CCK and satiation. *Peptides* 22:1251–63.

Geary, N., D. Trace, B. McEwen, and G. P. Smith. 1994. Cyclic estradiol replacement increases the satiety effect of CCK-8 in ovariectomized rats. *Physiol Behav* 56:281–9.

Gibbs, J., R. C. Young, and G. P. Smith. 1973. Cholecystokinin decreases food intake in rats. *J Comp Physiol Psychol* 84:488–95.

Goldstone, A. P., J. G. Mercer, I. Gunn, K. M. Moar, C. M. Edwards, M. Rossi, J. K. Howard, S. Rasheed, M. D. Turton, C. Small, M. M. Heath, D. O'Shea, J. Steere, K. Meeran, M. A. Ghatei, N. Hoggard, and S. R. Bloom. 1997. Leptin interacts with glucagon-like peptide-1 neurons to reduce food intake and body weight in rodents. *FEBS Lett* 415:134–8.

Gould, B. R., and H. H. Zingg. 2003. Mapping oxytocin receptor gene expression in the mouse brain and mammary gland using an oxytocin receptor-LacZ reporter mouse. *Neuroscience* 122:155–67.

Grill, H. J., A. B. Ginsberg, R. J. Seeley, and J. M. Kaplan. 1998. Brainstem application of melanocortin receptor ligands produces long-lasting effects on feeding and body weight. *J Neurosci* 18:10128–35.

Grill, H. J., M. W. Schwartz, J. M. Kaplan, J. S. Foxhall, J. Breininger, and D. G. Baskin. 2002. Evidence that the caudal brainstem is a target for the inhibitory effect of leptin on food intake. *Endocrinology* 143:239–46.

Guard, D. B., T. D. Swartz, R. C. Ritter, G. A. Burns, and M. Covasa. 2009. NMDA NR2 receptors participate in CCK-induced reduction of food intake and hindbrain neuronal activation. *Brain Res* 1266:37–44.

Harris, R. B. 2013a. Evidence that leptin-induced weight loss requires activation of both fore-brain and hindbrain receptors. *Physiol Behav* 120:83–92.

Harris, R. B. 2013b. Is leptin the parabiotic "satiety" factor? Past and present interpretations. *Appetite* 61:111–8.

Harris, R. B., T. J. Bartness, and H. J. Grill. 2007. Leptin responsiveness in chronically decer-ebrate rats. *Endocrinology* 148:4623–33.

Heldsinger, A., G. Grabauskas, I. Song, and C. Owyang. 2011. Synergistic interaction between leptin and cholecystokinin in the rat nodose ganglia is mediated by PI3K and STAT3 signaling pathways: Implications for leptin as a regulator of short term satiety. *J Biol Chem* 286:11707–15.

Hisadome, K., F. Reimann, F. M. Gribble, and S. Trapp. 2010. Leptin directly depolarizes preproglucagon neurons in the nucleus tractus solitarius: Electrical properties of glucagon-like Peptide 1 neurons. *Diabetes* 59:1890–8.

Hommel, J. D., R. Trinko, R. M. Sears, D. Georgescu, Z. W. Liu, X. B. Gao, J. J. Thurmon, M. Marinelli, and R. J. DiLeone. 2006. Leptin receptor signaling in midbrain dopamine neurons regulates feeding. *Neuron* 51:801–10.

Huo, L., K. M. Gamber, H. J. Grill, and C. Bjorbaek. 2008. Divergent leptin signaling in proglucagon neurons of the nucleus of the solitary tract in mice and rats. *Endocrinology* 149:492–7.

Huo, L., L. Maeng, C. Bjorbaek, and H. J. Grill. 2007. Leptin and the control of food intake: Neurons in the nucleus of the solitary tract are activated by both gastric distension and leptin. *Endocrinology* 148:2189–97.

Irving, A. J., and J. Harvey. 2014. Leptin regulation of hippocampal synaptic function in health and disease. *Philos Trans R Soc Lond B Biol Sci* 369:20130155.

Janowitz, H., and M. I. Grossman. 1948. Effect of parenteral administration of glucose and protein hydrolysate on food intake in the rat. *Am J Physiol* 155:28–32.

Janowitz, H. D., and M. I. Grossman. 1949. Some factors affecting the food intake of normal dogs and dogs with esophagostomy and gastric fistula. *Am J Physiol* 159:143–8.

Janowitz, H. D., M. E. Hanson, and M. I. Grossman. 1949. Effect of intravenously administered glucose on food intake in the dog. *Am J Physiol* 156:87–91.

Kahler, A., N. Geary, L. A. Eckel, L. A. Campfield, F. J. Smith, and W. Langhans. 1998. Chronic administration of OB protein decreases food intake by selectively reducing meal size in male rats. *Am J Physiol* 275:R180–5.

Kanoski, S. E., M. R. Hayes, H. S. Greenwald, S. M. Fortin, C. A. Gianessi, J. R. Gilbert, and H. J. Grill. 2011. Hippocampal leptin signaling reduces food intake and modulates food-related memory processing. *Neuropsychopharmacology* 36:1859–70.

Kanoski, S. E., E. K. Walls, and T. L. Davidson. 2007. Interoceptive "satiety" signals produced by leptin and CCK. *Peptides* 28:988–1002.

Kishi, T., C. J. Aschkenasi, C. E. Lee, K. G. Mountjoy, C. B. Saper, and J. K. Elmquist. 2003. Expression of melanocortin 4 receptor mRNA in the central nervous system of the rat. *J Comp Neurol* 457:213–35.

Kistler-Heer, V., M. F. Lauber, and W. Lichtensteiger. 1998. Different developmental patterns of melanocortin MC3 and MC4 receptor mRNA: Predominance of Mc4 in fetal rat nervous system. *J Neuroendocrinol* 10:133–46.

Koch, M., and T. L. Horvath. 2014. Molecular and cellular regulation of hypothalamic melanocortin neurons controlling food intake and energy metabolism. *Mol Psychiatry* 19:752–61.

Kopp, J., Z. Q. Xu, X. Zhang, T. Pedrazzini, H. Herzog, A. Kresse, H. Wong, J. H. Walsh, and T. Hokfelt. 2002. Expression of the neuropeptide Y Y1 receptor in the CNS of rat and of wild-type and Y1 receptor knock-out mice. Focus on immunohistochemical localization. *Neuroscience* 111:443–532.

Labouesse, M. A., U. Stadlbauer, E. Weber, M. Arnold, W. Langhans, and G. Pacheco-Lopez. 2012. Vagal afferents mediate early satiation and prevent flavour avoidance learning in response to intraperitoneally infused exendin-4. *J Neuroendocrinol* 24:1505–16.

Lachamp, P., M. Crest, and J. P. Kessler. 2006. Vesicular glutamate transporters type 1 and 2 expression in axon terminals of the rat nucleus of the solitary tract. *Neuroscience* 137:73–81.

Ladenheim, E. E., M. Emond, and T. H. Moran. 2005. Leptin enhances feeding suppression and neural activation produced by systemically administered bombesin. *Am J Physiol Regul Integr Comp Physiol* 289:R473–R477.

Maffei, M., J. Halaas, E. Ravussin, R. E. Pratley, G. H. Lee, Y. Zhang, H. Fei, S. Kim, R. Lallone, S. Ranganathan et al. 1995. Leptin levels in human and rodent: Measurement of plasma leptin and ob RNA in obese and weight-reduced subjects. *Nat Med* 1:1155–61.

Maniscalco, J. W., and L. Rinaman. 2014. Systemic leptin dose-dependently increases STAT3 phosphorylation within hypothalamic and hindbrain nuclei. *Am J Physiol Regul Integr Comp Physiol* 306:R576–85.

Marks, D. L., V. Hruby, G. Brookhart, and R. D. Cone. 2006. The regulation of food intake by selective stimulation of the type 3 melanocortin receptor (MC3R). *Peptides* 27:259–64.

Moran, T. H., and P. R. McHugh. 1988. Gastric and nongastric mechanisms for satiety action of cholecystokinin. *Am J Physiol* 254:R628–32.

Mountjoy, K. G., M. T. Mortrud, M. J. Low, R. B. Simerly, and R. D. Cone. 1994. Localization of the melanocortin-4 receptor (MC4-R) in neuroendocrine and autonomic control circuits in the brain. *Mol Endocrinol* 8:1298–308.

Nefti, W., C. Chaumontet, G. Fromentin, D. Tome, and N. Darcel. 2009. A high-fat diet attenuates the central response to within-meal satiation signals and modifies the receptor expression of vagal afferents in mice. *Am J Physiol Regul Integr Comp Physiol* 296:R1681–6.

Pavlov, I. P. 1910. *The work of the digestive glands*. Translated by W. H. Tompson. United Kingdom: Charles Griffin and Company.

Pavlov, I. P. 1928. "The food centre." In *Lectures on conditioned reflexes*, ed. W. Horsley Gantt, 147–155. New York: Liveright Publishing Corporation.

Peters, J. H., A. B. Karpiel, R. C. Ritter, and S. M. Simasko. 2004. Cooperative activation of cultured vagal afferent neurons by leptin and cholecystokinin. *Endocrinology* 145:3652–7.

Peters, J. H., S. J. McDougall, D. O. Kellett, D. Jordan, I. J. Llewellyn-Smith, and M. C. Andresen. 2008. Oxytocin enhances cranial visceral afferent synaptic transmission to the solitary tract nucleus. *J Neurosci* 28:11731–40.

Peters, J. H., B. M. McKay, S. M. Simasko, and R. C. Ritter. 2005. Leptin-induced satiation mediated by abdominal vagal afferents. *Am J Physiol Regul Integr Comp Physiol* 288:R879–84.

Peters, J. H., R. C. Ritter, and S. M. Simasko. 2006. Leptin and CCK selectively activate vagal afferent neurons innervating the stomach and duodenum. *Am J Physiol Regul Integr Comp Physiol* 290:R1544–9.

Phillips, R. J., and T. L. Powley. 1996. Gastric volume rather than nutrient content inhibits food intake. *Am J Physiol* 271:R766–9.

Ritter, R. C., and E. E. Ladenheim. 1985. Capsaicin pretreatment attenuates suppression of food intake by cholecystokinin. *Am J Physiol* 248:R501–4.

Rogers, R. C., and G. E. Hermann. 2008. Mechanisms of action of CCK to activate central vagal afferent terminals. *Peptides* 29:1716–25.

Roselli-Rehfuss, L., K. G. Mountjoy, L. S. Robbins, M. T. Mortrud, M. J. Low, J. B. Tatro, M. L. Entwistle, R. B. Simerly, and R. D. Cone. 1993. Identification of a receptor for gamma melanotropin and other proopiomelanocortin peptides in the hypothalamus and limbic system. *Proc Natl Acad Sci U S A* 90:8856–60.

Rowland, N. E., J. W. Schaub, K. L. Robertson, A. Andreasen, and C. Haskell-Luevano. 2010. Effect of MTII on food intake and brain c-Fos in melanocortin-3, melanocortin-4, and double MC3 and MC4 receptor knockout mice. *Peptides* 31:2314–7.

Ruiter, M., P. Duffy, S. Simasko, and R. C. Ritter. 2010. Increased hypothalamic signal transducer and activator of transcription 3 phosphorylation after hindbrain leptin injection. *Endocrinology* 151:1509–19.

Sassu, E. D., J. E. McDermott, B. J. Keys, M. Esmaeili, A. C. Keene, M. J. Birnbaum, and J. R. DiAngelo. 2012. Mio/dChREBP coordinately increases fat mass by regulating lipid synthesis and feeding behavior in Drosophila. *Biochem Biophys Res Commun* 426:43–8.

Schwartz, G. J., L. A. Netterville, P. R. McHugh, and T. H. Moran. 1991. Gastric loads potentiate inhibition of food intake produced by a cholecystokinin analogue. *Am J Physiol* 261:R1141–6.

Schwartz, M. W., R. J. Seeley, L. A. Campfield, P. Burn, and D. G. Baskin. 1996. Identification of targets of leptin action in rat hypothalamus. *J Clin Invest* 98:1101–6.

Schwartz, M. W., R. J. Seeley, S. C. Woods, D. S. Weigle, L. A. Campfield, P. Burn, and D. G. Baskin. 1997. Leptin increases hypothalamic pro-opiomelanocortin mRNA expression in the rostral arcuate nucleus. *Diabetes* 46:2119–23.

Sclafani, A. 2013. Gut-brain nutrient signaling. Appetition vs. satiation. *Appetite* 71:454–8.

Sclafani, A., and K. Ackroff. 2012. Role of gut nutrient sensing in stimulating appetite and conditioning food preferences. *Am J Physiol Regul Integr Comp Physiol* 302:R1119–33.

Sclafani, A., and F. Lucas. 1996. Abdominal vagotomy does not block carbohydrate-conditioned flavor preferences in rats. *Physiol Behav* 60:447–53.

Sclafani, A., S. Zukerman, and K. Ackroff. 2013. GPR40 and GPR120 fatty acid sensors are critical for postoral but not oral mediation of fat preferences in the mouse. *Am J Physiol Regul Integr Comp Physiol* 305:R1490–7.

Scott, M. M., J. L. Lachey, S. M. Sternson, C. E. Lee, C. F. Elias, J. M. Friedman, and J. K. Elmquist. 2009. Leptin targets in the mouse brain. *J Comp Neurol* 514:518–32.

Seeley, R. J., K. A. Yagaloff, S. L. Fisher, P. Burn, T. E. Thiele, G. van Dijk, D. G. Baskin, and M. W. Schwartz. 1997. Melanocortin receptors in leptin effects. *Nature* 390:349.

Smith, G. P. 1995. Pavlov and appetite. *Integr Physiol Behav Sci* 30:169–74.

Smith, G. P. 1996. The direct and indirect controls of meal size. *Neurosci Biobehav Rev* 20:41–6.

Smith, G. P., C. Jerome, and R. Norgren. 1985. Afferent axons in abdominal vagus mediate satiety effect of cholecystokinin in rats. *Am J Physiol* 249:R638–41.

South, E. H., and R. C. Ritter. 1988. Capsaicin application to central or peripheral vagal fibers attenuates CCK satiety. *Peptides* 9:601–12.

Stanic, D., P. Brumovsky, S. Fetissov, S. Shuster, H. Herzog, and T. Hokfelt. 2006. Characterization of neuropeptide Y2 receptor protein expression in the mouse brain. I. Distribution in cell bodies and nerve terminals. *J Comp Neurol* 499:357–90.

Sutton, G. M., B. Duos, L. M. Patterson, and H. R. Berthoud. 2005. Melanocortinergic modulation of cholecystokinin-induced suppression of feeding through extracellular signal-regulated kinase signaling in rat solitary nucleus. *Endocrinology* 146:3739–47.

Sutton, G. M., L. M. Patterson, and H. R. Berthoud. 2004. Extracellular signal-regulated kinase 1/2 signaling pathway in solitary nucleus mediates cholecystokinin-induced suppression of food intake in rats. *J Neurosci* 24:10240–7.

Uematsu, A., T. Tsurugizawa, H. Uneyama, and K. Torii. 2010. Brain-gut communication via vagus nerve modulates conditioned flavor preference. *Eur J Neurosci* 31:1136–43.

Valente, P., S. Casagrande, T. Nieus, A. M. Verstegen, F. Valtorta, F. Benfenati, and P. Baldelli. 2012. Site-specific synapsin I phosphorylation participates in the expression of post-tetanic potentiation and its enhancement by BDNF. *J Neurosci* 32:5868–79.

van de Wall, E. H., P. Duffy, and R. C. Ritter. 2005. CCK enhances response to gastric distension by acting on capsaicin-insensitive vagal afferents. *Am J Physiol Regul Integr Comp Physiol* 289:R695–703.

Vatier, C., J. F. Gautier, and C. Vigouroux. 2012. Therapeutic use of recombinant methionyl human leptin. *Biochimie* 94:2116–25.

Wan, S., K. N. Browning, F. H. Coleman, G. Sutton, H. Zheng, A. Butler, H. R. Berthoud, and R. A. Travagli. 2008. Presynaptic melanocortin-4 receptors on vagal afferent fibers modulate the excitability of rat nucleus tractus solitarius neurons. *J Neurosci* 28:4957–66.

Wang, Y. H., Y. Tache, A. B. Sheibel, V. L. Go, and J. Y. Wei. 1997. Two types of leptin-responsive gastric vagal afferent terminals: An in vitro single-unit study in rats. *Am J Physiol* 273:R833–7.

Welch, M. G., H. Tamir, K. J. Gross, J. Chen, M. Anwar, and M. D. Gershon. 2009. Expression and developmental regulation of oxytocin (OT) and oxytocin receptors (OTR) in the enteric nervous system (ENS) and intestinal epithelium. *J Comp Neurol* 512:256–70.

Williams, K. W., and B. N. Smith. 2006. Rapid inhibition of neural excitability in the nucleus tractus solitarii by leptin: Implications for ingestive behaviour. *J Physiol* 573:395–412.

Williams, D. L., J. M. Kaplan, and H. J. Grill. 2000. The role of the dorsal vagal complex and the vagus nerve in feeding effects of melanocortin-3/4 receptor stimulation. *Endocrinology* 141:1332–7.

Wright, J., C. Campos, T. Herzog, M. Covasa, K. Czaja, and R. C. Ritter. 2011. Reduction of food intake by cholecystokinin requires activation of hindbrain NMDA-type glutamate receptors. *Am J Physiol Regul Integr Comp Physiol* 301:R448–55.

Yang, L., K. A. Scott, J. Hyun, K. L. Tamashiro, N. Tray, T. H. Moran, and S. Bi. 2009. Role of dorsomedial hypothalamic neuropeptide Y in modulating food intake and energy balance. *J Neurosci* 29:179–90.

Yox, D. P., and R. C. Ritter. 1988. Capsaicin attenuates suppression of sham feeding induced by intestinal nutrients. *Am J Physiol* 255:R569–74.

Yox, D. P., H. Stokesberry, and R. C. Ritter. 1991. Vagotomy attenuates suppression of sham feeding induced by intestinal nutrients. *Am J Physiol* 260:R503–8.

Zhang, X., T. Shi, K. Holmberg, M. Landry, W. Huang, H. Xiao, G. Ju, and T. Hokfelt. 1997. Expression and regulation of the neuropeptide Y Y2 receptor in sensory and autonomic ganglia. *Proc Natl Acad Sci U S A* 94:729–34.

Zhao, H., J. H. Peters, M. Zhu, S. J. Page, R. C. Ritter, and S. M. Appleyard. 2015. Frequency-dependent facilitation of synaptic throughput via postsynaptic NMDA receptors in the nucleus of the solitary tract. *J Physiol* 593:111–25.

Zheng, H., L. M. Patterson, C. B. Phifer, and H. R. Berthoud. 2005. Brain stem melanocortinergic modulation of meal size and identification of hypothalamic POMC projections. *Am J Physiol Regul Integr Comp Physiol* 289:R247–58.

Zheng, H., L. M. Patterson, C. J. Rhodes, G. W. Louis, K. P. Skibicka, H. J. Grill, M. G. Myers, Jr., and H. R. Berthoud. 2010. A potential role for hypothalamomedullary POMC projections in leptin-induced suppression of food intake. *Am J Physiol Regul Integr Comp Physiol* 298:R720–8.

12 Energy Metabolism and Appetite Control

Separate Roles for Fat-Free Mass and Fat Mass in the Control of Food Intake in Humans

Mark Hopkins and John E. Blundell

CONTENTS

12.1 INTRODUCTION

Concepts for the control of food intake and the idea of regulation of body weight have been proposed for well over 50 years (Kennedy 1953, Mayer 1953, Mellinkoff et al. 1956). The debate has been based mainly on animal experiments (usually rodents) often using brain interventions. The proposed central mechanisms purported to control food intake have undergone a series of progressive refinements arising from technical advances in neuroscience. The mechanisms discussed in scientific circles today bear little resemblance to the simple notions of "hunger and satiety centers" that were the pinnacle of scientific understanding over 60 years ago.

259

A major feature of early hypotheses was the influence of the notion of homeostasis and its parallel in cybernetics or control theory. Both of these positions focused on the identity of feedback signals that monitored some deviation from an ideal value and stimulated compensatory adjustments via a central controller. This gave rise to a strong emphasis on the notion of regulation with body weight itself identified as the regulated variable. One view was that the organization of the body's physiology was similar, in principle, to the control of ambient temperature in a thermostatically controlled room. Indeed, some physiological systems do appear to work in this way, and it was assumed that it applied equally to the relationship of the control of food intake and the "regulation" of body weight. If true regulation does occur, it is not clear if the regulated variable is gross body weight, adipose tissue or fat-free mass (FFM). It is in the light of this background that we have interpreted certain relationships among body composition, energy expenditure and food intake in humans.

12.2 COMMENT ON THE LIPOSTATIC THEORY OF APPETITE CONTROL

Early theoretical approaches to the regulation of food intake and body weight were based on the notion that the regulatory mechanisms stemmed from peripheral signals arising from glucose metabolism (e.g., the glucostatic theory; Mayer 1953), amino acids (e.g., the aminostatic theory; Mellinkoff et al. 1956), or adipose tissue (e.g. the lipostatic theory; Kennedy 1957). The discovery of leptin by Zhang et al. (1994) provided a molecular basis and apparent proof of the authenticity of the lipostatic theory. This hypothesis was based on Kennedy's (1953) classic ventromedial hypothalamus lesions studies in rats, in which he proposed that "lipostasis" was regulated by circulating metabolites that acted on a hypothalamic "calorimetric satiety" center to inhibit feeding (Kennedy 1953, 1966). Interestingly, it is worth noting that Kennedy's (1953) original lipostatic hypothesis was only concerned with "the prevention of an overall surplus of energy intake over expenditure," rather than a universal "thermostat" that defended both upper and lower limits of fat mass (FM). Subsequently Hervey (Hervey 1969, Hervey and Hervey 1969) proposed a mechanism for lipostatic regulation based on a fat-soluble hormone, with findings from parabiotic rat studies suggesting that the exchange of a blood-borne factor differentially affected food intake in lean and obese animals (Hervey and Hervey 1969). Similar experiments in the late 1970s using genetically obese rodents (Coleman and Hummel 1969, Coleman 1973) created the conceptual basis for the studies that led to the identification of leptin (Zhang et al. 1994).

12.2.1 LEPTIN AND ENERGY HOMEOSTASIS

There is now considerable experimental data to support the view that leptin affects many central structures known to be involved in the neural control of food intake (Sainsbury and Zhang 2010), and it is commonly accepted that leptin is a signal that conveys information from the periphery to the brain regarding the long-term state of the body's energy stores (Badman and Flier 2005, Morton et al. 2006, Woods and Ramsay 2011). Based on animal and in vitro molecular studies, changes to circulating leptin concentrations are thought to alter the hypothalamic expression of anorexigenic and orexigenic neuropeptide effector molecules, which promote corrective responses in energy intake (EI) and expenditure to minimize perturbation to energy balance (Morton et al. 2006). For example, a reduction in leptin is thought to promote increased motivation to eat via a down-regulation in the hypothalamic expression of anorexigenic neuropeptides such as proopiomelanocortin (POMC) and alpha melanocyte-stimulating hormone (α-MSH) and an up-regulation in the expression of orexigenic neuropeptides such as neuropeptide Y (NPY) and agouti-related protein (AgRP) (Lenard and Berthoud 2008, Sainsbury and Zhang 2010). As a consequence, leptin is now viewed as central to the hypothalamic control of energy homeostasis and has become inextricably linked with support for the lipostatic theory of appetite control. Indeed, it has been suggested that EI and energy expenditure are actually controlled in the interests of regulating body weight and, specifically, fat mass (FM) (Rosen and Spiegelman 2006), with leptin central to this coordination. This approach has encouraged the view that adipose tissue is the main driver of day-to-day food intake (Badman and Flier 2005, Morton et al. 2006, Woods and Ramsay 2011).

However, despite recent advances in our understanding of the neural pathways underpinning feeding, a unifying theory of how these central neural signals are integrated with peripheral signals of nutrient intake and energy status (and cognitive and environmental factors) remains elusive (Borer 2014). Importantly, a number of questions exist regarding the applicability of this lipostatic control system to the regulation of appetite and food intake in humans under normal physiological conditions, i.e., in those free from congenital leptin deficiency (Jequier 2002). Secular trends in obesity prevalence (Finucane 2011, Ng et al. 2014) suggest that adipose tissue accumulation does not exert strong negative feedback to restore energy balance (at least from the point of excess EI). Furthermore, despite the apparent acceptance that leptin plays a key role in appetite control, there is surprisingly little evidence in humans on the extent to which changes in adipose tissue (and associated adipokines) exert feedback on food intake.

As leptin is secreted by adipocytes in proportion to the degree of adipose tissue (Schwartz et al. 2000), leptin's primary role in appetite control maybe as a putative tonic inhibitory peptide. In this role, it could act as an enduring or continual inhibitory (dampening) influence on the drive to eat. Early studies demonstrated that leptin deficiency is associated with profound hyperphagia (Farooqi et al. 2007), which is abated with exogenous leptin administration (Farooqi et al. 1999). However, the administration of physiological doses of leptin in lean or obese humans has little or no effect on food intake or body weight (Heymsfield et al. 1999). Rather, the effect of leptin on energy homeostatis appears to be closely coupled to the body's short- and long-term energy status (Sainsbury and Zhang 2010). Acute and short-term (2–7 days) energy restriction has been shown to result in significant and often disproportionate reductions in circulating leptin relative to the associated change in FM (Weigle et al. 1997, Dubuc et al. 1998, Chin-Chance, Polonsky, and Schoeller 2000, Mars et al. 2005a,b, Pasiakos et al. 2011). However, there is limited and contradictory evidence that acute or short-term changes in circulating leptin influence subjective appetite and food intake (Chin-Chance, Polonsky, and Schoeller 2000, Mars et al. 2005a,b). Similarly, there is only sparse evidence demonstrating that peripheral changes in leptin are associated with changes in appetite and food intake following long-term energy restriction and weight loss (Heini et al. 1998, Keim, Stern, and Havel 1998, Doucet et al. 2000).

It has also been argued that the effect of leptin on energy homeostasis is asymmetrical. While a decline in circulating leptin is thought to promote increased EI and decreased energy expenditure, an increase in leptin does not appear to exert a proportional down-regulation in food intake or up-regulation in energy expenditure (Leibel 2002). This attenuated catabolic response following sustained elevations in circulating leptin concentrations is thought to reflect "leptin resistance" in the obese state. Low leptin concentrations, indicative of energy deficit or reduced FM, therefore appear to be of greater biological importance than elevated leptin concentrations, with leptin playing little role in appetite control or body weight regulation in the overfed or obese state (Ravussin, Leibel, and Ferrante 2014). Such findings have led some to suggest leptin acts primarily as a "starvation signal" involved in the defense of body weight, rather than a satiation or satiety signal involved in control of day-to-day food intake (Leibel 2002, Chan et al. 2003).

12.3 ENERGY EXPENDITURE AND ENERGY INTAKE

An alternative view of appetite control that did not involve the dominating theme of "regulation" was proposed over 50 years ago based on the relationship between food intake and energy expenditure (Mayer et al. 1954, Edholm et al. 1955a, Mayer, Roy, and Mitra 1956, Edholm 1977). This approach questioned whether food intake is controlled by the dynamics of adipose tissue (as postulated in the lipostatic hypothesis) and proposed instead that food intake might be driven by the body's demand for energy. However, despite its apparent fundamental importance to our understanding of appetite control, the question of whether energy expenditure influences EI has been rarely investigated and has yet to be fully resolved. Consequently, it remains unclear whether the physiological demand for energy arising from the biological processes and behavioral activities of daily living influence appetite and food intake.

12.4 ROLE OF ENERGY EXPENDITURE AND BODY COMPOSITION IN THE CONTROL OF FOOD INTAKE

Over 50 years ago, Jean Mayer questioned whether an increase in energy expenditure causes an automatic (compensatory) increase in EI (Mayer et al. 1954), stating that "the regulation of food intake functions with such flexibility that an increase in energy output due to exercise is automatically followed by an equivalent increase in caloric intake." This issue was systematically examined by Edholm and colleagues, who sought to examine whether energy expenditure created a demand for food in a series of studies employing army cadets (Edholm et al. 1955b, 1970, Edholm 1977). While Edholm et al. (1955b) proposed that "the differences in intakes of food must originate in the differences in energy expenditure," no relationship was found between daily energy expenditure and daily food intake in lean males undergoing infantry training within a single day ($n = 12$). These findings are consistent with more recent studies demonstrating that acute increases in energy expenditure (via exercise)

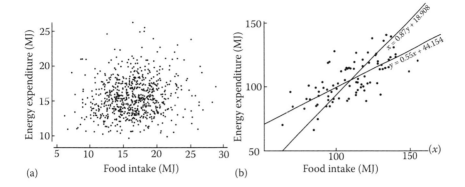

FIGURE 12.1   Data of Edholm (1977) demonstrating no relationship between food intake and daily energy expenditure within a single day intake in lean males undergoing infantry training. However, a strong relationship was found when daily energy expenditure and food intake were averaged across one week. (From Edholm, O.G., *J. Hum. Nutr.*, 31, 413–431, 1977.)

are not accompanied by immediate (within one day) increases in EI to restore energy balance (King and Blundell 1995, King et al. 1996, 1997, Blundell and King 1998, Hopkins, King, and Blundell 2010).

The fact that body weight can remain relatively stable in some individuals over long periods of time has been taken to suggest that energy expenditure must be coupled (at least loosely) to EI (Bessesen 2011). Indeed, it has been shown that there is a "time lag" in the corrective responses elicited by energy depletion or surfeit, with Bray et al. (2008) reporting that compensatory changes in EI are evident 2–3 days after dietary manipulation of food intake. This would suggest that energy balance is not regulated across a single day, but that attempts are made to restore energy balance over subsequent days. It is interesting to note that while Edholm et al. (1955b) failed to find any relationship between daily energy expenditure and EI within a single day, a strong relationship was found when daily energy expenditure and EI were averaged across 1 week (Edholm 1977) (see Figure 12.1). These findings are consistent with those of Mayer, Roy, and Mitra (1956), who demonstrated a relationship between occupational physical energy expenditure and daily EI. Mayer, Roy, and Mitra (1956) reported that EI was greater in Bengali jute mill workers who performed physically demanding jobs as opposed to those who performed sedentary jobs, consistent with the view that daily energy expenditure does create a demand for food intake.

12.5   FAT FREE MASS AS AN OREXIGENIC DRIVER

Recently, a number of studies have examined the specific role that body composition and energy expenditure play in the control of food intake in humans (Blundell et al. 2011, Caudwell et al. 2013, Weise et al. 2013). These studies demonstrate that FFM, but not FM, is a strong determinant of day-to-day food intake (Blundell et al. 2011, Weise et al. 2013). Blundell et al. (2011) reported that self-selected meal size and total daily EI (measured objectively in a laboratory environment) were positively associated with FFM in 92 overweight and obese individuals. However, in contrast, no such associations were found between FM and food intake. These findings have been confirmed by Weise et al. (2013), who reported the FFM index was positively associated with ad libitum EI in 184 lean and obese individuals. A number of earlier observation have also demonstrated associations between FFM and food intake, with Lissner et al. (1989) reporting that lean body mass (but not FM) predicted EI in 63 nonobese and obese women whose EI and body composition were objectively measured in a laboratory environment. The authors argued that "the emphasis of research that focuses on the relationship between EI and obesity is misplaced because energy requirement appears to be a direct function of lean mass rather than of adiposity." Similarly, Cugini et al. (1998), in a little known and rarely cited body of research, also reported that daily hunger was positively associated with FFM (and negatively related to FM) in lean (Cugini et al. 1998), but not overweight and obese (Cugini et al. 1999), individuals.

It is worth noting that such findings are in keeping with previous research demonstrating that lean tissue acts as an orexigenic feedback signal during periods of weight loss and weight regain (Dulloo, Jacquet, and Girardier 1997, Dulloo, Jacquet, and Montani 2012). Based on findings from semistarvation studies and, in particular, Ancel Key's Minnesota semistarvation experiment (Keys et al. 1950), Dulloo, Jacquet, and Girardier (1997) have noted that FM and FFM losses during significant weight loss (approximately 25% of initial body weight) independently predicted the poststarvation hyperphagic response. Furthermore, during recovery from weight loss, the restoration of FFM was found to be incomplete at the point at which body mass and FM were fully restored to prestarvation levels. Importantly, hyperphagia was evident despite the full restoration of body mass and FM and persisted until FFM levels were fully restored to prestarvation levels. These data were interpreted as evidence of a "proteinostatic" mechanism in the control of food intake, with feedback signals arising from both FM and FFM that acted to stimulating appetite and food intake in order to restore body weight (Dulloo, Jacquet, and Girardier 1997, Dulloo, Jacquet, and Montani 2012).

While the demands imposed by semistarvation on body weight regulation clearly exceed those experienced under normal free-living conditions, the idea of a physiological drive for food intake stemming from FFM is consistent with the "protein-stat" (Millward 1995) and "amino-static" (Mellinkoff et al. 1956) theories of lean tissue and appetite regulation, respectively. Millward's protein-stat theory suggests that lean mass, and skeletal muscle in particular, is under tight regulation and food intake is directed to meet the needs of lean tissue growth and maintenance (Millward 1995). The basis of this theory is the existence of an "aminostatic" appetite control mechanism, in which food intake is adjusted in response to amino acid availability to meet the protein demands of lean tissue growth and maintenance. However, it should be noted that evidence of such regulation, or the existence of a "protein-stat," is not extensive, mainly because the concept has not been a target for investigation.

It has also been suggested that day-to-day food intake is regulated via nutrient-specific appetite control mechanisms rather than an energy-based regulatory system reliant on the energy content of the diet. In particular, the protein-leverage hypothesis

(Simpson and Raubenheimer 2005) proposes that dietary protein intake is (i) tightly regulated, (ii) independent of the regulation of dietary fat and carbohydrate intake, and (iii) prioritized over the energy content of the diet. It has been proposed that such regulatory control can lead to excess EI when a diet is low in protein as fat and carbohydrate are consumed in excess to "compensate" for the perceived protein deficit by "leveraging" dietary fat and carbohydrate intake (Sørensen et al. 2008). Evidence for "nutrient-specific appetites" exists in a range of animal models (see Morrison and Laeger 2015 for a review) Furthermore, experimental and cross-sectional survey data suggest that humans also compensate for reductions in dietary protein via increased food intake and, in so doing, consume excessive amounts of dietary fats and carbohydrates (Gosby et al. 2014). While such data fit with the notion of a protein-stat or amino-stat, such leverage by appetites for specific nutrients suggests that EI is not linked to "energy sensing" mechanisms (that reflect energy need). However, the underlying mechanisms behind such nutrient-specific appetite control mechanisms in humans remain poorly defined (Morrison and Laeger 2015). Furthermore, it is quite feasible that a nutrient-specific protein-sensing mechanism could function alongside a regulatory mechanism that reflects energy need.

12.6   RESTING METABOLIC RATE AND TOTAL DAILY ENERGY EXPENDITURE AS DRIVERS OF FOOD INTAKE

The reported associations between FFM and food intake (Lissner et al. 1989, Cugini et al. 1998, Blundell et al. 2011, Weise et al. 2013) may have important implications for day-to-day appetite control. It is well established that FFM is the primary determinant of resting metabolic rate (RMR) (Ravussin et al. 1986a), which in turn is the largest component of daily total energy expenditure (TEE) (Ravussin et al. 1986b). The findings of Edholm et al. (1955b) that energy expenditure and EI were not coupled within a single day (Edholm 1977) would initially suggest that daily energy expenditure is not a determinant of food intake. However, it is almost inevitable that the high degree of day-to-day variability in sedentary and active behaviors contributes to the high variability in daily energy expenditure (Ravussin et al. 1982) and could mask such a relationship. By contrast, RMR is relatively stable between days and typically accounts for 60%–75% of total daily energy expenditure (Ravussin et al. 1986a). Its enduring stability is in part due to the fact that FFM is the main determinant of RMR, accounting for 50%–60% of the between-subject variance (Johnstone et al. 2005). Therefore, given the more constant energetic demand arising from RMR (or FFM as its main determinant), it is possible that RMR may provide a more stable signal of energy demand.

In line with this proposal, Caudwell et al. (2013) demonstrated that RMR (but again, not FM) was a strong determinant of daily hunger, self-selected meal size, and daily EI in overweight and obese individuals. RMR and daily EI under conditions of high and low energy density were objectively measured in 41 overweight and obese individuals during a 12-week exercise intervention. A higher RMR was associated with greater daily hunger, self-selected meal size, and daily EI (independent of sex and energy density). Furthermore, Westerterp-Plantenga et al. (2003) have also demonstrated a positive association between RMR and self-reported meal frequency (derived from food diaries) in 12 older men (62 ± 4.0 years), with RMR explaining 40% of the between-subject variance in meal frequency. Interestingly, a negative association between RMR and meal frequency was noted in 19 young men (23.1 ± 3.9 years), with RMR explaining 85% of the variance in meal frequency. While it was suggested that meal frequency might represent a method of "tuning" EI to energy expenditure, it is unclear why the direction of association differed between young and older participants. However, it is certainly possible that RMR could influence either meal size or meal frequency according to the constraints imposed by the experimental design.

Based on the findings that FFM and RMR (but not FM) are associated with day-to-day food intake, Blundell et al. (2011) have proposed that energy expenditure arising from FFM (as the main determinant of RMR) represents a physiological source of hunger that drives food intake at a level proportional to basal energy requirements. This long-term (tonic) signal of energy demand would help "tune" EI to energy expenditure and help ensure the maintenance and execution of key biological and behavioral processes. This signal would appear to be robust, with FFM (Blundell et al. 2011) and RMR (Caudwell et al. 2013) remaining strong determinants of hunger, meal size, and daily EI even when total daily energy expenditure was strongly perturbed during 12 weeks of aerobic exercise (Blundell et al. 2011).

This proposal has recently been supported by results from Hopkins et al. (2016) in a study that modeled the associations between body composition, energy expenditure, and EI in the context of total energy balance in order to determine whether it was body composition per se or energy expenditure that drives food intake. Measures of RMR (indirect calorimetry), total daily energy expenditure (doubly labeled water), body composition (deuterium dilution), and daily EI (laboratory weighed intakes) were taken in 59 individuals during a 14-day stay in a residential feeding behavior suite. During days 1 and 2, participants consumed a fixed diet designed to maintain energy balance. On days 3–14, food intake was covertly measured in subjects who had ad libitum access to a wide variety of foods typical of their normal diets. Consequently, although the study was scientifically controlled, the subjects followed a near-normal pattern of daily activities. After controlling for age and sex, both FFM and RMR (but not FM) were found to predict daily EI. However, a mediation model using path analysis indicated that the effect of FFM (and FM) on EI was fully mediated by RMR (Figure 12.2); i.e., FFM had no direct effect on food intake but rather indirectly influenced food intake via its effect on RMR. However, it should be noted that this model cannot distinguish between the effects of FFM-associated energy expenditure and the effects of any molecular signaling arising from lean tissue that may also covary with RMR.

A similar approach was adopted by Piaggi et al. (2015), who examined whether 24-hour energy expenditure or substrate oxidation predicted the overconsumption of food (independent of FFM) in 107 individuals. Twenty-four-hour energy expenditure was measured in a whole room calorimeter, with ad libitum food intake measured during the subsequent 3 days using a computerized vending machine procedure. Twenty-four-hour energy expenditure and respiratory quotient were found to independently predict food intake, with a 100 kcal surplus in 24-hour energy expenditure associated with a 175 kcal increase in EI, while a 1% change in 24-hour respiratory quotient was associated with a 204 kcal change in EI. In line with Hopkins

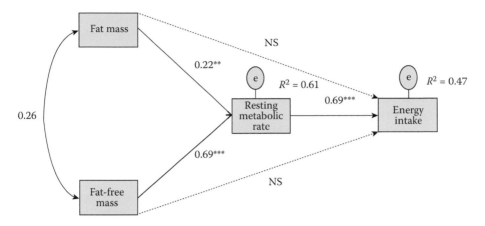

FIGURE 12.2 Path diagram illustrating the direct and indirect effects of FM, FFM, and RMR on EI in 59 individuals during a 14-day stay in a residential feeding behavior suite. As can be seen, the effect of FFM (and FM) on EI was fully mediated by RMR. (From Hopkins, M., Finlayson, G., Duarte, C., Whybrow, S., Horgan, G.W., Blundell, J.E., Stubbs, R.J. *Int. J. Obes.*, 2015.)

et al. (2015), mediation analysis indicated that FFM did not have any direct effect on EI, with 24-hour energy expenditure accounting for 80% of the observed effect FFM exerted on EI. However, it should be noted that participants overconsumed by approximately 60% during the 3-day ad libitum measurement period of this study, with EI equal to 159% ± 40% of weight maintenance needs. As such, this paper provides insight into overconsumption rather than the mechanisms that control more normal day-to-day food intake under conditions close to energy balance.

The studies of Piaggi et al. (2015) and Hopkins et al. (2016) raise the question of whether the relationship between RMR and food intake is a function of, or independent of, total daily energy expenditure. While Piaggi et al. (2015) reported that 24-hour energy expenditure independently predicted EI, RMR was not measured in this study. Interestingly, sleeping metabolic rate, which equates to approximately 95% of RMR (Goldberg et al. 1988), failed to predict EI (although sleeping metabolic rate was adjusted for age, sex ethnicity, FM, and FFM). However, 24-hour energy expenditure was restricted in the respiratory chamber and equivalent to only 1.4 times sleeping metabolic rate. Therefore, it still remains to be seen whether RMR and total daily energy expenditure independently predict food intake in conditions when total daily energy expenditure can vary more freely. However, such an effect of TEE would be unlikely to be mediated by FFM, as individuals can exhibit a wide range of TEE (depending on the amount of volitional active or sedentary behaviors carried out) for a given level of body composition or RMR.

12.7 IMPLICATIONS FOR THE CONTROL OF APPETITE

Studies demonstrating that FFM or RMR (rather than FM) are the main predictors of day-to-day food intake (Lissner et al. 1989, Cugini et al. 1998, Blundell et al. 2011, Caudwell et al. 2013, Weise et al. 2013) are not consistent with the traditional "adipocentric" view of appetite control. However, this should not be taken to imply that FM does not play an important role in appetite control. Indeed, consistent with an inhibitory action, a negative association between the FM index and daily EI was reported by some of these studies (Cugini et al. 1998). Furthermore, the mediation analyses performed by Hopkins et al. (2016) and Piaggi et al. (2015) indicated that FM indirectly influenced EI via its effect on RMR and daily energy expenditure, respectively (albeit to a lesser extent than FFM). It is also worth noting that studies demonstrating a relationship between FFM or RMR and food intake have been carried out under conditions close to energy balance (Weise et al. 2013, Hopkins et al. 2015, 2016, Piaggi et al. 2015). As such, they may not provide insight into the mechanisms controlling EI during dynamic periods of substantial energy or weight change. It is possible that FM and other regulatory signals (such as leptin) may influence appetite control more strongly during sustained weight loss (Rosenbaum et al. 2010). This highlights the need to examine the roles of FM and FFM (and associated putative signals) under varying conditions of energy balance. Indeed, the majority of studies examining the relationship between FFM/RMR and EI are cross-sectional in nature (Lissner et al. 1989, Cugini et al. 1998, 1999, Westerterp-Plantenga et al. 2003, Weise et al. 2013, Hopkins et al. 2015, 2016, Piaggi et al. 2013), and therefore, inferences cannot be made regarding how systematic changes in body composition or RMR influence EI.

It is important to note that if energy expenditure and EI are linked as part of a biologically regulated system, a mechanism must exist that tunes EI to the rate of energy expenditure (Hall et al. 2012). However, how the demand for energy is translated into motivated behavior (i.e., food intake) is unclear, but the first step in seeking signals that "translate" a physiological state into a behavioral action is to demonstrate the reliability and robustness of the underlying relationships. It has previously been suggested that the energy demand of tissues such as the liver might be translated into tonic signals of hunger, creating a constant drive to eat (Halford and Blundell 2000). This notion fits with a proposed energostatic control of food intake (Friedman 1995), in which changes in hepatic energy status have been suggested to influence EI through the stimulation of vagal afferent nerve activity (Leonhardt and Langhans 2004). It is also becoming clear that skeletal muscle is a major endocrine organ, capable of producing and secreting a large number of myokines (Pedersen and Febbraio 2012). These myokines provide a molecular basis through which skeletal muscle can communicate bidirectionally with organs such as the liver, the brain, and adipose tissue (Trayhurn, Drevon, and Eckel 2011). A number of myokines such as interleukin 6 (Ropelle et al. 2010) and irisin (Swick, Orena, and O'Connor 2013) have been linked to food intake and energy expenditure, but the specific role that these myokines (and others) play in appetite control is unclear.

It may be worth recognizing that a signal linking energy demand with brain activity (and ultimately behavior) may not be a single circulating molecule. The signal may reflect the degree of intracellular metabolism; however, there is no reason why this should not be sensed via biochemical pathways. Interestingly, a recent study used positron emission tomography (PET) technology to investigate how energy needs (arising from FFM) could be sensed by the brain and translated into homeostatically relevant behavior (Weise et al. 2015). The study demonstrated significant associations between FFM and several brain regions, but no associations with FM. Moreover the study indicated a link between FFM, hunger, and brain activity (cerebral blood flow) in the periacqueductal gray. As the authors point out, this area is a key station on the ascending homeostatic pathways, and neural activity here can plausibly be envisaged as part of a system that transforms FFM-induced energy demand into motivated feeding behavior.

A further issue concerns the role of FFM and FM in EI in people under varying conditions of FM. Would it be expected that the relationship between body composition variables and EI would remain uniform during the progressive increase in FM during the development of obesity? Interestingly, Cugini et al. (1998, 1999) reported that the relationship between body composition and hunger varied between lean and obese individuals, with FM being negatively associated with hunger in lean individuals, but not obese individuals. Consistent with this, it has been reported that in young, lean active men and women FM is inversely associated with EI (Blundell et al. 2015). This evidence fits with the interpretation that the influence of FM on appetite varies according to the amount of fat (and therefore its biological function) in the body. Considering these data, it can be envisaged that a threshold exists at which the level of FM changes from being inhibitory to becoming disinhibitory as an individual passes from leanness to fatness. However, such a threshold would necessarily be an individual parameter, and it is not conceivable that "average" FM would possess such functional potential.

Figure 12.3 displays a conceptual model that highlights the tonic drive to eat arising from body composition and resting energy expenditure, the tonic inhibition

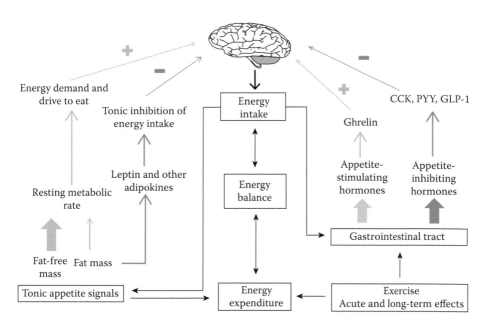

FIGURE 12.3 Conceptual model illustrating the major tonic and episodic processes that influence appetite control using an energy balance framework. Tonic signals of energy need arising from body composition (primarily FFM) are mediated by RMR. FM also indirectly influences EI via the action of leptin. The overall strength of the drive for food is the balance between the tonic excitatory and inhibitory processes, intermittently modulated by episodic signals.

arising from signals of energy storage, and the signals involved in the short-term (episodic) regulation of food intake. This model provides a theoretical approach to the biology of appetite control in which the influence of FFM and RMR is incorporated alongside signals stemming from adipose tissue and gastrointestinal (GI) peptides. FFM, as the main determinant of RMR, provides a tonic drive to eat that reflects basal energy requirements. This excitatory drive is under tonic inhibition from adiposity signals such as leptin, whose action reflects the size of stored energy reserves in the body. However, as the amount of adipose tissue increases, leptin and insulin insensitivity develop, and this tonic inhibition is reduced. This attenuation in tonic inhibition can contribute to overconsumption in obese individuals (despite the abundance of stored energy), as the tonic drive to eat stemming from FFM (which is elevated in the obese) remains unabated.

12.8 SUMMARY

Modern theories of appetite control embody the view that episodic and tonic inhibitory signals arising from adipose tissue and GI peptides modulate a constant excitatory drive to eat (Blundell and Gillett 2001). However, the source of this excitatory drive has been poorly defined, with current models of appetite control better able to account for the inhibition rather than initiation of feeding (Halford and Blundell 2000). Recent data indicate that FFM and FM play important (but distinct) roles in the control of appetite and food intake (Blundell et al. 2011, Caudwell et al. 2013, Weise et al. 2013, Hopkins et al. 2016). While FFM (as the main determinant of RMR) represents a potential physiological source of hunger that drives day-to-day food intake at a level proportional to basal energy requirements, FM (and associated adipokines such as leptin) appears not to strongly influence day-to-day food intake under conditions of energy balance. Indeed, despite the commonly held view that FM (and leptin) plays a key role in the control appetite, evidence indicating that peripheral leptin concentrations influence appetite and food intake is not as strong as commonly assumed (and confined to conditions of negative energy balance).

Recent findings suggesting that FFM and RMR play important roles in day-to-day food intake suggest that the classic adipocentric model of appetite control could easily be revised to reflect the influence of RMR and energy demands. Acting conjointly, the influence of RMR (and other components of EE) and signals stemming from adipose tissue and GI peptides appear to better account for the role of whole-body peripheral signals involved in human appetite control. These data may help to further our understanding of the relationship between an excitatory drive to eat and the intermittent suppression of eating (i.e., episodic satiety signaling and tonic inhibition). However, there is a need to examine how FM and FFM (and the associated putative signals) operate conjointly under varying conditions of energy balance. Indeed, while the energy expenditure associated with FFM and RMR appear to be stronger determinants of food intake under conditions of energy balance, it is possible that FM and other regulatory signals (such as leptin) may influence appetite control more strongly during sustained weight loss. It is likely that future studies will indicate how different components of the energy balance budget influence eating patterns in different groups of individuals under different physiological and environmental conditions. Such studies will inevitably provide a more comprehensive account of the relationship between energy demands and EI.

CONFLICT OF INTEREST

The authors declare no conflict of interest.

FUNDING

Research relating to this study was funded by the Biotechnology and Biological Sciences Research Council, grant numbers BBS/B/05079 and BB/G005524/1 (DRINC).

LITERATURE CITED

Badman, M.K., and J.S. Flier. 2005. The gut and energy balance: Visceral allies in the obesity wars. *Science* 307:1909.

Bessesen, D.H. 2011. Regulation of body weight: What is the regulated parameter? *Physiol Behav* 104:599–607.

Blundell, J.E., and A. Gillett. 2001. Control of food intake in the obese. *Obes Res* 9:263S–270S.

Blundell, J.E., and N.A. King. 1998. Effects of exercise on appetite control: Loose coupling between energy expenditure and energy intake. *Intl J Obesity Relat Metab Dis* 22:S22–S29.

Blundell, J.E., P. Caudwell, C. Gibbons, M. Hopkins, E. Näslund, N.A. King, and G. Finlayson. 2011. Body composition and appetite: Fat-free mass (but not fat mass or BMI) is positively associated with self-determined meal size and daily energy intake in humans. *Br J Nutr* 107:445–449.

Blundell, J.E., G. Finlayson, C. Gibbons, P. Caudwell, and M. Hopkins. 2015. The biology of appetite control: Do resting metabolic rate and fat-free mass drive energy intake? *Physiol Behav* 152:473–478.

Borer, K.T. 2014. Counterregulation of insulin by leptin as key component of autonomic regulation of body weight. *World J Diab* 5:606.

Bray, G.A., J.P. Flatt, J. Volaufova, J.P. DeLany, and C.M. Champagne. 2008. Corrective responses in human food intake identified from an analysis of 7-d food-intake records. *Am J Clin Nutr* 88:1504.

Caudwell, P., G. Finlayson, C. Gibbons, M. Hopkins, N. King, E. Naslund, and J. Blundell. 2013. Resting metabolic rate is associated with hunger, self-determined meal size, and daily energy intake and may represent a marker for appetite. *Am J Clin Nutr* 97:7–14.

Chan, J.L., K. Heist, A.M. DePaoli, J.D. Veldhuis, and C.S. Mantzoros. 2003. The role of falling leptin levels in the neuroendocrine and metabolic adaptation to short-term starvation in healthy men. *J Clin Invest* 111:1409–1421.

Chin-Chance, C., K.S. Polonsky, and D.A. Schoeller. 2000. Twenty-four-hour leptin levels respond to cumulative short-term energy imbalance and predict subsequent intake. *J Clin Endocrinol Metab* 85:2685.

Coleman, D.L. 1973. Effects of parabiosis of obese with diabetes and normal mice. *Diabetalogia* 9:294–298.

Coleman, D.L., and K.P. Hummel. 1969. Effects of parabiosis of normal with genetically diabetic mice. *Am J Physiol* 217:1298–1304.

Cugini, P., A. Salandri, M. Cilli, P. Ceccotti, A. Di Marzo, A. Rodio, S. Fontana, A.M. Pellegrino, G.P. De Francesco, and S. Coda. 1999. Daily hunger sensation and body compartments: II. Their relationships in obese patients. *Eat Weight Dis* 4:81–88.

Cugini, P., A. Salandri, M. Cilli, P. Ceccotti, A. Di Marzo, A. Rodio, F. MarcianÃ, S. Fontana, A.M. Pellegrino, and K. Vacca. 1998. Daily hunger sensation and body composition: I. Their relationships in clinically healthy subjects. *Eat Weight Dis* 3:168–172.

Doucet, E., P. Imbeault, S. St-Pierre, N. Almeras, P. Mauriege, D. Richard, and A. Tremblay. 2000. Appetite after weight loss by energy restriction and a low-fat diet-exercise follow-up. *Int J Obesity* 24:906–914.

Dubuc, G.R., S.D. Phinney, J.S. Stern, and P.J. Havel. 1998. Changes of serum leptin and endocrine and metabolic parameters after 7 days of energy restriction in men and women. *Metabolism* 47:429–434.

Dulloo, A.G., J. Jacquet, and L. Girardier. 1997. Poststarvation hyperphagia and body fat overshooting in humans: A role for feedback signals from lean and fat tissues. *Am J Clin Nutr* 65:717–723.

Dulloo, A.G., J. Jacquet, and J.P. Montani. 2012. How dieting makes some fatter: From a perspective of human body composition autoregulation. *Proc Nutr Soc* 71:379–389.

Edholm, O.G. 1977. Energy balance in man. Studies carried out by the Division of Human Physiology, National Institute for Medical Research. *J Hum Nutr* 31:413–431.

Edholm, O.G., J.M. Adam, M.J.R. Healy, H.S. Wolff, R. Goldsmith, and T.W. Best. 1970. Food intake and energy expenditure of army recruits. *Br J Nutr* 24:1091–1107.

Edholm, O.G., J.G. Fletcher, E.M. Widdowson, and R.A. McCance. 1955a. The energy expenditure and food intake of individual men. *Br J Nutr* 9:286–300.

Edholm, O.G., J.G. Fletcher, E.M. Widdowson, and R.A. McCance. 1955b. The energy expenditure and food intake of individual men. *Br J Nutr* 9:286–300.

Farooqi, I.S., S.A. Jebb, G. Langmack, E. Lawrence, C.H. Cheetham, A.M. Prentice, I.A. Hughes, M.A. McCamish, and S. O'Rahilly. 1999. Effects of recombinant leptin therapy in a child with congenital leptin deficiency. *New Engl J Med* 341:879–884.

Farooqi, I.S., T. Wangensteen, S. Collins, W. Kimber, G. Matarese, J.M. Keogh, E. Lank, B. Bottomley, J. Lopez-Fernandez, and I. Ferraz-Amaro. 2007. Clinical and molecular genetic spectrum of congenital deficiency of the leptin receptor. *New Engl J Med* 356:237–247.

Finucane, M.M., G.A. Stevens, M.J. Cowan, G. Danaei, J.K. Lin, C.J. Paciorek et al. 2011. National, regional, and global trends in body-mass index since 1980: Systematic analysis of health examination surveys and epidemiological studies with 960 country-years and 9.1 million participants. *Lancet* 377:557–567.

Friedman, M.I. 1995. Control of energy intake by energy metabolism. *Am J Clin Nutr* 62:1096S.

Goldberg, G.R., A.M. Prentice, H.L. Davies, and P.R. Murgatroyd. 1988. Overnight and basal metabolic rates in men and women. *Eur J Clin Nutr* 42:137–144.

Gosby, A.K., A.D. Conigrave, D. Raubenheimer, and S.J. Simpson. 2014. Protein leverage and energy intake. *Obes Rev* 15:183–191.

Halford, J.C.G., and J.E. Blundell. 2000. Separate systems for serotonin and leptin in appetite control. *Ann Med* 32:222–232.

Hall, K.D., S.B. Heymsfield, J.W. Kemnitz, S. Klein, D.A. Schoeller, and J.R. Speakman. 2012. Energy balance and its components: Implications for body weight regulation. *Am J Clin Nutr* 95:989–994.

Heini, A.F., C. Lara-Castro, K.A. Kirk, R.V. Considine, J.F. Caro, and R.L. Weinsier. 1998. Association of leptin and hunger-satiety ratings in obese women. *Intl J Obesity* 22:1084–1087.

Hervey, G.R. 1969. Regulation of energy balance. *Nature* 222:629–631.

Hervey, E., and G.R. Hervey. 1969. Energy storage in female rats treated with progesterone in the absence of increased intake of food. *J Physiol* 200:118P–119P.

Heymsfield, S.B., A.S. Greenberg, K. Fujioka, R.M. Dixon, R. Kushner, T. Hunt, J.A. Lubina, J. Patane, B. Self, and P. Hunt. 1999. Recombinant leptin for weight loss in obese and lean adults: A randomized, controlled, dose-escalation trial. *JAMA* 282:1568–1575.

Hopkins, M., G. Finlayson, C. Duarte, S. Whybrow, G.W. Horgan, J.E. Blundell, and R.J. Stubbs. 2015. What is the role of fat-free mass and resting metabolic rate in the control of food intake. *Obesity Facts* 8:49.

Hopkins, M., G. Finlayson, C. Duarte, S. Whybrow, G.W. Horgan, J.E. Blundell, and R.J. Stubbs. 2016. Modelling the associations between fat-free mass, resting metabolic rate and energy intake in the context of total energy balance. *Intl J Obes (Lond)* 40:312–318.

Hopkins, M., N.A. King, and J.E. Blundell. 2010. Acute and long-term effects of exercise on appetite control: Is there any benefit for weight control? *Curr Opin Clin Nutr Metab Care* 13:635.

Jequier, E. 2002. Leptin signaling, adiposity, and energy balance. *Ann NY Acad Sci* 967:379–388.

Johnstone, A.M., S.D. Murison, J.S. Duncan, K.A. Rance, and J.R. Speakman. 2005. Factors influencing variation in basal metabolic rate include fat-free mass, fat mass, age, and circulating thyroxine but not sex, circulating leptin, or triiodothyronine. *Am J Clin Nutr* 82:941–948.

Keim, N.L., J.S. Stern, and P.J. Havel. 1998. Relation between circulating leptin concentrations and appetite during a prolonged, moderate energy deficit in women. *Am J Clin Nutr* 68:794–801.

Kennedy, G.C. 1953. The role of depot fat in the hypothalamic control of food intake in the rat. *Proc Royal Soc London. Series B-Biol Sci* 140:578.

Kennedy, G.C. 1957. The development with age of hypothalamic restraint upon the appetite of the rat. *J Endocrinol* 16:9–17.

Kennedy, G.C. 1966. The hypothalamus and obesity. *Proc R Soc Med* 59:1276.

Keys, A., J. Brožek, A. Henschel, O. Mickelsen, and H.L. Taylor. 1950. *The Biology of Human Starvation.* Minnesota: University of Minnesota Press.

King, N.A., and J.E. Blundell. 1995. High-fat foods overcome the energy expenditure induced by high-intensity cycling or running. *Eur J Clin Nutr* 49:114–123.

King, N.A., A. Lluch, R.J. Stubbs, and J.E. Blundell. 1997. High dose exercise does not increase hunger or energy intake in free living males. *Eur J Clin Nutr* 51:478–483.

King, N.A., L. Snell, R.D. Smith, and J.E. Blundell. 1996. Effects of short-term exercise on appetite responses in unrestrained females. *Eur J Clin Nutr* 50:663.

Leibel, R.L. 2002. The role of leptin in the control of body weight. *Nutr Rev* 60:S15–S19.

Lenard, N.R., and H.R. Berthoud. 2008. Central and peripheral regulation of food intake and physical activity: Pathways and genes. *Obesity* 16:S11.

Leonhardt, M., and W. Langhans. 2004. Fatty acid oxidation and control of food intake. *Physiol Behav* 83:645–651.

Lissner, L., J.P. Habicht, B.J. Strupp, D.A. Levitsky, J.D. Haas, and D.A. Roe. 1989. Body composition and energy intake: Do overweight women overeat and underreport? *Am J Clin Nutr* 49:320–325.

Mars, M., C. de Graaf, L.C. de Groot, and F.J. Kok. 2005a. Decreases in fasting leptin and insulin concentrations after acute energy restriction and subsequent compensation in food intake. *Am J Clin Nutr* 81:570–577.

Mars, M., C. De Graaf, L.C. De Groot, C. Van Rossum, and F.J. Kok. 2005b. Fasting leptin and appetite responses induced by a 4-day 65% energy restricted diet. *Intl J Obes* 30:122–128.

Mayer, J. 1953. Glucostatic mechanism of regulation of food intake. *New Engl J Med* 249:13.

Mayer, J., N.B. Marshall, J.J. Vitale, J.H. Christensen, M.B. Mashayekhi, and F.J. Stare. 1954. Exercise, food intake and body weight in normal rats and genetically obese adult mice. *Am J Physiol* 177:544.

Mayer, J., P. Roy, and K.P. Mitra. 1956. Relation between caloric intake, body weight, and physical work: Studies in an industrial male population in West Bengal. *Am J Clin Nutr* 4:169.

Mellinkoff, S.M., M. Frankland, D. Boyle, and M. Greipel. 1956. Relationship between serum amino acid concentration and fluctuations in appetite. *J Appl Physiol* 8:535.

Millward, D.J. 1995. A protein-stat mechanism for regulation of growth and maintenance of the lean body mass. *Nutr Res Rev* 8:93–120.

Morrison, C.D., and T. Laeger. 2015. Protein-dependent regulation of feeding and metabolism. *Trends Endocrinol Metab* 26:256–262.

Morton, G.J., D.E. Cummings, D.G. Baskin, G.S. Barsh, and M.W. Schwartz. 2006. Central nervous system control of food intake and body weight. *Nature* 443:289–295.

Ng, M., T. Fleming, M. Robinson, B. Thomson, N. Graetz, C. Margono, E.C. Mullany, S. Biryukov, C. Abbafati, and S.F. Abera. 2014. Global, regional, and national prevalence of overweight and obesity in children and adults during 1980–2013: A systematic analysis for the Global Burden of Disease Study 2013. *The Lancet*

Pasiakos, S.M., C.M. Caruso, M.D. Kellogg, F.M. Kramer, and H.R. Lieberman. 2011. Appetite and endocrine regulators of energy balance after 2 days of energy restriction: Insulin, leptin, ghrelin, and DHEA-S. *Obesity* 19:1124–1130.

Pedersen, B.K., and M.A. Febbraio. 2012. Muscles, exercise and obesity: Skeletal muscle as a secretory organ. *Nat Rev Endocrinol* 8:457–465.

Piaggi, P., M.S. Thearle, C. Bogardus, and J. Krakoff. 2013. Lower energy expenditure predicts long-term increases in weight and fat mass. *J Clin Endocrinol Metab* 98:E703–E707.

Piaggi, P., M.S. Thearle, J. Krakoff, and S.B. Votruba. 2015. Higher daily energy expenditure and respiratory quotient, rather than fat free mass, independently determine greater ad libitum overeating. *J Clin Endocrinol Metab* 100:3011–3020.

Ravussin, E., B. Burnand, Y. Schutz, and E. Jequier. 1982. Twenty-four-hour energy expenditure and resting metabolic rate in obese, moderately obese, and control subjects. *Am J Clin Nutr* 35:566–573.

Ravussin, E., S. Lillioja, T.E. Anderson, L. Christin, and C. Bogardus. 1986a. Determinants of 24-hour energy expenditure in man. Methods and results using a respiratory chamber. *J Clin Invest* 78:1568–1578.

Ravussin, E., S. Lillioja, T.E. Anderson, L. Christin, and C. Bogardus. 1986b. Determinants of 24-hour energy expenditure in man. Methods and results using a respiratory chamber. *J Clin Invest* 78:1568–1578.

Ravussin, Y., R.L. Leibel, and A.W. Ferrante. 2014. A missing link in body weight homeostasis: The catabolic signal of the overfed state. *Cell Metab* 20:565–572.

Ropelle, E.R., M.B. Flores, D.E. Cintra, G.Z. Rocha, J.R. Pauli, J. Morari, C.T. de Souza, J.C. Moraes, P.O. Prada, and D. Guadagnini. 2010. IL-6 and IL-10 anti-inflammatory activity links exercise to hypothalamic insulin and leptin sensitivity through IKKβ and ER stress inhibition. *PLoS Biol* 8:e1000465.

Rosen, E.D., and B.M. Spiegelman. 2006. Adipocytes as regulators of energy balance and glucose homeostasis. *Nature* 444:847–853.

Rosenbaum, M., H.R. Kissileff, L.E.S. Mayer, J. Hirsch, and R.L. Leibel. 2010. Energy intake in weight-reduced humans. *Brain Res* 1350:95–102.

Sainsbury, A., and L. Zhang. 2010. Role of the arcuate nucleus of the hypothalamus in regulation of body weight during energy deficit. *Mol Cell Endocrinol* 316:109–119.

Schwartz, M.W., S.C. Woods, D. Porte, R.J. Seeley, and D.G. Baskin. 2000. Central nervous system control of food intake. *Nature* 404:661–671.

Simpson, S.J., and D. Raubenheimer. 2005. Obesity: The protein leverage hypothesis. *Obes Rev* 6:133–142.

Sørensen, A., D. Mayntz, D. Raubenheimer, and S.J. Simpson. 2008. Protein-leverage in mice: The geometry of macronutrient balancing and consequences for fat deposition. *Obesity* 16:566–571.

Swick, A.G., S. Orena, and A. O'Connor. 2013. Irisin levels correlate with energy expenditure in a subgroup of humans with energy expenditure greater than predicted by fat free mass. *Metabolism* 63:1070–1073.

Trayhurn, P., C.A. Drevon, and J. Eckel. 2011. Secreted proteins from adipose tissue and skeletal muscle—Adipokines, myokines and adipose/muscle cross-talk. *Arch Physiol Biochem* 117:47–56.

Weigle, D.S., P. Barton Duell, W.E. Connor, R.A. Steiner, M.R. Soules, and J.L. Kuijper. 1997. Effect of fasting, refeeding, and dietary fat restriction on plasma leptin levels 1. *J Clin Endocrinol Metab* 82:561–565.

Weise, C.M., P. Thiyyagura, E.M. Reiman, K. Chen, and J. Krakoff. 2015. A potential role for the midbrain in integrating fat-free mass determined energy needs: An H215O PET study. *Hum Brain Mapp* 36:2406–2415.

Weise, C.M., M.G. Hohenadel, J. Krakoff, and S.B. Votruba. 2013. Body composition and energy expenditure predict ad-libitum food and macronutrient intake in humans. *Intl J Obesity* 38:243–251

Westerterp-Plantenga, M.S., A.H.C. Goris, E.P. Meijer, and K.R. Westerterp. 2003. Habitual meal frequency in relation to resting and activity-induced energy expenditure in human subjects: The role of fat-free mass. *Br J Nutr* 90:643–649.

Woods, S.C., and D.S. Ramsay. 2011. Food intake, metabolism and homeostasis. *Physiol Behav* 104:4–7.

Zhang, Y., R. Proenca, M. Maffei, M. Barone, L. Leopold, and J.M. Friedman. 1994. Positional cloning of the mouse obese gene and its human homologue. *Nature* 372:425–432.

13 Pharmacotherapy for Weight Loss

Thomas A. Lutz and Lori Asarian

CONTENTS

13.1 INTRODUCTION

"Disease will always be with us, but we may look forward confidently to a time when epidemics shall be no more" (Osler, 1891). Such an optimistic attitude has carried the world forward through many epidemics and likely will also help us prevail in the case of obesity. An important component of the effort is the development of improved pharmaceutical therapy for obesity. Ideally, this should have a widespread use, being available from overweight to morbidly obese people, at a lower cost and with fewer side effects than bariatric surgery. In this chapter, we review the latest pharmaceutical approaches to treat obesity through therapies targeting the control of eating.

The energy input refers to the regulation of an adequate and readily available supply of energy metabolites in the circulation. Differences between energy input and output are buffered by the control of adipose-tissue mass, which is the major energy store. These are among the most important biological functions of any living organism.

These aspects of energy homeostasis are linked to the control of eating. Eating, however, not only is under the control of physiological processes but is also affected by social stimuli, experience, learning, and a multitude of other exogenous factors. From a physiological standpoint, understanding the controls of eating remains an unsolved problem in behavioral neuroscience that is a prerequisite to the development of specific and more effective obesity therapy.

13.2   APPROACHES TO THE TREATMENT OF OBESITY

The peripheral physiological controls of eating can be understood as positive and negative feedbacks arising from preabsorptive and postabsorptive food stimuli. Positive feedback arises from the sight and smell of food, in preparation for meal-taking and from the ingesta, in the form of flavor hedonics, which begins with the onset of eating. Negative feedback increases in strength gradually, as eating continues (Smith, 2000). Research has dissected various sources and consequences of these feedbacks and several pharmacological attempts to control their output have been made (Table 13.1).

TABLE 13.1
Single Drug Therapies

Therapy	Dose (mg/day)	Duration (week)	Mechanism	Reference
Dinitrophenol	3 to 5	10	Interferes with ATP synthesis	Cutting and Tainter, 1932
Amphetamine	10	6 to 25	Increases NE and DA	Lesses and Myerson, 1938
Phentermine	30	24	Increases NE	Weintraub et al., 1984
Fenfluramine	39 to 120	4 to 18	Blocks 5-HT reuptake	Haddock et al., 2002
Dexfenfluramine	30	52	Blocks 5-HT reuptake	Guy-Grand et al., 1989
Ephedrine	20	24	Increases NE	Astrup et al., 1992
Y5 receptor antagonist	1	52	Blocks the effect of NPY	Erondu et al., 2006
MC4R agonist	400 to 800	12 to 18	Increases release of α-MSH	Krishna et al., 2009
Leptin	0.7 to 21	4 to 20	Translocation of JAK-STAT system	Heymsfield et al., 1999
DA1/5 R antagonist	30 to 100	12 to 52	Stimulates adenyl cyclase	Astrup et al., 2007
Fluoxetine	60	36 to 60	SSRI	Goldstein et al., 1995
Topiramate	175	16	AMPA/kainate glutamate R	Rosenstock et al., 2007
Zonisamine	200 to 400	52	Increases DA and 5-HT	Gadde et al., 2012
CB1 R antagonist	5 to 20	52	Blocks effects of endogenous CB	Pi-Sunyer et al., 2006
CNTF	0.3 to 2[a]	12	Translocation of JAK-STAT system	Ettinger et al., 2003
PYY (3-36)	2 nmol[b]	Acute (meal)	Gut peptide	Batterham et al., 2003

Abbreviations: AMPA, alpha-amino-3-hydroxy-5-methyl-4-isoxazoleproprionic acid; aMSH, alpha melanocyte stimulating hormone; ATP, adenosine triphosphate; CB, cannabinoid; CNTF, ciliary neurotrophic factor; DA, dopamine; JAK-STAT, janus kinase–signal transducer; NE, norepinephrine; NPY, neuropeptide Y; PYY, peptide YY; R, receptor; SSRI, selective serotonin reuptake inhibitor; 5-HT, serotonin.

[a] Dose is mg/kg.
[b] Dose is nmol/m^2 of body surface area.

These pharmacological targets, however, were not sufficiently strong to produce truly effective weight-loss outcomes (e.g., leptin; see Heymsfield et al., 1999), and some, such as dinitrophenol, had major toxic effects (Tainter et al., 1935).

Two milestones shaped contemporary approaches to obesity treatment. First, the pioneering clinical work by Weintraub and colleagues (1992) reported a series of systematically designed clinical trials showing that the combination of D,L-fenfluramine (a serotonergic drug) and phentermine (a noradrenergic drug) led to more weight loss than either drug alone. Although this drug combination was withdrawn from the market because of dangerous cardiovascular side effects, their work set a standard in the field both in terms of the use of combination-therapy approach, as well as the improved experimental design and evaluation of safety and efficacy of the drugs.

Second, the advent of molecular and pharmacogenetic techniques increased our knowledge of the peripheral and central physiological controls of eating and facilitated the production of drugs targeting specific receptors involved in the neural processing of what elicits meal-ending satiation.

In the next section, we describe examples of both pharmacological approaches, which are now approved therapies for the treatment of obesity. The approved drug Xenical (Orlistat; Roche Pharma) will not be discussed here because the compound reduces intestinal fat digestion and does not interact with the peripheral and central control mechanisms of eating.

13.3 CURRENT PHARMACOTHERAPIES FOR OBESITY

13.3.1 COMBINATION THERAPIES

13.3.1.1 Naltrexone/Bupropion

13.3.1.1.1 Clinical

Contrave (Orexigen Therapeutics, United States), an extended-release formula containing naltrexone (32 mg) and bupropion (360 mg), was approved for use in the United States and Europe in September 2014 and March 2015, respectively. Contrave (United States) or Mysimba (Europe) was designed on the basis of animal and human studies to affect both homeostatic and hedonic aspects of eating (Greenway et al., 2009; Billes and Greenway, 2011). Several Phase II and III clinical studies were completed (Table 13.2) as part of the Contrave Obesity Research trials. These trials

---

TABLE 13.2
Currently Approved Therapies for Obesity

Drug	Number of Studies	Dose (mg)	Percentage Change Weight Loss (1 year)	% Subjects with >5% Weight Loss, Drug vs. Placebo
Bupropion/naltrexone	4	32/360	3.2–5.2	44–67 vs. 16–25
Phentermine/topiramate	2	15/92	8.6–9.3	67–70 vs. 17–21
Locarserin	3	10, 20	3–3.6	45–67 vs. 16–25
Liraglutide	3	1.2–3	5.4–6.1	50–73 vs. 22–28

resulted in weight loss of ≥8% over 56 weeks when combined with lifestyle interventions. The drug was well tolerated and also led to improvements in several cardiovascular and metabolic indices. Thus, currently available data suggest that Contrave/Mysimba is a safe and moderately effective tool for combating obesity.

13.3.1.1.2   Mechanism of Action: Naltrexone

Naltrexone is a high-affinity μ-opioid receptor antagonist, which is also used for the treatment of alcoholism and opioid addiction (Ginzburg and Glass, 1984; Johansson et al., 2006; Anton, 2008). This opioid-receptor subtype, however, has also been implicated in the control of eating through hypothalamic effects that target both the homeostatic and reward pathways. First, mice that lack the μ-opioid receptor are resistant to high-fat-diet-induced obesity (Tabarin et al., 2005). That naltrexone (1) increases proopiomelanocortin (POMC) mRNA (Bronstein et al., 1993) and (2) blocks β-endorphin action at the μ-opioid receptor (Cowley et al., 2001) suggests that its inhibitory effect on eating is due to releasing the POMC neurons from the inhibitory effect of β-endorphin (Cowley et al., 2001). Second, naltrexone acts on neural networks that underlie hedonic eating. For example, dopamine levels in the nucleus accumbens are decreased by naltrexone, leading to a decrease in food seeking and, critically, binge-like eating (Taber et al., 1998; Giuliano et al., 2012; Blasio et al., 2014). This decrease in dopamine is probably responsible for reducing the preference for highly palatable, high-fat, and high-sugar foods (Kelley et al., 1996; Zhang et al., 1998; Shin et al., 2010).

It is important to mention that naltrexone monotherapy did not lead to the same degree of success in humans as obtained in animal models. Initial evidence that naltrexone was effective as a monotherapy came from studies that were not placebo-controlled or double-blinded and which were not substantiated in well-controlled studies (Maggio et al., 1985; Malcolm et al., 1985; Greenway et al., 2009).

13.3.1.1.3   Mechanism of Action: Bupropion

Bupropion is used for the treatment of major depressive disorder and seasonal-affective disorder (Jefferson et al., 2006; Dhillon et al., 2008). It acts by inhibiting dopamine and norepinephrine (NE) transporters and thus retards their reuptake (Ascher et al., 1995; Fava et al., 2005). The resultant increases in synaptic dopamine and NE stimulate the melanocortin system (Khan et al., 1998; Fraley and Ritter, 2003; Greenway et al., 2009) and increase α-melanocyte stimulating hormone (α-MSH) secretion from the POMC neurons. This results in decreased eating and increased energy expenditure in both lean and obese rodent models (Liu et al., 2002, 2004; Hasegawa et al., 2005; Billes and Cowley, 2007; Wright and Rodgers, 2013).

In overweight and obese humans, bupropion therapy (300–400 mg/day) for up to 6 months resulted in modest placebo-subtracted weight loss of 2%–4% in an intent-to-treat analysis and 3%–5% in study completers (Gadde et al., 2001; Anderson et al., 2002; Jain et al., 2002; Greenway et al., 2009). The effects of bupropion on food intake and energy expenditure in humans have never been studied directly.

13.3.1.1.4   Mechanism of Combined Action: Naltrexone and Bupropion

A model for the combined action of naltrexone and bupropion on the POMC neurons is depicted in Figure 13.1 (Greenway et al., 2009) and is based on the idea that the eating

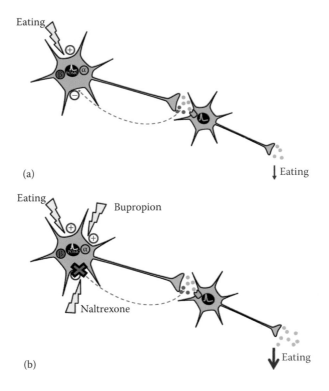

FIGURE 13.1 (a) POMC neurons control eating by releasing α-melanocyte-stimulating hormone (α-MSH; blue vesicles) and β-endorphin (brown vesicles). α-MSH activates downstream neurons, leading to a decrease in eating. At the same time, β-endorphin acts perhaps via interneurons to inhibit the POMC neurons and decrease the α-MSH release. This feedback loop ensures that normal meals are taken and energy homeostasis is maintained. (b) Bupropion/naltrexone therapy decreases eating in obese subjects by stimulating the POMC neurons (bupropion), which results in more α-MSH release and by eliminating the inhibitory effect of β-endorphin (naltrexone) and thus releasing the POMC neuron from autoinhibition.

inhibitory effects of the naltrexone/bupropion combination arise from an increase in POMC neuronal activity. That is, bupropion stimulates POMC neurons, and naltrexone augments this effect by removing the autoinhibitory effect of β-endorphin on POMC neurons. In addition to the POMC signaling system, the naltrexone/bupropion combination acts on the neurons in the ventral tegmental area (VTA) and the nucleus accumbens to decrease the reward value of food, in part by decreasing the dopaminergic input to the nucleus accumbens from the ventral tegmental area.

13.3.1.2 Phentermine/Topiramate

13.3.1.2.1 Clinical

Phentermine/topiramate (PHEN/TPM) extended release (Qsymia, Vivus, United State; 7.5 mg phentermine/46 mg topiramate extended release) was approved as a therapy for weight management in the United States in July 2012 (Cosentino et al., 2011;

Cameron et al., 2012; Garvey, 2013; Shin and Gadde, 2013; Smith et al., 2013). This was based on three trials of 52–108 week duration (Gadde et al., 2011; Allison et al., 2012; Garvey et al., 2012) (Table 13.2). All three trials documented successful percentage weight loss and percentage of patients achieving at least 5% weight loss. Two-year data suggest that no additional weight loss is achieved after week 40 and that patients will likely need to remain on PHEN/TPM long-term to maintain their weight loss. Equally importantly, PHEN/TPM is well tolerated. PHEN/TPM also has been shown to be beneficial for patients with sleep apnea (Winslow et al., 2012).

PHEN/TPM exemplifies the use of combination therapy to reduce the adverse effects produced by the agents alone without losing therapeutic efficacy. Phentermine monotherapy or together with fenfluramine was used in the United States from 1959 to 1997 (Ioannides-Demos et al., 2011). According to a meta-analysis, obese patients treated with phentermine for 2–24 weeks lost an average of 3.6 kg additional body weight compared to placebo (95% confidence interval [CI], 0.6–6.0 kg) and maintained 2.4 kg weight loss after discontinuation of the drug (Haddock et al., 2002). Phentermine is a psychomotor stimulant, whereas topiramate was initially introduced in 1996 as an anticonvulsant. Topiramate was also found to reduce body weight (Astrup et al., 2004). A meta-analysis of six studies indicated that topiramate led to a 6.5% (95% CI, 4.8%–8.3%) weight loss in 24 weeks (Li et al., 2005). Unfortunately, topiramate monotherapy for obesity was abandoned due to dose-dependent neuropsychiatric and cognitive adverse effects, including memory and concentration impairment, language difficulties, and mood changes (Nathan et al., 2011; Sommer et al., 2013).

13.3.1.2.2 Mechanism of Action: Phentermine

Phentermine is a sympathomimetic with pharmacologic activity similar to that of amphetamine. One effect is to increase levels of NE in the hypothalamus (Alexander et al., 2005; Rothman et al., 2001) and the resultant increase in the stimulation of β2-adrenergic receptors apparently leads to decreased eating (Ioannides-Demos et al., 2011; Witkamp, 2011). An increase in resting energy expenditure may also contribute to its weight-loss effects (Bays, 2010).

Phentermine increases NE in the synapse by a mechanism characteristic of a substrate-type releaser, not a reuptake inhibitor (Rothman et al., 2001). Substrate-type releasers bind to membrane proteins and are transported into the cytoplasm of the nerve bouton, where they interfere with vesicular storage and increase extracellular NE levels by reversing the process of transporter-mediated exchange (Rudnick and Clark, 1993; Wall et al., 1995). Substrate-type releasers are more effective than reuptake inhibitors in increasing extracellular monoamines because the former increase the pool of neurotransmitters available for release by transporter-mediated exchange. Moreover, the effectiveness in increasing extracellular monoamines is not dependent upon the basal rate of neurotransmitter release. In contrast, the effectiveness of reuptake inhibitors is nerve impulse-dependent and therefore limited by the tone of presynaptic activity (Rudnick and Clark, 1993; Wall et al., 1995).

13.3.1.2.3 Mechanism of Action: Topiramate

Topiramate is a non-specific drug, and several cellular targets have been proposed to mediate its anticonvulsant effect (Porter et al., 2012). These include

(1) voltage-gated sodium channels, (2) high-voltage-activated calcium channels, (3) gamma-aminobutyric acid (GABA-A) receptors, (4) α-amino-3-hydroxy-5-methyl-4-isoxazolepropionic acid (AMPA)/kainate (AMPA/KA) receptors, and (5) carbonic anhydrase isoenzymes (see Figure 13.2). Whether these or other actions of topiramate lead to weight loss is unclear. Topiramate's antagonism of AMPA/KA receptors may reduce compulsive or addictive food cravings (Khazaal and Zullino, 2007) because topiramate seems to improve binge-eating disorder (McElroy et al., 2003) and reduce other addictive behaviors (Khazaal and Sullino, 2006). Topiramate's activation of GABA-A receptors is likely to decrease nocturnal and deprivation-induced eating in rats (Turenius et al., 2009), which stabilizes weight loss due to a reduced food intake. Animal studies suggest that topiramate increases hypothalamic levels of neuropeptide Y (NPY), corticotropin-releasing hormone, and galanin (Husum et al., 2003), but these effects have not been linked to reductions in eating or body weight. Topiramate may reduce leptin levels less than expected for the weight loss that is achieved (Theisen et al., 2008; Schütt et al., 2010), which could contribute to its therapeutic effect, but this has never been formally tested. Decreases in eating are associated with reduced hunger (Tremblay et al., 2007). In addition, topiramate may increase energy expenditure (Tremblay et al., 2007), and due to inhibition of adipocyte mitochondrial carbonic anhydrase isozyme V (Winum et al., 2005), carbonic anhydrase-mediated lipogenesis is decreased (Vullo et al., 2004; Poulsen et al., 2008). Moreover, lipoprotein lipase activity in white and brown adipose tissue is decreased, limiting the availability of free fatty acid as substrates for lipogenesis and increasing thermogenesis (Richard et al., 2000).

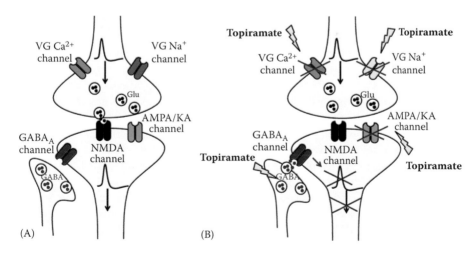

FIGURE 13.2 (A) As action potentials travel down the neuron, glutamate is released in the synapse exciting the postsynaptic neuron. (B) Topiramate acts to (a) inhibit the glutamate vesicle release in the presynaptic neurons by blocking the Na^+ and Ca^{2+} voltage gated channels. Postsynaptic NMDA receptors are no longer activated; (b) block the AMPA/KA receptors and (c) activate GABAergic neurons and postsynaptic GABA receptors. Topiramate therefore decreases the neuronal excitability.

13.3.2 Monotherapies

13.3.2.1 Lorcaserin

Lorcaserin (Belviq, Arena Pharmaceuticals, Switzerland), approved in the United States in 2012, reduces appetite by selectively stimulating serotonin (5-HT) 2C ($5-HT_{2C}$) receptors.

13.3.2.1.1 Preclinical and Clinical Trials

In rats, a single oral dose of lorcaserin decreased eating during the first 2 hours, with the effect maintained over the following 22 hours (Smith et al., 2008), and a 4-week trial of locaserin in diet-obese rats resulted in reduced food intake and a selective loss of fat mass (Thomsen et al., 2008). Tests with selective 5-HT receptor subtype antagonists indicated that lorcaserin's eating-inhibitory effect depends on $5-HT_{2C}$ receptors (Thomsen et al., 2008). In humans, the efficacy and safety of lorcaserin were evaluated in three separate phase III trials (Table 13.2). Lorcaserin produced only modest weight loss, as summarized in a recent meta-analysis taking into account five randomized controlled studies, with a mean weight loss of 3.2 kg at 1 year and body mass index reduction of 1.2 kg/m^2 compared with placebo (Chan et al., 2013).

13.3.2.1.2 Mechanism of Action

5-HT is synthesized both peripherally (enterochromaffin cells and mast cells) and centrally (neurons in the raphe nuclei and mast cells) (Silver et al., 1996; Azmitia, 2007; Gershon, 2013). Peripheral exogenous 5-HT administration leads to satiation and reduced meal size in rats (Edwards and Stevens, 1991). Because of poor blood–brain barrier penetration, it is unlikely that peripheral serotonin elicits satiation by acting directly in the brain, but rather indirectly, by activating ascending vagal afferent fibers (Mazda et al., 2004; Hayes and Covasa, 2006; Savastano et al., 2007). These effects, however, appeared to be mediated by $5-HT_3$ receptors rather than $5-HT_{2C}$ receptors.

Central 5-HT is primarily released by the 5-HT-synthesizing neurons in the raphe nuclei which, project to most regions of the brain. Neuropharmacological work by Blundell and his colleagues led to the hypothesis that central 5-HT has an important, physiological role in eliciting satiety (Blundell and Latham, 1980; Halford et al., 1998). To date, a variety of serotonergic drugs have been implicated in satiation: (i) D-fenfluramine, which inhibits 5-HT reuptake apparently via $5-HT_{2C}$ receptors; (ii) the selective 5-HT reuptake inhibitors fluoxetine and sertraline; (iii) the 5-HT/NE reuptake inhibitor sibutramine, whose hypophagic effect is mediated by $5-HT_{2C}$ receptors; and (iv) the direct agonists of several 5-HT receptors, including $5-HT_{2C}$ receptors, whose actions can be reversed by their specific antagonists (Kennett and Curzon, 1988, 1991; Clifton et al., 1989; Simansky and Viadya, 1990; Kitchener and Dourish, 1994; Halford and Blundell, 1996; Jackson et al., 1997; Lee and Simansky, 1997; Vickers et al., 2001; Lee et al., 2002; Hewitt et al., 2002; Heisler et al., 2006; Higgs et al., 2011). Two of these, D-fenfluramine and sibutramine, were approved for weight loss in the United States but later withdrawn due to adverse cardiovascular effects. Nevertheless, their potent hypophagic and weight-lowering effects support a role for 5-HT and $5-HT_{2C}$ receptors, in particular, in the inhibitory control of eating and validates them as targets for antiobesity drug development.

Perhaps the first evidence for a specific action of 5-HT_{2C} receptors on eating and body weight was the report that transgenic mice lacking these receptors ($5\text{-HT}_{2C}\text{R}$ knockout [KO] mice) were hyperphagic and developed obesity (Tecott et al., 1995; Nonogaki et al., 1998; Xu et al., 2008). These mice have decreased responses to dexfenfluramine (Vickers et al., 1999), glucagon-like peptide-1 (GLP-1), and cholecystokinin (CCK) (Asarian, 2009).

Which population of 5-HT_{2C} receptors is crucial for the control of eating is unclear and may be situationally dependent. For example, CCK increased neuronal activity, as gauged by c-Fos expression, in the nucleus tractus solitarii (NTS) of wild-type (WT) mice, but not $5\text{-HT}_{2C}\text{R}$ KO mice, but induced similar degrees of c-Fos expression in their paraventricular (PVN) and arcuate (Arc) nuclei of the hypothalamus, suggesting that hindbrain but not hypothalamic 5-HT_{2C} signaling was involved in the phenotype (Asarian, 2009). In contrast, GLP-1 increased c-Fos expression similarly in the NTS of both genotypes but increased c-Fos expression more in the PVN and Arc of $5\text{-HT}_{2C}\text{R}$ KO mice than WT mice, suggesting a hypothalamic action. Similarly, m-chlorophenyl-piperazine and dexfenfluramine also seem to decrease eating via Arc 5-HT_{2C} receptors (Heisler et al., 2002). Selective rescue of Arc 5-HT_{2C} receptors reversed the obesity phenotype of $5\text{-HT}_{2C}\text{R}$ KO mice (Xu et al., 2008), and because the reexpression occurred only in Arc POMC neurons, these data strongly suggest that 5-HT signals via downstream melanocortin pathways to decrease eating (Xu et al., 2008). Serotonergic terminals synaptically contact POMC and agouti-related peptide (AgRP) neurons in the Arc (Kiss et al., 1984; Heisler et al., 2006), confirming that 5-HT neurons are anatomically positioned to influence melanocortin neuron activity.

Important for the development of drugs targeting the 5-HT receptors is that two or more Arc 5-HT receptor subtypes may interact to produce the full eating-inhibitory effect, namely, 5-HT_{2C} receptors on POMC neurons and 5-HT_{1B} receptors on AgRP neurons (Heisler et al., 2002; Heisler et al., 2006; Lam et al., 2008). Thus, the GABA-mediated inhibitory action of 5-HT action on 5-HT_{1B} receptors may decrease AgRP release, thereby decreasing the local inhibitory input onto POMC neurons. The combined effect of these actions may lead to an increase in α-MSH release and a decrease in AgRP release, reducing the competitive antagonism at melanocortin 3 and 4 receptor-expressing target cells and leading to a decrease in eating.

13.3.2.2 Liraglutide

A number of hormones have also been considered as pharmacological targets for obesity therapies (Korner et al., 2013; Hay et al., 2015). For example, liraglutide is an acylated form of GLP-1 that is resistant to breakdown by the enzyme dipeptidyl peptidase-4 (DPP-4) and therefore has a greatly prolonged half-life compared to native GLP-1. Liraglutide was originally developed for the management of type 2 diabetes mellitus (T2DM), but after it was found to produce modest weight loss, it was approved for treatment of obesity in the United States in December 2014 and in Europe in March 2015 (Saxenda, NovoNordisk, Denmark).

13.3.2.2.1 Clinical Studies

A meta-analysis of the effects of GLP-1 receptor (GLP-1R) agonists on weight loss in 6411 overweight or obese subjects with or without T2DM indicated only a modest effect, i.e., a decrease of 2.9 kg (95% CI, 2.2–3.6 kg) (Vilsbøll et al., 2012). However, weight was a secondary endpoint in most of these trials. In an influential trial, Pi-Sunyer and colleagues (2015) found that, when carried over 56 weeks, patients lost on average 8.4 kg compared with 2.8 kg in the placebo group. A summary of clinical trials using liraglutide tailored to detect effects on body weight at 1 year posttreatment are summarized in Table 13.2.

13.3.2.2.2   Mechanisms of Action

GLP-1 is a hormone released following the posttranslational processing of prepro-glucagon (Holst, 2006; Campbell and Drucker, 2013). Endocrine GLP-1 is secreted by enteroendocrine L-cells both during and after a meal. GLP-1 is also produced by a population of neurons in the caudal brainstem (Merchenthaler et al., 1999; Zheng et al., 2015). The GLP-1R is widely expressed in the periphery and brain (Thorens, 1992; Bullock et al., 1996; Pyke et al., 2014).

The physiological role of GLP-1 in eating is unclear. Acute GLP-1 antagonism increased eating in some rat studies, but this has not been replicated in humans (Steinert et al., 2014). Interestingly, global KO of the GLP-1R produced no body weight or food intake phenotype in chow-fed mice (Scrocchi et al., 1996) but decreased the obesify-ing effect of feeding a high-fat diet (Hansotia et al., 2007; Wilson-Perez et al., 2013). Similarly, although some surgical vagotomy studies indicated that the vagus mediates the eating-inhibitory effect of peripherally injected GLP-1, liraglutide, or exendin-4 (another GLP-1 analog) (Abbott et al., 2005; Rüttimann et al., 2009; Kanoski et al., 2011), liraglutide still reduced eating and body weight in mice with transgenic deletion of GLP-1R in vagal afferent nerves (Sisley et al., 2014). Part of the resolution of these apparently conflicting results may lie in the fact that exogenous GLP-1 can act in a number of brain sites to inhibit eating, including the NTS, VTA, lateral parabrachial nucleus, nucleus accumbens, and Arc (Mietlicki-Baase et al., 2013, 2014; Alhadeff et al., 2014; Richard et al., 2015). Furthermore, the sites of action of native GLP-1 and liraglutide may differ, as indicated by a recent report (Secher et al., 2014) showing that most peripherally administered liraglutide gains access to the Arc and median emi-nence, with smaller amounts entering the PVN. Hence, it is important that different pharmacokinetic and, in particular, brain penetrating properties of the different com-pounds are taken into account. In the Arc, GLP-1 directly stimulated POMC cells and indirectly inhibited NPY/AgRP (Secher et al., 2014). GLP-1 also acted postsynaptically on ghrelin-sensitive neurons in the Arc, suggesting yet another possible mechanism contributing to its effects on eating (Riediger et al., 2010).

13.4   PHARMACOTHERAPY IN PHASE II AND III CLINICAL TRIALS

Although many pharmacological targets have been proposed based on animal mod-els with various degrees of obesity, only a few of these are now being tested in non-human primates or in human clinical trials. Current information on ongoing clinical trials recorded by the National Institutes of Health is given at www.clinicaltrials .gov. We considered only the purely pharmacological studies (i.e., no behavioral interventions) that had weight loss as a primary outcome. As of August 2015, only six Phase III monotherapy studies and no Phase III polytherapy studies were listed

TABLE 13.3
Past and Current Monotherapy Clinical Trials (CTs)

CT ID	Drug	Sponsor	Status
NCT01535014	Dietressa	Materia Medica	Completed
NCT00131430	Taranabant	Merck	Terminated
NCT00092872	MK0557	Merck	Completed
NCT00856609	Exenatide	NIDDK	Recruiting
NCT00134199	CP-945,598	Pfizer	Completed
NCT00073242	Leptin	NIDDK	Recruiting

Source: Data from trials in Phase III (http://www.clinicaltrials.gov).

TABLE 13.4
Past and Current Polytherapy Clinical Trials (CTs)

CT ID	Drug	Sponsor	Status
NCT02313220	Dapagliflozin/exenatide	Astra Zeneca	Active (not recruiting)
NCT00339014	Zonisamide/bupropion	Orexigen Therapeutics	Completed
NCT00402077	Pramlintide/sibutramine/ phentermine	Astra Zeneca	Completed
NCT01126970	Velneperit/orlistat	Shionogi	Completed
NCT00349635	Metformin/fenofibrate	Solvay	Completed
NCT00392925	Pramlintide/metreleptin	Astra Zeneca	Completed
NCT00819234	Pramlintide/metreleptin	Astra Zeneca	Completed
NCT02075281	HM11260C	Hanmi	Not yet recruiting
NCT02412631	Lorcaserin/varenicline	Mayo Clinic	Not yet recruiting

Source: Data from trials in Phase II (http://www.clinicaltrials.gov).

(Table 13.3). Nine Phase II combination therapies were listed, involving a number of targets not included in currently approved medications (Table 13.4).

13.5 DISCUSSION

In reviewing obesity treatments in 1959, Stunkard and McLaren-Hume (1959) observed that "The current widespread concern with weight reduction rests on at least two assumptions: first, that weight reduction programs are effective; second that they are harmless. Recent studies indicate that such programs may be far from harmless. This report documents their ineffectiveness." This gloomy observation was indeed true. In his analysis of literature going back to the 1930s, Stunkard found only eight studies that, among other criteria, provided figures of the outcome of the experiment and did not exclude from reports the outcome for patients who dropped-out or were "otherwise uncooperative," i.e., used the now-standard intention-to-treat analytic approach. The science behind obesity treatment has come a long way since then. This is due not only to an explosion of pharmaceutical targets being tested but also to an improvement in nutrition counseling and in behavioral and more recently surgical therapy for obese patients. At the same time, it has become clear that the responsibility for treating obese individuals is shared among government support for obesity research, the pharmaceutical industry, the food industry, and the clinician.

There is no doubt that much lies ahead for the pharmaceutical industry. For example, as reviewed here, monoamines are a major target of obesity therapeutics. But drugs that increase the availability of monoamines in the synapse cannot be highly selective because of the number of monoamine transmitters. Thus, targeting particular receptors may decrease side effects with no loss of therapeutic potency.

Further development of combination therapies is also imperative. Hormones that act as physiological eating controls are one attractive target. More and more studies are published showing increased effects of drugs targeting two or more hormones, sometimes in single-molecule drugs (Finan et al., 2015). Another rational strategy to identify novel obesity-therapy targets is to better understand the mechanism of action of successful therapies, i.e., of the four currently approved pharmaceutical options reviewed above and of bariatric surgery, and try to mimic them using pharmacology. One success story is liraglutide, which, as discussed earlier, was developed in investigations of the apparent role of GLP-1 in the beneficial effects of bariatric surgery. Other targets are emerging, such as bile acids, exemplified by the farnesoid X receptor, TGR5 and FGF15/19, which also were identified in investigations of the effects of bariatric surgery on bile/acid physiology (Li and Chiang, 2015). A third source of candidates should be the molecules shown in animal and human research to have reliable physiological effects, for example, CCK and amylin. Combinations of pharmacological and nonpharmacological treatments seem most likely to be the optimal approach and should be examined in all phases of drug development. To quote Thomas Insel, director of the National Institute for Mental Health of the USA, "For complex, chronic disorders, from diabetes to hypertension, the search for a magic bullet is giving way to combinatorial or convergent solutions. Medications, devices, mobile health apps, social support, education, and team care are all part of the package." It is hoped that these modalities will eventually surpass and replace bariatric surgery, which is best viewed as an effective but necessarily stopgap strategy.

Another important aspect concerns subject classification in clinical trials. For example, sex and race are rarely taken into account. The marked variability in obesity prevalence across men and women and across racial groups living in the United States, and many other Western countries, suggests the importance of these variables. Ignoring them may obscure some important results.

Regarding clinical practice, probably the most important goals are, first, for primary care physicians to be better informed about the best available therapeutic modalities; second, to recognize that obesity treatment is likely to be long and difficult; and, third, to treat obese patients with respect and to include their aspirations in any treatment plan. In a 2003 study, 75% of physicians interviewed stigmatized patients and did not recognize the importance of improving patients' self-image and mental health along with their obesity comorbidities (Foster et al., 2003). We give Stunkard and McLaren-Hume (1959) the last word:

How may the medical profession regain its proper role in the treatment of obesity? We can begin by looking at the situation as it exists and not as we would like it to be. We can acknowledge that treatment for obesity is a terribly difficult business, one in which our experts achieve only modest success, and the rest of us, even less. It is a treatment, which can be fraught with danger, a treatment not to be undertaken lightly by any obese person and by some perhaps not at all. Certainly weight reduction is not a matter to be left to unqualified practitioners. Lowering our level of aspiration may go far toward achieving our aims. If we do not expect weight reduction as a matter of course we may be able to accord due recognition to success. If we do not feel obliged to excuse our failures we may be able to investigate them. Learning to respect the complexities of their illnesses will help us to respect our patients. And the patient who has the respect of his physician has little reason to seek elsewhere for treatment.

ACKNOWLEDGMENT

LA is supported by NIH NIDDK DK092638.

LITERATURE CITED

Abbott, C.R., M. Monteiro, C.J. Small, A. Sajedi, K.L. Smith, J.R. Parkinson, M.A. Ghatei, and S.R. Bloom. 2005. The inhibitory effects of peripheral administration of peptide YY(3-36) and glucagon-like peptide-1 on food intake are attenuated by ablation of the vagal–brainstem–hypothalamic pathway. *Brain Res.* 1044(1):127–31.

Alexander, M., R.B. Rothman, M.H. Baumann, C.J. Endres, J.R. Brasić, and D.F. Wong. 2005. Noradrenergic and dopaminergic effects of (+)-amphetamine-like stimulants in the baboon *Papio anubis*. *Synapse.* 56(2):94–9.

Alhadeff, A.L., J.P. Baird, J.C. Swick, M.R. Hayes, and H.J. Grill. 2014. Glucagon-like peptide-1 receptor signaling in the lateral parabrachial nucleus contributes to the control of food intake and motivation to feed. *Neuropsychopharmacology.* 39(9):2233–43.

Allison, D.B., K.M. Gadde, W.T. Garvey, C.A. Peterson, M.L. Schwiers, T. Najarian, P.Y. Tam, B. Troupin, and W.W. Day. 2012. Controlled-release phentermine/topiramate in severely obese adults: A randomized controlled trial (EQUIP). *Obesity* (Silver Spring). 20(2):330–42.

Anderson, J.W., F.L. Greenway, K. Fujioka, K.M. Gadde, J. McKenney, and P.M. O'Neil. 2002. Bupropion SR enhances weight loss: A 48-week double-blind, placebo- controlled trial. *Obes Res.* 10(7):633–41.

Anton, R.F. 2008. Naltrexone for the management of alcohol dependence. *N Engl J Med.* 359(7):715–21.

Asarian, L. 2009. Loss of cholecystokinin and glucagon-like peptide-1-induced satiation in mice lacking serotonin 2C receptors. *Am J Physiol Regul Integr Comp Physiol.* 296(1):R51–6.

Ascher, J.A., J.O. Cole, J.N. Colin, J.P. Feighner, R.M. Ferris, H.C. Fibiger, R.N. Golden, P. Martin, W.Z. Potter, E. Richelson et al. 1995. Bupropion: A review of its mechanism of antidepressant activity. *J Clin Psychiatry.* 56(9):395–401.

Astrup, A., I. Caterson, P. Zelissen, B. Guy-Grand, M. Carruba, B. Levy, X. Sun, and M. Fitchet. 2004. Topiramate: Long-term maintenance of weight loss induced by a low-calorie diet in obese subjects. *Obes Res.* 12(10):1658–69.

Azmitia, E.C. 2007. Serotonin and brain: Evolution, neuroplasticity, and homeostasis. *Int Rev Neurobiol.* 77:31–56.

Bays, H. 2010. Phentermine, topiramate and their combination for the treatment of adiposopathy ('sick fat') and metabolic disease. *Expert Rev Cardiovasc Ther.* 8(12):1777–801.

Billes, S.K. and M.A. Cowley. 2007. Inhibition of dopamine and norepinephrine reuptake produces additive effects on energy balance in lean and obese mice. *Neuropsychopharmacology.* 32(4):822–34.

Billes, S.K. and F.L. Greenway. 2011. Combination therapy with naltrexone and bupropion for obesity. *Expert Opin Pharmacother.* 12(11):1813–26.

Blasio, A., L. Steardo, V. Sabino, and P. Cottone. 2014. Opioid system in the medial prefrontal cortex mediates binge-like eating. *Addict Biol.* 19(4):652–62.

Blundell, J.E. and C.J. Latham. 1980. Characterisation of adjustments to the structure of feeding behaviour following pharmacological treatment: Effects of amphetamine and fenfluramine and the antagonism produced by pimozide and methergoline. *Pharmacol Biochem Behav.* 12(5):717–22.

Bronstein, D.M., N.C. Day, H.B. Gutstein, K.A. Trujillo, and H. Akil. 1993. Pre- and post-translational regulation of beta-endorphin biosynthesis in the CNS: Effects of chronic naltrexone treatment. *J Neurochem.* 60(1):40–9.

Bullock, B.P., R.S. Heller, and J.F. Habener. 1996. Tissue distribution of messenger ribonucleic acid encoding the rat glucagon-like peptide-1 receptor. *Endocrinology.* 137:2968–78.

Cameron, F., G. Whiteside, and K. McKeage. 2012. Phentermine and topiramate extended release (Qsymia™): First global approval. *Drugs.* 72(15):2033–42.

Campbell, J.E. and D.J. Drucker. 2013. Pharmacology, physiology, and mechanisms of incretin hormone action. *Cell Metab.* 17:819–37.

Chan, E.W., Y. He, C.S. Chui, A.Y. Wong, W.C. Lau, and I.C. Wong. 2013. Efficacy and safety of lorcaserin in obese adults: A meta-analysis of 1-year randomized controlled trials (RCTs) and narrative review on short-term RCTs. *Obes Rev.* 14(5):383–92.

Clifton, P.G., A.M. Barnfield, and L. Philcox. 1989. A behavioural profile of fluoxetine-induced anorexia. *Psychopharmacology* (Berl). 97(1):89–95.

Cosentino, G., A.O. Conrad, and G.I. Uwaifo. 2011. Phentermine and topiramate for the management of obesity: A review. *Drug Des Dev Ther.* 7:267–78.

Cowley, M.A., J.L. Smart, M. Rubinstein, M.G. Cerdán, S. Diano, T.L. Horvath, R.D. Cone, and M.J. Low. 2001. Leptin activates anorexigenic POMC neurons through a neural network in the arcuate nucleus. *Nature.* 411(6836):480–4.

Dhillon, S., L.P. Yang, and M.P. Curran. 2008. Bupropion: A review of its use in the management of major depressive disorder. *Drugs.* 68(5):653–89.

Edwards, S. and R. Stevens. 1991. Peripherally administered 5-hydroxytryptamine elicits the full behavioural sequence of satiety. *Physiol Behav.* 50(5):1075–7.

Fava, M., A.J. Rush, M.E. Thase, A. Clayton, S.M. Stahl, J.F. Pradko, and J.A. Johnston. 2005. 15 years of clinical experience with bupropion HCl: From bupropion to bupropion SR to bupropion XL. *Prim Care Companion J Clin Psychiatry.* 7(3):106–13.

Finan, B., B. Yang, N. Ottaway, D.L. Smiley, T. Ma, C. Clemmensen, J. Chabenne, L. Zhang, K.M. Habegger, K. Fischer, J.E. Campbell, D. Sandoval, R.J. Seeley, K. Bleicher, S. Uhles, W. Riboulet, J. Funk, C. Hertel, S. Belli, E. Sebokova, K. Conde-Knape, A. Konkar, D.J. Drucker, V. Gelfanov, P.T. Pfluger, T.D. Müller, D. Perez-Tilve, R.D. DiMarchi, and M.H. Tschöp. 2015. A rationally designed monomeric peptide triagonist corrects obesity and diabetes in rodents. *Nat Med.* 21(1):27–36.

Foster, G.D., T.A. Wadden, A.P. Makris, D. Davidson, R.S. Sanderson, D.B. Allison, and A. Kessler. 2003. Primary care physicians' attitudes about obesity and its treatment. *Obes Res.* 11(10):1168–77.

Fraley, G.S. and S. Ritter. 2003. Immunolesion of norepinephrine and epinephrine afferents to medial hypothalamus alters basal and 2-deoxy-D-glucose-induced neuropeptide Y and agouti gene-related protein messenger ribonucleic acid expression in the arcuate nucleus. *Endocrinology.* 144(1):75–83.

Gadde, K.M., C.B. Parker, L.G. Maner, and H.R. Wagner 2nd, E.J. Logue, M.K. Drezner, K.R. Krishnan. 2001. Bupropion for weight loss: An investigation of efficacy and tolerability in overweight and obese women. *Obes Res.* 9(9):544–51.

Gadde, K.M., D.B. Allison, D.H. Ryan, C.A. Peterson, B. Troupin, M.L. Schwiers, and W.W. Day. 2011. Effects of low-dose, controlled-release, phentermine plus topiramate combination on weight and associated comorbidities in overweight and obese adults (CONQUER): A randomised, placebo-controlled, phase 3 trial. *Lancet.* 377(9774):1341–52.

Garvey, W.T. 2013. Phentermine and topiramate extended-release: A new treatment for obesity and its role in a complications-centric approach to obesity medical management. *Expert Opin Drug Saf.* 12(5):741–56.

Garvey, W.T., D.H. Ryan, M. Look, K.M. Gadde, D.B. Allison, C.A. Peterson, M. Schwiers, W.W. Day, and C.H. Bowden. 2012. Two-year sustained weight loss and metabolic benefits with controlled-release phentermine/topiramate in obese and overweight adults (SEQUEL): A randomized, placebo-controlled, phase 3 extension study. *Am J Clin Nutr.* 95(2):297–308.

Gershon, M.D. 2013. 5-Hydroxytryptamine (serotonin) in the gastrointestinal tract. *Curr Opin Endocrinol Diabetes Obes.* 20(1):14–21.

Ginzburg, H.M. and W.J. Glass. 1984. The role of the National Institute on Drug Abuse in the development of naltrexone. *J Clin Psychiatry.* 45(9 Pt 2):4–6.

Giuliano, C., T.W. Robbins, P.J. Nathan, E.T. Bullmore, and B.J. Everitt. 2012. Inhibition of opioid transmission at the μ-opioid receptor prevents both food seeking and binge-like eating. *Neuropsychopharmacology.* 37(12):2643–52.

Greenway, F.L., M.J. Whitehouse, M. Guttadauria, J.W. Anderson, R.L. Atkinson, K. Fujioka, K.M. Gadde, A.K. Gupta, P. O'Neil, D. Schumacher, D. Smith, E. Dunayevich, G.D. Tollefson, E. Weber, and M.A. Cowley. 2009. Rational design of a combination medication for the treatment of obesity. *Obesity* (Silver Spring). 17(1):30–9.

Haddock, C.K., W.S. Poston, P.L. Dill, J.P. Foreyt, M. Ericsson. 2002. Pharmacotherapy for obesity: A quantitative analysis of four decades of published randomized clinical trials. *Int J Obes Relat Metab Disord.* 26(2):262–73.

Halford, J.C. and J.E. Blundell. 1996. Metergoline antagonizes fluoxetine-induced suppression of food intake but not changes in the behavioural satiety sequence. *Pharmacol Biochem Behav.* 54(4):745–51.

Halford, J.C., S.C. Wanninayake, and J.E. Blundell. 1998. Behavioral satiety sequence (BSS) for the diagnosis of drug action on food intake. *Pharmacol Biochem Behav.* 61(2):159–68.

Hansotia, T., A. Maida, G. Flock, Y. Yamada, K. Tsukiyama, Y. Seino, and D.J. Drucker. 2007. Extrapancreatic incretin receptors modulate glucose homeostasis, body weight, and energy expenditure. *J Clin Invest.* 117(1):143–52.

Hasegawa, H., R. Meeusen, S. Sarre, M. Diltoer, M.F. Piacentini, and Y. Michotte. 2005. Acute dopamine/norepinephrine reuptake inhibition increases brain and core temperature in rats. *J Appl Physiol.* 99(4):1397–401.

Hay, D.L., S. Chen, T.A. Lutz, D.G. Parkes, and J.D. Roth. 2015. Amylin: Pharmacology, physiology, and clinical potential. *Pharmacol Rev.* 67(3):564–600.

Hayes, M.R. and M. Covasa. 2006. Dorsal hindbrain 5-HT3 receptors participate in control of meal size and mediate CCK-induced satiation. *Brain Res.* 1103(1):99–107.

Heisler, L.K., M.A. Cowley, L.H. Tecott, W. Fan, M.J. Low, J.L. Smart, M. Rubinstei, J.B. Tatro, J.N. Marcus, H. Holstege, C.E. Lee, R.D. Cone, J.K. Elmquist. 2002. Activation of central melanocortin pathways by fenfluramine. *Science.* 297(5581):609–11.

Heisler, L.K., E.E. Jobst, G.M. Sutton, L. Zhou, E. Borok, Z. Thornton-Jones, H.Y. Liu, J.M. Zigman, N. Balthasar, T. Kishi, C.E. Lee, C.J. Aschkenasi, C.Y. Zhang, J. Yu, O. Boss, K.G. Mountjoy, P.G. Clifton, B.B. Lowell, J.M. Friedman, T. Horvath, A.A. Butler,

M.A. Cowley. 2006. Serotonin reciprocally regulates melanocortin neurons to modulate food intake. Neuron. 51(2):239–49.

Heisler, L.K., R.B. Kanarek, and A. Gerstein. 1997. Fluoxetine decreases fat and protein intakes but not carbohydrate intake in male rats. Pharmacol Biochem Behav. 58:767–73.

Hewitt, K.N., M.D. Lee, C.T. Dourish, and P.G. Clifton. 2002. Serotonin 2C receptor agonists and the behavioural satiety sequence in mice. Pharmacol Biochem Behav. 71(4):691–700.

Heymsfield, S.B., A.S. Greenberg, K. Fujioka, R.M. Dixon, R. Kushner, T. Hunt, J.A. Lubina, J. Patane, B. Sclf, P. Hunt, M. McCamish. 1999. Recombinant leptin for weight loss in obese and lean adults: A randomized, controlled, dose-escalation trial. JAMA. 282(16):1568–75.

Higgs, S., A.J. Cooper, and N.M. Barnes. 2011. Reversal of sibutramine-induced anorexia with a selective 5-HT(2C) receptor antagonist. Psychopharmacology (Berl). 214:941–7.

Holst, J.J. 2006. Glucagon-like peptide-1: From extract to agent. The Claude Bernard Lecture, 2005. Diabetologia. 49:253–60.

Husum, H., D. Van Kammen, E. Termeer, G. Bolwig, and A. Mathé. 2003. Topiramate normalizes hippocampal NPY-LI in flinders sensitive line 'depressed' rats and upregulates NPY, galanin, and CRH-LI in the hypothalamus: Implications for mood-stabilizing and weight loss-inducing effects. Neuropsychopharmacology. 28(7):1292–9.

Ioannides-Demos, L.L., L. Piccenna, and J.J. McNeil. 2011. Pharmacotherapies for obesity: Past, current, and future therapies. J Obes. 2011:179674.

Jackson, H.C., M.C. Bearham, L.J. Hutchins, S.E. Mazurkiewicz, A.M. Needham, and D.J. Heal. 1997. Investigation of the mechanisms underlying the hypophagic effects of the 5-HT and noradrenaline reuptake inhibitor, sibutramine, in the rat. Br J Pharmacol. 121(8):1613–8. PubMed PMID: 9283694; PubMed Central PMCID: PMC1564868.

Jain, A.K., R.A. Kaplan, K.M. Gadde, T.A. Wadden, D.B. Allison, E.R. Brewer, R.A. Leadbetter, N. Richard, B. Haight, B.D. Jamerson, K.S. Buaron, and A. Metz. 2002. Bupropion SR vs. placebo for weight loss in obese patients with depressive symptoms. Obes Res. 10(10):1049–56.

Jefferson, J.W., A.J. Rush, J.C. Nelson, S.A. VanMeter, A. Krishen, K.D. Hampton, D.S. Wightman, and J.G. Modell. 2006. Extended-release bupropion for patients with major depressive disorder presenting with symptoms of reduced energy, pleasure, and interest: Findings from a randomized, double-blind, placebo-controlled study. J Clin Psychiatry. 67(6):865–73.

Johansson, B.A., M. Berglund, and A. Lindgren. 2006. Efficacy of maintenance treatment with naltrexone for opioid dependence: A meta-analytical review. Addiction. 101(4):491–503.

Kanoski, S.E., S.M. Fortin, M. Arnold, H.J. Grill, and M.R. Hayes. 2011. Peripheral and central GLP-1 receptor populations mediate the anorectic effects of peripherally administered GLP-1 receptor agonists, liraglutide and exendin-4. Endocrinology. 152(8):3103–12.

Kelley, A.E., E.P. Bless, and C.J. Swanson. 1996. Investigation of the effects of opiate antagonists infused into the nucleus accumbens on feeding and sucrose drinking in rats. J Pharmacol Exp Ther. 278(3):1499–507.

Kennett, G.A. and G. Curzon. 1988. Evidence that mCPP may have behavioural effects mediated by central 5-HT1C receptors. Br J Pharmacol. 94(1):137–47.

Kennett, G.A. and G. Curzon. 1991. Potencies of antagonists indicate that 5-HT1C receptors mediate 1-3(chlorophenyl)piperazine-induced hypophagia. Br J Pharmacol. 103:2016–20.

Khan, Z.U., A. Gutiérrez, R. Martín, A. Peñafiel, A. Rivera, and A. De La Calle. 1998. Differential regional and cellular distribution of dopamine D2-like receptors: An immunocytochemical study of subtype-specific antibodies in rat and human brain. J Comp Neurol. 402(3):353–71.

Khazaal, Y. and D.F. Zullino. 2006. Topiramate in the treatment of compulsive sexual behavior: Case report. BMC Psychiatry. 6:22.

Khazaal, Y. and D.F. Zullino. 2007. Topiramate-induced weight loss is possibly due to the blockade of conditioned and automatic processes. *Eur J Clin Pharmacol.* 63(9):891–2; author reply 893.

Kiss, J., C. Léránth, and B. Halász. 1984. Serotoninergic endings on VIP-neurons in the suprachiasmatic nucleus and on ACTH-neurons in the arcuate nucleus of the rat hypothalamus. A combination of high resolution autoradiography and electron microscopic immunocytochemistry. *Neurosci Lett.* 44(2):119–24.

Kitchener, S.J. and C.T. Dourish. 1994. An examination of the behavioural specificity of hypophagia induced by 5-HT1B, 5-HT1C and 5-HT2 receptor agonists using the post-prandial satiety sequence in rats. *Psychopharmacology* (Berl). 113(3–4):369–77.

Korner, J., R. Conroy, G. Febres, D.J. McMahon, I. Conwell, W. Karmally, and L.J. Aronne. 2013. Randomized double-blind placebo-controlled study of leptin administration after gastric bypass. *Obesity* (Silver Spring). 21(5):951–6.

Lam, D.D., M.J. Przydzial, S.H. Ridley, G.S. Yeo, J.J. Rochford, S. O'Rahilly, and L.K. Heisler. 2008. Serotonin 5-HT2C receptor agonist promotes hypophagia via downstream activation of melanocortin 4 receptors. *Endocrinology.* 149(3):1323–8.

Lee, M.D. and K.J. Simansky. 1997. CP-94, 253: A selective serotonin1B (5-HT1B) agonist that promotes satiety. *Psychopharmacology* (Berl). 131(3):264–70.

Lee, M.D., G.A. Kennett, C.T. Dourish, and P.G. Clifton. 2002. 5-HT1B receptors modulate components of satiety in the rat: Behavioural and pharmacological analyses of the selective serotonin1B agonist CP-94,253. *Psychopharmacology* (Berl). 164(1):49–60.

Li, T. and J.Y. Chiang. 2015. Bile acids as metabolic regulators. *Curr Opin Gastroenterol.* 31(2):159–65.

Li, Z., M. Maglione, W. Tu, W. Mojica, D. Arterburn, L.R. Shugarman, L. Hilton, M. Suttorp, V. Solomon, P.G. Shekelle, and S.C. Morton. 2005. Meta-analysis: Pharmacologic treatment of obesity. *Ann Intern Med.* 142(7):532–46.

Liu, Y.L., I.P. Connoley, J. Harrison, D.J. Heal, and M.J. Stock. 2002. Comparison of the thermogenic and hypophagic effects of sibutramine's metabolite 2 and other monoamine reuptake inhibitors. *Eur J Pharmacol.* 452(1):49–56.

Liu, Y.L., I.P. Connoley, D.J. Heal, and M.J. Stock. 2004. Harmacological characterisation of the thermogenic effect of bupropion. *Eur J Pharmacol.* 498(1–3):219–25.

Maggio, C.A., E. Presta, E.F. Bracco, J.R. Vasselli, H.R. Kissileff, D.N. Pfohl, and S.A. Hashim. 1985. Naltrexone and human eating behavior: A dose-ranging inpatient trial in moderately obese men. *Brain Res Bull.* 14(6):657–61.

Malcolm, R., P.M. O'Neil, J.D. Sexauer, F.E. Riddle, H.S. Currey, and C. Counts. 1985. A controlled trial of naltrexone in obese humans. *Int J Obes.* 9(5):347–53

Mazda, T., H. Yamamoto, M. Fujimura, and M. Fujimiya. 2004. Gastric distension-induced release of 5-HT stimulates c-fos expression in specific brain nuclei via 5-HT3 receptors in conscious rats. *Am J Physiol Gastrointest Liver Physiol.* 287(1):G228–35.

McElroy, S.L., L.M. Arnold, N.A. Shapira, P.E. Keck Jr, N.R. Rosenthal, M.R. Karim, M. Kamin, and J.I. Hudson. 2003. Topiramate in the treatment of binge eating disorder associated with obesity: A randomized, placebo-controlled trial. *Am J Psychiatry.* 160(2):255–61.

Merchenthaler, I., M. Lane, and P. Shughrue. 1999. Distribution of pre-pro-glucagon and glucagon-like peptide-1 receptor messenger RNAs in the rat central nervous system. *J Comp Neurol.* 403:261–80.

Mietlicki-Baase, E.G., P.I. Ortinski, L.E. Rupprecht, D.R. Olivos, A.L. Alhadeff, R.C. Pierce, and M.R. Hayes. 2013. The food intake-suppressive effects of glucagon-like peptide-1 receptor signaling in the ventral tegmental area are mediated by AMPA/kainate receptors. *Am J Physiol Endocrinol Metab.* 305(11):E1367–74.

Mietlicki-Baase, E.G., P.I. Ortinski, D.J. Reiner, C.G. Sinon, J.E. McCutcheon, R.C. Pierce, M.F. Roitman, and M.R. Hayes. 2014. Glucagon-like peptide-1 receptor activation in the nucleus accumbens core suppresses feeding by increasing glutamatergic AMPA/ kainate signaling. *J Neurosci.* 34(20):6985–92.

Nathan, P.J., B.V. O'Neill, A. Napolitano, and E.T. Bullmore. 2011. Neuropsychiatric adverse effects of centrally acting antiobesity drugs. *CNS Neurosci Ther.* 17(5):490–505.

Nonogaki, K., A.M. Strack, M.F. Dallman, and L.H. Tecott. 1998. Leptin-independent hyperphagia and type 2 diabetes in mice with a mutated serotonin 5-HT2C receptor gene. *Nat Med.* 4(10):1152–6.

Osler, W. 1891. Recent advances in medicine. *Science.* 17(425):170–1.

Pi-Sunyer, X., A. Astrup, K. Fujioka, F. Greenway, A. Halpern, M. Krempf, D.C. Lau, C.W. le Roux, R. Violante Ortiz, C.B. Jensen, and J.P. Wilding. 2015. SCALE Obesity and Prediabetes NN8022-1839 Study Group. A randomized, controlled trial of 3.0 mg of liraglutide in weight management. *N Engl J Med.* 373(1):11–22.

Porter, R.J., A. Dhir, R.L. Macdonald, and M.A. Rogawski. 2012. Mechanisms of action of antiseizure drugs, In: *Handbook of Clinical Neurology, Volume 108.* H. Stefan and W.H. Theodore, eds, 663–81. Cambridge: Elsevier.

Poulsen, S.A., B.L. Wilkinson, A. Innocenti, D. Vullo, and C.T. Supuran. 2008. Inhibition of human mitochondrial carbonic anhydrases VA and VB with para-(4-phenyltriazole-1-yl)-benzenesulfonamide derivatives. *Bioorg Med Chem Lett.* 15;18(16):4624–7.

Pyke, C., R.S. Heller, R.K. Kirk, C. Ørskov, S. Reedtz-Runge, P. Kaastrup, A. Hvelplund, L. Bardram, D. Calatayud, and L.B. Knudsen. 2014. GLP-1 receptor localization in monkey and human tissue: novel distribution revealed with extensively validated monoclonal antibody. *Endocrinology.* Apr;155(4):1280–90.

Richard, J.E., R.H. Anderberg, A. Göteson, F.M. Gribble, F. Reimann, and K.P. Skibicka. 2015. Activation of the GLP-1 receptors in the nucleus of the solitary tract reduces food reward behavior and targets the mesolimbic system. *PLoS One.* 20;10(3):e0119034.

Richard, D., J. Ferland, J. Lalonde, P. Samson, and Y. Deshaies. 2000. Influence of topiramate in the regulation of energy balance. *Nutrition.* 16(10):961–6.

Riediger, T., N. Eisele, C. Scheel, and T.A. Lutz. 2010. Effects of glucagon-like peptide 1 and oxyntomodulin on neuronal activity of ghrelin-sensitive neurons in the hypothalamic arcuate nucleus. *Am J Physiol Regul Integr Comp Physiol.* 298(4):R1061–7.

Rothman, R.B., M.H. Baumann, C.M. Dersch, D.V. Romero, K.C. Rice, F.I. Carroll, and J.S. Partilla. 2001. Amphetamine-type central nervous system stimulants release norepinephrine more potently than they release dopamine and serotonin. *Synapse.* 39(1):32–41.

Rudnick, G. and J. Clark. 1993. From synapse to vesicle: The reuptake and storage of biogenic amine neurotransmitters. *Biochim Biophys Acta.* 4;1144(3):249–63.

Rüttimann, E.B., M. Arnold, J.J. Hillebrand, N. Geary, and W. Langhans. 2009. Intrameal hepatic portal and intraperitoneal infusions of glucagon-like peptide-1 reduce spontaneous meal size in the rat via different mechanisms. *Endocrinology.* 150(3):1174–81.

Savastano, D.M., M.R. Hayes, and M. Covasa. 2007. Serotonin-type 3 receptors mediate intestinal lipid-induced satiation and Fos-like immunoreactivity in the dorsal hindbrain. *Am J Physiol Regul Integr Comp Physiol.* 292(3):R1063–70.

Schütt, M., J. Brinkhoff, M. Drenckhan, H. Lehnert, and C. Sommer. 2010. Weight reducing and metabolic effects of topiramate in patients with migraine—an observational study. *Exp Clin Endocrinol Diabetes.* 118(7):449–52.

Scrocchi, L.A., T.J. Brown, N. MaClusky, P.L. Brubaker, A.B. Auerbach, A.L. Joyner, and D.J. Drucker. 1996. Glucose intolerance but normal satiety in mice with a null mutation in the glucagon-like peptide 1 receptor gene. *Nat Med.* 2(11):1254–8.

Secher, A., J. Jelsing, A.F. Baquero, J. Hecksher-Sørensen, M.A. Cowley, L.S. Dalbøge, G. Hansen, K.L. Grove, C. Pyke, K. Raun, L. Schäffer, M. Tang-Christensen, S. Verma, B.M. Witgen, N. Vrang, and L. Bjerre Knudsen. 2014. The arcuate nucleus mediates GLP-1 receptor agonist liraglutide-dependent weight loss. *J Clin Invest.* 124(10):4473–88.

Shin, J.H. and K.M. Gadde. 2013. Clinical utility of phentermine/topiramate (Qsymia™) combination for the treatment of obesity. *Diabetes Metab Syndr Obes.* 6:131–9.

Shin, A.C., P.J. Pistell, C.B. Phifer, and H.R. Berthoud. 2010. Reversible suppression of food reward behavior by chronic mu-opioid receptor antagonism in the nucleus accumbens. *Neuroscience.* 170(2):580–8.

Silver, R., A.J. Silverman, L. Vitković, and I.I. Lederhendler. 1996. Mast cells in the brain: Evidence and functional significance. *Trends Neurosci.* 19(1):25–31. Review. PubMed PMID: 8787137.

Simansky, K.J. and A.H. Vaidya. 1990. Behavioral mechanisms for the anorectic action of the serotonin (5-HT) uptake inhibitor sertraline in rats: Comparison with directly acting 5-HT agonists. *Brain Res Bull.* 25(6):953–60. PubMed PMID: 2149668.

Sisley, S., R. Gutierrez-Aguilar, M. Scott, D.A. D'Alessio, D.A. Sandoval, and R.J. Seeley. 2014. Neuronal GLP1R mediates liraglutide's anorectic but not glucose-lowering effect. *J Clin Invest.* 124(6):2456–63.

Smith, G.P. 2000. The controls of eating: A shift from nutritional homeostasis to behavioral neuroscience. *Nutrition.* 16(10):814–20.

Smith, S.M., M. Meyer, and K.E. Trinkley. 2013. Phentermine/topiramate for the treatment of obesity. *Ann Pharmacother.* 47(3):340–9.

Smith, B.M., J.M. Smith, J.H. Tsai, J.A. Schultz, C.A. Gilson, S.A. Estrada, R.R. Chen, D.M. Park, E.B. Prieto, C.S. Gallardo, D. Sengupta, P.I. Dosa, J.A. Covel, A. Ren, R.R. Webb, N.R. Beeley, M. Martin, M. Morgan, S. Espitia, H.R. Saldana, C. Bjenning, K.T. Whelan, A.J. Grottick, F. Menzaghi, and W.J. Thomsen. 2008. Discovery and structure-activity relationship of (1R)-8-chloro-2,3,4,5-tetrahydro-1-methyl-1H-3-benzazepine (Lorcaserin), a selective serotonin 5-HT2C receptor agonist for the treatment of obesity. *J Med Chem* 51:305–13.

Sommer, B.R., E.L. Mitchell, and T.E. Wroolie. 2013. Topiramate: Effects on cognition in patients with epilepsy, migraine headache and obesity. *Ther Adv Neurol Disord.* 6(4):211–27.

Steinert, R.E., J. Schirra, A.C. Meyer-Gerspach, P. Kienle, H. Fischer, F. Schulte, B. Goeke, and C. Beglinger. 2014. Effect of glucagon-like peptide-1 receptor antagonism on appetite and food intake in healthy men. *Am J Clin Nutr.* 100(2):514–23.

Stunkard, A. and M. McLaren-Hume. 1959. The results of treatment for obesity: A review of the literature and report of a series. *AMA Arch Intern Med.* 103(1):79–85.

Tabarin, A., Y. Diz-Chaves, C. Carmona Mdel, B. Catargi, E.P. Zorrilla, A.J. Roberts, D.V. Coscina, S. Rousset, A. Redonnet, G.C. Parker, K. Inoue, D. Ricquier, L. Pénicaud, B.L. Kieffer, and G.F. Koob. 2005. Resistance to diet-induced obesity in mu-opioid receptor-deficient mice: Evidence for a "thrifty gene". *Diabetes.* 54(12):3510–6.

Taber, M.T., G. Zernig, and H.C. Fibiger. 1998. Opioid receptor modulation of feeding-evoked dopamine release in the rat nucleus accumbens. *Brain Res.* 785(1):24–30.

Tainter, M.L., A.B. Stockton, and W.C. Cutting. 1935. Dinitrophenol in the treatment of obesity: Final report. *JAMA.* 105(5): 332–336.

Tecott, L.H., L.M. Sun, S.F. Akana, A.M. Strack, D.H. Lowenstein, M.F. Dallman, and D. Julius. 1995. Eating disorder and epilepsy in mice lacking 5-HT2c serotonin receptors. *Nature.* 374(6522):542–6.

Theisen, F.M., S. Beyenburg, S. Gebhardt, M. Kluge, W.F. Blum, H. Remschmidt, C.E. Elger, and J. Hebebrand. 2008. A prospective study of body weight and serum leptin levels in patients treated with topiramate. *Clin Neuropharmacol.* 31(4):226–30.

Thomsen, W.J., A.J. Grottick, F. Menzaghi, H. Reyes-Saldana, S. Espitia, D. Yuskin, K. Whelan, M. Martin, M. Morgan, W. Chen, H. Al-Shamma, B. Smith, D. Chalmers, and D. Behan. 2008. Lorcaserin, a novel selective human 5-hydroxytryptamine2C agonist: In vitro and in vivo pharmacological characterization. *J Pharmacol Exp Ther.* 325(2):577–87.

Thorens, B. 1992. Expression cloning of the pancreatic beta cell receptor for the gluco-incretin hormone glucagon-like peptide 1. *Proc Natl Acad Sci USA*. 89:8641–5.

Tremblay, A., J.P. Chaput, S. Bérubé-Parent, D. Prud'homme, C. Leblanc, N. Alméras, and J.P. Déprés. 2007. The effect of topiramate on energy balance in obese men: A 6-month double-blind randomized placebo-controlled study with a 6-month open-label extension. *Eur J Clin Pharmacol*. 63(2):123–34.

Turenius, C.I., M.M. Htut, D.A. Prodon, P.L. Ebersole, P.T. Ngo, R.N. Lara, J.L. Wilczynski, and B.G. Stanley. 2009. GABA(A) receptors in the lateral hypothalamus as mediators of satiety and body weight regulation. *Brain Res*. 1262:16–24.

Vickers, S.P., P.G. Clifton, C.T. Dourish, and L.H. Tecott. 1999. Reduced satiating effect of d-fenfluramine in serotonin 5-HT(2C) receptor mutant mice. *Psychopharmacology* (Berl). 143(3):309–14.

Vickers, S.P., C.T. Dourish, and G.A. Kennett. 2001. Evidence that hypophagia induced by D-fenfluramine and D-norfenfluramine in the rat is mediated by 5-HT2C receptors. *Neuropharmacology*. 41(2):200–9.

Vilsbøll, T., M. Christensen, A.E. Junker, F.K. Knop, and L.L. Gluud. 2012. Effects of glucagon-like peptide-1 receptor agonists on weight loss: Systematic review and meta-analyses of randomised controlled trials. *BMJ*. 10;344:d7771.

Vullo, D., M. Franchi, E. Gallori, J. Antel, A. Scozzafava, and C.T. Supuran. 2004. Carbonic anhydrase inhibitors. Inhibition of mitochondrial isozyme V with aromatic and hetero-cyclic sulfonamides. *J Med Chem*. 47(5):1272–9.

Wall SC, H. Gu, and G. Rudnick. 1995. Biogenic amine flux mediated by cloned transport-ers stably expressed in cultured cell lines: Amphetamine specificity for inhibition and efflux. *Mol Pharmacol*. 47:544–50.

Weintraub, M. 1992. Long-term weight control study: Conclusions. *Clin Pharmacol Ther*. 51(5):642–6.

Wilson-Pérez, H.E., A.P. Chambers, K.K. Ryan, B. Li, D.A. Sandoval, D. Stoffers, D.J. Drucker, D. Pérez-Tilve, and R.J. Seeley. 2013. Vertical sleeve gastrectomy is effective in two genetic mouse models of glucagon-like peptide 1 receptor deficiency. *Diabetes*. 62(7):2380–5.

Winslow, D.H., C.H. Bowden, K.P. DiDonato, and P.A. McCullough. 2012. A randomized, double-blind, placebo-controlled study of an oral, extended-release formulation of phentermine/topiramate for the treatment of obstructive sleep apnea in obese adults. *Sleep*. 35(11):1529–39.

Winum, J.Y., A. Scozzafava, J.L. Montero, and C.T. Supuran. 2005. Sulfamates and their therapeutic potential. *Med Res Rev*. 25(2):186–228.

Witkamp, R.F. 2011. Current and future drug targets in weight management. *Pharm Res*. 28(8):1792–818.

Wright, F.L. and R.J. Rodgers. 2013. Acute behavioural effects of bupropion and naltrexone, alone and in combination, in non-deprived male rats presented with palatable mash. *Psychopharmacology* (Berl). 228(2):291–307.

Xu, Y., J.E. Jones, D. Kohno, K.W. Williams, C.E. Lee, M.J. Choi, J.G. Anderson, L.K. Heisler, J.M. Zigman, B.B. Lowell, and J.K. Elmquist. 2008. 5-HT2CRs expressed by pro-opiomelanocortin neurons regulate energy homeostasis. *Neuron* 60(4):582–9.

Zhang, M., B.A. Gosnell, and A.E. Kelley. 1998. Intake of high-fat food is selectively enhanced by mu opioid receptor stimulation within the nucleus accumbens. *J Pharmacol Exp Ther*. 285(2):908–14.

Zheng, C., W. Zhou, T. Wang, P. You, Y. Zhao, Y. Yang, X. Wang, J. Luo, Y. Chen, M. Liu, and H. Chen . 2015. A novel TGR5 activator WB403 promotes GLP-1 secretion and preserves pancreatic β-cells in type 2 diabetic mice. *PLoS One*. 10:e0134051.

Index

Page numbers followed by f and t indicate figures and tables, respectively.